The Research Guide: A primer for residents, other health care trainees, and practitioners

Editors

Bart J. Harvey, MD, PhD, MEd, FACPM, FRCPC
Eddy S. Lang, MDCM, CCFP(EM), CSPQ
Jason R. Frank, MD, MA(Ed), FRCPC

Table of Contents

Preamble

■ The motivation to create this guide

arose from our efforts as clinician-educators to support and supervise trainees—predominantly, residents from a variety of medical specialty training programs—who wished or were required to complete a formal research project. Our experiences repeatedly highlighted the fact that many health trainees lack formal education in the design and conduct of research. As a result, a large portion of the initial stages of each trainee's research project was spent addressing a variety of knowledge gaps, often through a series of one-to-one tutorials. Moreover, as we endeavoured to provide effective guidance on a diverse range of research efforts we often became aware of the limitations of our own knowledge. Over the course of our careers, it has become clear that this individualized teaching of the fundamentals of research is neither efficient nor sustainable. Even more important, we became only too aware that, for a variety of reasons, many promising research initiatives are never completed. This is regrettable on at least two levels. First, progress in research is a keystone of contemporary health care: patients and health care providers alike demand continual, evidence-based improvement in the quality and effectiveness of care. Second, the ability to critically appraise research, along with at least a basic familiarity with the conduct of research, is an important dimension of the competencies of all health care professionals. Within the domain of medical practice, these research competencies have been articulated in terms of the CanMEDS Scholar Role.

Assembling a guide such as this one is not a challenge to be undertaken idly, and so our first step was to determine whether the kind of resource we envisioned already existed. Was there a text that could guide health care trainees through all the steps of successfully designing and completing a research project? Although several excellent textbooks on research methods are available—and many are referenced in this guide—none offered the kind of "self-study" resource we had in mind. To test our impression of the scope of existing resources we also contacted several Canadian and American health training programs and specialty associations. Although our discussions did not result in the discovery of a suitable resource, many of the clinician-educators we spoke with highlighted the potential value of such a resource. At the same time, we were encouraged by the example of some successes in research training, such as the well-received two-day "introduction to research" course that has been offered for several years to residents in Obstetrics and Gynaecology by the Association of Professors of Obstetrics & Gynaecology of Canada. The organization and content of this course informed our thoughts about the possibility of creating a one-stop, comprehensive guide to research for trainees in all health care professions and specialties. We are grateful to that course's key faculty members, Robert Reid and Phil Hahn, for their helpful discussions, their generous input throughout the development of this guide, and their contribution as co-authors, collectively, of three of its chapters.

Once we were persuaded of the merits—and feasibility—of creating a research guide for health professions trainees, we drafted an outline, a working table of contents and a prospective "abstract" for each of the proposed chapters. We then set out to identify and invite potential authors or co-authors of what would eventually become a complement of 32 chapters. Clearly, the final product—The Research Guide: A primer for residents, other health care trainees, and practitioners—would not have been possible without the generous contributions of this capable and diverse group of authors! We are also very grateful to the dozens of reviewers who kindly provided feedback on early drafts and helped to strengthen the organization, content and relevance of each chapter. The names and affiliations of these chapter authors and reviewers are listed on pages vi–vii and 294–295, respectively . We are particularly appreciative of the contributions of Tom Lang, David Streiner and Ross Upshur, who not only served as chapter authors but also provided rapid and informative peer review of several chapters.

The Research Guide is organized into seven sections, each comprising up to eight chapters. Core components recur through the book to facilitate reading: thus, where appropriate, each chapter begins with an illustrative case, a set of learning objectives and a list of "key terms" to set the context and relevance of the topic being addressed, and concludes with a "postscript" to the illustrative case, one or more exercises, and a summary checklist. For readers who would like to explore some aspects of a topic further, an annotated list of additional resources is included at the end of each chapter.

If you are new to research, The Research Guide will ease you into the journey. Each chapter is intended to walk you through what you need to know and what you need to do to ensure success in your project. The sections of the Guide are meant to present a logical progression in step with the development of your project, but each stands alone. You can use the Guide as a personal modular curriculum for the development of research skills, or as an introductory reference to be consulted as needed. The universe of research could not possibly be compressed into a brief text, and so we have designed this book to be accessible, practical and succinct. We wish you an eye-opening, informative and rewarding experience. This is your opportunity to better understand and even contribute to progress in the vast world of modern health care.

If you are a supervisor of new researchers, this guide is also for you, and has been written by your peers, who know what it takes to support and mentor those less experienced in the process of a scholarly inquiry. If you need an accessible curriculum to help your trainees understand what needs to be done, this text can form the basis of a research handbook. If you need short readings to make your supervision more efficient, you can direct your trainee to the relevant chapters in the Guide.

This project would not have been possible without the support and "home" provided by the CanMEDS Office at the Royal College of Physicians and Surgeons of Canada. We are particularly indebted to Wendy Jemmett from the CanMEDS Office, who very capably managed this project throughout. We would also like to express our gratitude to Anne Marie Todkill for her editorial support and expertise in helping to transform each draft chapter into a more efficient, readable and satisfying form.

The Research Guide is meant to make the lives of novice researchers and their supervisors easier. We would like to hear from you, the reader, about how well we have achieved this goal. Please tell us how future editions of this guide could be improved. Are there gaps to address? Ways to make the Guide more relevant and easy to use? We welcome all comments and suggestions at canmeds@royalcollege.ca

In the meantime, we hope you will enjoy the guide and your research journey!

Bart J. Harvey, Toronto
Eddy S. Lang, Calgary
Jason R. Frank, Ottawa

September 1, 2011

Contributors

Stacy Ackroyd-Stolarz, MSc, PhD
Queen Elizabeth II Health Sciences Centre Halifax Infirmary
Dalhousie University
Halifax, Nova Scotia

Susan J. Bondy, BA, MSc, PhD, FACE
Dalla Lana School of Public Health
University of Toronto
Toronto, Ontario

Carolyn Brown, ELS
Science and medicine writer and editor
   and publishing consultant
Ottawa, Ontario

G. Mark Brown, MSc
University of Calgary
Calgary, Alberta

June C. Carroll, MD, CCFP, FCFP
Department of Family and Community Medicine
Mount Sinai Hospital, University of Toronto
Toronto, Ontario

Steve Choi, MD, FRCPC
Department of Emergency Medicine
The Ottawa Hospital, University of Ottawa
Ottawa, Ontario

Kaberi Dasgupta, MD, MSc, FRCPC
Department of Internal Medicine and Endocrinology
McGill University Health Centre, McGill University
Montreal, Quebec

Jason R. Frank, MD, MA(Ed), FRCPC
Office of Education
Royal College of Physicians and Surgeons of Canada
Ottawa, Ontario

Scott Garrison, MD
Department of Family Practice
University of British Columbia
Vancouver, British Columbia

Ian D. Graham, PhD
Canadian Institutes of Health Research
Ottawa, Ontario

Stefan Grzybowski, MD, FCFP, MClSc
Department of Family Practice
University of British Columbia
Vancouver, British Columbia

Philip M. Hahn, MSc
Department of Obstetrics and Gynecology
Queen's University
Kingston, Ontario

Bart J. Harvey, MD, PhD, MEd, FACPM, FRCPC
Dalla Lana School of Public Health
University of Toronto
Toronto, Ontario

Grant Innes, MD, FRCPC
Emergency Medicine
Alberta Health Services
University of Calgary
Calgary, Alberta

Monika Kastner, PhD
Li Ka Shing Knowledge Institute
St. Michael's Hospital, University of Toronto
Toronto, Ontario

Karim Khan, MD, PhD
Department of Family Practice
University of British Columbia
Vancouver, British Columbia

Terry P. Klassen, MD, MSc, FRCPC
Manitoba Institute Child Health
Winnipeg, Manitoba

Lorie A. Kloda, MLIS, AHIP, PhD (candidate)
McGill Life Sciences Library
McGill University
Montreal, Quebec

Eddy S. Lang, MDCM, CCFP(EM), CSPQ
Alberta Health Services
University of Calgary
Calgary, Alberta

Thomas A. Lang, MA
Tom Lang Communications and Training
Kirkland, Washington

A. Curtis Lee, PhD
Educational Evaluation and Analysis
Royal College of Physicians and Surgeons of Canada
Ottawa, Ontario

Sarah Jane Lusina, MSc
Centre for Hip Health and Mobility
University of British Columbia
Vancouver, British Columbia

Fiona Alice Miller, MA, PhD
Department of Health Policy, Management and Evaluation
University of Toronto
Toronto, Ontario

Jeffrey J. Perry, MSC, MD, CCFP-EM
Department of Emergency Medicine
Department of Epidemiology and Community Medicine
University of Ottawa
Ottawa, Ontario

Robert L. Reid, MD, FRCSC
Division of Reproductive Endocrinology and Infertility
Department of Obstetrics and Gynecology
Kingston General Hospital, Queen's University
Kingston, Ontario

David L. Sackett, OC, MD, FRSC, FRCP
Kilgore Trout Research and Education Centre
Hamilton, Ontario

Julie M. Spence, MD, MSc, FRCPC
Department of Emergency Medicine
St. Michael's Hospital, University of Toronto
Toronto, Ontario

Sharon E. Straus, MD, MSc, FRCPC
Li Ka Shing Knowledge Institute
St. Michael's Hospital, University of Toronto
Toronto, Ontario

David L. Streiner, PhD, CPsych
Department of Psychiatry and Behavioural Neurosciences
McMaster University, Hamilton, Ontario
Department of Psychiatry
University of Toronto, Toronto, Ontario

Vicky Tagalakis, MD, MSc
Department of General Internal Medicine
Jewish General Hospital, McGill University
Montreal, Quebec

Jacqueline Tetroe, MA
Canadian Institutes of Health Research
Ottawa, Ontario

Ross E.G. Upshur, MD, MA, MSc, CCFP, FRCPC
Department of Family and Community Medicine
Sunnybrook Health Sciences Centre, University of Toronto
Toronto, Ontario

Christian Vaillancourt, MD, MSc, FRCPC, CSPQ
Department of Emergency Medicine and
Ottawa Hospital Research Institute
The Ottawa Hospital, University of Ottawa
Ottawa, Ontario

Carl van Walraven, MD, MSc, FRCPC
Department of Medicine
The Ottawa Hospital, University of Ottawa
Ottawa, Ontario

Andrew Worster, MD, MSc, CCFP(EM), FCFP
Division of Emergency Medicine
McMaster University
Hamilton, Ontario

Starting

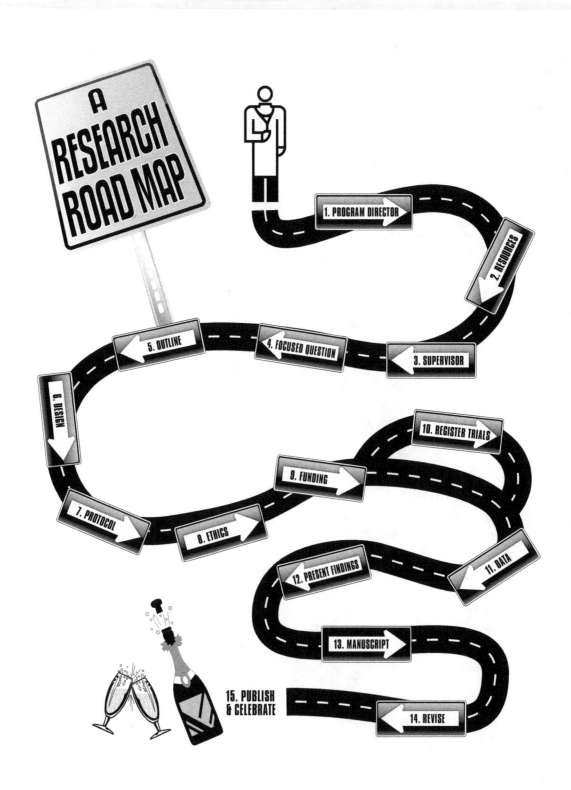

1

A research road map:
Fifteen steps to a successful research project
(and ten pitfalls to avoid)

Philip M. Hahn, MSc

Are you thinking about starting a research project, either because of a particular interest or to satisfy a requirement of your training program? If so, reading this chapter is a good way to begin. It offers a road map to research, outlining what is involved in conducting a research project, how to get started, what to anticipate at each phase and how to stay on track to finish your project within a reasonable time. Remember that successful research begins with careful planning: you won't be able to fix at the analysis stage any shortcomings in your study design.

1. Meet with your program director or departmental research coordinator as soon as possible.

- Find out what is expected by your program or department.
- Talk about potential research areas and suitable faculty members who might be available to support you in the completion of a research project.

2. Look for resources that provide an introduction to the basic concepts of research methodology and critical appraisal.

- Read through this guide.
- Attend local or national resource courses or training programs.
- Consult the references and additional resources listed at the end of this chapter.

3. Find a research supervisor (ch. 3).

- Look for someone whose expertise is relevant to your field of interest and who is able to devote sufficient time and effort to supporting and supervising your work. Most health trainees and junior practitioners have limited research experience and will need someone to guide and advise them along the way. Finding a suitable supervisor is one of the most important steps to success in planning and completing a research project.

- Consider the following in your selection of a research supervisor:
  - publication record
  - access to research funding
  - availability to provide timely advice
  - reports from current and former research trainees

- Agree on expectations, including those with regard to authorship of any publications that result from your project

4. Pose a focused and specific research question (ch. 6).

- Make sure your research question is novel, answerable and feasible
- Consider the PICOT approach to framing a research question.[1] This involves describing the **P**opulation involved in the study and, as applicable, the **I**ntervention, **C**omparator, **O**utcome and **T**ime frame. For example, in women expected to deliver before term (**P**) do corticosteroids (**I**) compared to placebo (**C**) decrease the incidence of neonatal death (**O**) at delivery (**T**)?
- Also consider the FINER criteria.[1] Is your research question **F**easible, **I**nteresting, **N**ovel, **E**thical and **R**elevant?

Starting

5. Develop a research outline.[2]

- Conduct a thorough literature search (ch. 7).
- If your project is designed to examine a therapeutic intervention, check for applicable systematic reviews in The Cochrane Library.[a]
- Collaborate with content and methodological experts. Your supervisor should be able to suggest suitable individuals and to facilitate an introduction to them.
- Determine which study design is the best fit and the most practical approach to framing your research project (ch. 9).
- Write an outline.
  — Focus on the primary objective or question of the proposed research.
  — Include a brief background statement highlighting the importance of your research question.
  — Estimate how much time you will need to complete each of the anticipated stages of the research.
  — List available and required resources and, if applicable, provide a budget estimate.
  — If you already have a variety of interesting ideas to talk about, be sure to keep track of them, but for the purposes of your study outline you will need to boil them down to a single, focused, primary study objective.
  — Make sure your outline is concise—a maximum of two pages is best at this point.
  — With the outline of your proposed research project in hand, arrange to meet with methodological specialists (Step 6) in preparation for writing a more detailed protocol (Step 7).

6. Meet with methodological (especially biostatistical) specialists with particular expertise in your area of study.

- Refine the study's primary objective.
- Discuss pertinent design issues, focusing on the primary study objective.
- Be realistic.
  — Bear in mind that planning and completing a retrospective study (such as a systematic review, case-control study, chart review or practice audit,

for which the data already exist) generally takes less time and fewer resources than a prospective study (such as a cohort study or randomized trial, for which primary data collection will be required).
  — Consider conducting a clinical audit, systematic review or survey as a manageable project for your first venture into research.

- As necessary, estimate an appropriate sample size.[3,4]
  — Focus your energy on addressing the primary research objective/question with just the right number of subjects. A study with too many subjects can expose participants needlessly to potential risks. A study with too few subjects might not have sufficient statistical power to detect a clinically important difference.
  — Design an appropriately sized, simple study rather than a small, complicated one.[5]

- Discuss the anticipated data collection and analysis methods (chs 22, 24 & 25).
- Select the tools (calculators, databases, and statistical and data-entry software) that will be appropriate for your analysis of the study data.
- Investigate which file formats for data recording will allow your study data to be imported into an appropriate application for statistical analysis (e.g., Excel spreadsheet for import into SPSS).

7. Develop the research protocol[6] (ch. 17).

- Create an expanded version of the outline created at Step 5.
- Include details on:
  — research team members and their roles (chs 3 & 4)
  — recruitment of study participants (ch. 20)
  — inclusion and exclusion criteria
  — design features such a criterion standard for a clinical practice audit,[7] the sampling technique for a survey,[8] or the random allocation technique and creation of placebos for a randomized controlled trial.[9]
  — any secondary objectives, questions and outcomes
  — statistical issues such as estimating sample size and methods to analyze the data (chs 24 & 25)

— your timetable for starting and finishing the project, as well as the anticipated time frame for each phase of the research project.

— ethical considerations such as safety, confidentiality and informed consent[10] (ch. 18).

• The proposal should contain as much detail as possible and provide the framework for ethics submission (ch. 18) and ultimately drafting a manuscript (ch. 29).

8. As applicable, obtain institutional and research ethics approval (ch. 18).

• Obtain approvals specific to your institution or research centre.

• Seek help from your research supervisor and other university and hospital personnel who are knowledgeable about and experienced with approval processes and requirements.

• Find out whether your project is eligible for an expedited review, which will take less time than a full Research Ethics Board (REB) review. A clinical practice audit, for example, might be eligible for an expedited review.

• If your research involves humans or human tissues, review the Tri-Council policy statement[11] and complete the Tri-Council tutorial on the ethical conduct for research involving humans.[12]

9. Seek necessary funding (ch. 19)

• Consult with your research supervisor and collaborators to identify potential funding sources for your project.

• Seek departmental and university resources first.

• If appropriate, submit a grant to an external funding agency such as the Physicians' Services Incorporated Foundation,[b] or the Canadian Institutes of Health Research.[c]

10. If you are conducting a clinical trial, ensure that it is registered with ClinicalTrials.gov[d] (ch. 18).

• Member journals of the International Committee of Medical Journal Editors (ICMJE), also called the Vancouver Group, require, as a condition of consideration for publication, registration of all clinical trials in a public trials registry.[13] Complete the trial registration before any study participants are recruited and enrolled.

11. Collect and analyze the data (chs 22, 24 & 25).

• Follow the data collection and analysis plan described in the research protocol.

• Report confidence intervals, if appropriate, in addition to *P* values for the results of the primary and any secondary research questions. As Martin Gardner and Douglas Altman note, "Overemphasis on hypothesis testing—and the use of *P* values to dichotomise significant or non-significant results—has detracted from more useful approaches to interpreting study results … . In medical studies investigators are usually interested in determining the size of difference of a measured outcome between groups, rather than a simple indication of whether or not it is statistically significant."[14]

12. Present your findings (chs 27 & 28).

• Remember that one of your responsibilities as a researcher is to communicate your results.

• Find appropriate venues in which to present your work as soon as possible, such as your department's annual research day and relevant local, national and international meetings.

13. Prepare and submit a manuscript describing the study and its results to a suitable journal (ch. 29).

• Be prepared for some hard work on preparing your research report for publication. In an excellent review on preparing manuscripts for submission to medical journals, Gill Welch outlines a systematic approach

---

b See the PSI Foundation website at www.psifoundation.org/ResidentResearchPrizes.html

c See the CIHR website at www.cihr.ca/

---

d The registry can be accessed at www.clinicaltrials.gov/

Starting

for making it easier to prepare a readable paper.[15] His take-home points are:

— Start writing before your project is completed.

— Focus your attention on what readers are most likely to look at: the title, abstract, tables and figures.

— Develop a systematic approach to the introduction, methods, results and discussion.

— Improve the paper by learning how to obtain and incorporate useful feedback.

- Familiarize yourself with the guidelines and checklists that you will need to follow in reporting your methods and results and in disclosing competing interests. An awareness of these standards before you begin will guard you against any deficiencies that could make your report ineligible for publication.

  — For examples of guidelines for the reporting of findings, see the CONSORT Statement on the reporting of randomized controlled trials as well as its extensions for other study types; the PRISMA Statement for the reporting of systematic reviews and meta-analyses; and the STARD Statement on the reporting of diagnostic accuracy studies.[e]

  — For an example of a checklist for reporting competing interests, see the Financial Conflicts of Interest Checklist 2010 for Clinical Research Studies developed by Rochon and colleagues.[16]

  — A fuller list of reporting guidelines is available on the website of the EQUATOR Network, an international initiative to improve the reporting of health sciences research.[f]

- Familiarize yourself with the Uniform Requirements for Manuscripts Submitted to Biomedical Journals outlined by the ICMJE;[g] these requirements are applied by most peer-reviewed medical journals.

- Establish authorship, and the order of authorship.

  — As early as possible, establish authorship credits, including the order in which authors will be listed. The first author is generally the individual who has, overall, contributed the most, while the last (or second) author is generally the project supervisor.

  — The ICMJE criteria for authorship credit state that authorship requires: (1) substantial contributions to conception and design, or acquisition of data, or analysis and interpretation of data; (2) drafting the article or revising it critically for important intellectual content; and (3) final approval of the version to be published.[17]

  — Be prepared to describe the contribution of each author. Many journals require on submission a description of each author's contribution and publish a contributors' statement at the end of each article.

  — Also consider those whose contribution should be acknowledged in the published article. Many journals require written permission from anyone identified in an acknowledgement.

14. If your manuscript is accepted, revise it according to the editors' and reviewers' comments.

- If your manuscript is rejected, take into account the editors' and reviewers' comments and consider submitting the revised paper to another appropriate journal (ch. 29).

15. Celebrate with your coauthors.

- You have just completed a research project and have contributed to the creation and dissemination of new health science knowledge. Don't let this accomplishment pass without taking time to celebrate with your co-investigators and others who have supported you and the project.

---

e The most recent guidelines for CONSORT, PRISMA and STARD can be viewed at www.consort-statement.org/consort-statement/, www.prisma-statement.org/ and www.stard-statement.org/

f See the EQUATOR website at www.equator-network.org/resource-centre

g Available at www.icmje.org/urm_main.html

Starting

TEN COMMON RESEARCH PITFALLS

1. Not establishing a focused, answerable question.
2. Enlisting a research supervisor who doesn't make sufficient time to advise and help you throughout the stages of the project.
3. Picking a topic about which you have little interest.
4. Planning a small, complicated study that attempts to answer many questions, rather than an appropriately sized, simple study focused on one primary objective/question.
5. Not taking the time to draft a research outline to keep your research team coordinated and on schedule.
6. Not being realistic about how much time and effort your project will take (see "Tips for Staying on Track").
7. Basing a prospective study on outcomes that are rare or take a long time to occur.
8. Entering your data into an Excel spreadsheet using formats that are not compatible for importing into a statistical application such as SPSS. The only thing worse than entering data is having to enter it twice.
9. Not meeting with a statistician to talk about the analysis before you begin collecting the data.
10. Waiting too long to begin (see "Tips for Staying on Track").

TIPS FOR STAYING ON TRACK

As you've no doubt already recognized, your biggest obstacle to successfully completing a research project will likely be finding the time.[18–20] Here are some tips for staying on track to finish a research project.

1. Carving out one or more blocks of protected time is key.[18] Use this time to develop your research proposal and start off on the right foot; additional blocks of time can be used for data collection, analysis or write-up.
2. If you are in a two- or three-year program, consider a study design that will allow you to finish on time, such as a medical record review or practice audit, for which the data should be comparatively easy to access and for which an expedited ethics review might be feasible.
3. If you are in a longer program, such as a five-year medical or surgical specialty, consider the following timelines and milestones.
   - In your first year, introduce yourself to the basic concepts of research methodology by taking a dedicated course or intensive workshop. Identify a research supervisor.
   - Identify a methodological specialist to help you develop your research question, study design and research protocol in your second year. Submit your study for ethics approval and funding opportunities. If you are conducting a clinical trial, remember to register your study before you begin to enrol participants.
   - Collect and analyze your data, and then present your findings locally, nationally or beyond by the end of your third or fourth year.
   - Begin drafting your manuscript, aiming for completion in year four.
   - Submit your manuscript to a suitable journal early in year five, leaving your final term free to prepare for your certification exam and life after graduation.

Starting

REFERENCES

1. Thabane L, Thomas T, Ye C, Paul J. Posing the research question: not so simple. *Can J Anaesth.* 2009;56(1):71–9.

2. Hulley SB, Cummings SR, Browner WS, Grady DG, Newman TB. *Designing clinical research: an epidemiologic approach.* 3rd ed. Philadelphia: Lippincott Williams & Wilkins; 2007. Appendix 1.1; p. 15.

3. Altman DG. Statistics and ethics in medical research: III How large a sample? *Br Med J.* 1980;281(6251):1336–8.

4. Schulz KF, Grimes DA. Sample size calculations in randomised trials: mandatory and mystical. *Lancet.* 2005;365(9467):1348–53.

5. McAlister FA, Straus SE, Sackett DL. Why we need large, simple studies of the clinical examination: the problem and a proposed solution. CARE-COAD1 group. Clinical Assessment of the Reliability of the Examination-Chronic Obstructive Airways Disease Group. *Lancet.* 1999;354(9191):1721–4.

6. Cummings SR, Hulley SB. Writing and funding a research proposal. In: Hulley SB, Cummings SR, Browner WS, Grady DG, Newman TB, editors. *Designing clinical research: an epidemiologic approach.* 3rd ed. Philadelphia: Lippincott Williams & Wilkins; 2007. p. 301–16.

7. Godwin M. 2001. Conducting a clinical practice audit. Fourteen steps to better patient care. *Can Fam Phys.* 2001;47(11):2331–3.

8. Salant P, DA Dillman. *How to conduct your own survey.* New York: John Wiley & Sons; 1994. Chapter 5, When and how to select a sample; p. 53–72.

9. Pocock SJ. *Clinical trials: a practical approach.* Toronto: John Wiley & Sons; 1983. Chapter 5, Methods of randomization, and chapter 6, Blinding and Placebos; p. 66–89, 90–9.

10. Pocock SJ. *Clinical trials: a practical approach.* Toronto: John Wiley & Sons; 1983. Chapter 7, Ethical issues; p. 100–9.

11. Canadian Institutes of Health Research, Natural Sciences and Engineering Council of Canada, Social Sciences and Humanities Research Council of Canada. *Tri-Council policy statement: ethical conduct for research involving humans* (December 2010). Ottawa: Interagency Secretariat on Research Ethics; 1998. Available from: www.pre.ethics.gc.ca/pdf/eng/tcps2/TCPS_2_FINAL_Web.pdf

12. Panel on Research Ethics. *Introductory tutorial for the Tri-Council policy statement: ethical conduct for research involving humans* [last modified 2009 Aug 30; cited 2009 Aug 30]. Available from: http://pre.ethics.gc.ca/english/tutorial/

13. DeAngelis C, Drazen JM, Frizelle FA, Haug C, Hoey J, Horton R, et al. 2004. Clinical trial registration: a statement from the International Committee of Medical Journal Editors. *CMAJ.* 2004;171(6):606–7.

14. Gardner MJ, Altman DG. Confidence intervals rather than P values: estimation rather than hypothesis testing. *BMJ.* 1986;292(6522):746–50.

15. Welch HG. Preparing manuscripts for submission to medical journals: the paper trail. *Eff Clin Pract.* 1999;2(3):131–7.

16. Rochon PA, Hoey J, Chan AW, Ferris LE, Lexchin J, Kalkar SR, et al. Financial conflicts of interest checklist 2010 for clinical research studies. *Open Med.* 2010;4(1):69–91. Available from: www.openmedicine.ca/article/view/356/318

17. Hoey J. Who wrote this paper anyway? The new Vancouver Group statement refines the definition of authorship. *CMAJ.* 2000;163(6):716–7.

18. Chan RK, Lockyer J, Hutchison C. Block to succeed: the Canadian orthopedic resident research experience. *Can J Surg.* 2009;52(3):187–95.

19. Silcox LC, Ashbury TL, VanDenKerkhof EG, Milne B. Residents' and program directors' attitudes toward research during anesthesiology training: a Canadian perspective. *Anesth Analg.* 2006;102(3):859–64.

20. Gill S, Levin A, Djurdjev O, Yoshida EM. Obstacles to residents' conducting research and predictors of publication. *Acad Med.* 2001;76(5):477.

ADDITIONAL RESOURCES

I recommend the following books to busy professionals who want to improve their understanding of key concepts in biostatistics and epidemiology.

Biostatistics

Altman DG. *Practical statistics for medical research.* London (UK): Chapman & Hall; 1991.

- Douglas Altman is Director of the Centre for Statistics in Medicine in Oxford, England. By discussing both the use and misuse of statistics this book equips the reader to judge the appropriateness of the methods and interpretations presented in papers published in medical journals.

Altman DG, Machin D, Bryant TN, Gardner JM, editors. *Statistics with confidence: confidence intervals and statistical guidelines.* 2nd ed. London (UK): BMJ Books; 2000.

- As Gardner and Altman say elsewhere,[14] "Overemphasis on hypothesis testing—and the use of P values to dichotomise significant or non-significant results—has detracted from more useful approaches to interpreting study results, such as estimation and confidence intervals." This book gives guidelines for calculating and using confidence intervals around just about any point estimate.

Norman GR, Streiner DL. *PDQ statistics.* 3rd ed. Hamilton (ON): B.C. Decker; 2003.

- That's PDQ for "pretty darn quick": with this book, you can rapidly find concise descriptions of statistical tests that you might come across while reading journal articles.

Epidemiology

Sackett DL, Haynes RB, Guyatt GH, Tugwell P. *Clinical epidemiology: a basic science for clinical medicine.* 2nd ed. Toronto (ON): Little Brown and Company; 1991.

- This text applies the principles learned in epidemiology to the complex clinical decisions that must be made every day.

Streiner DL, Norman GR. *PDQ epidemiology.* 2nd ed. Hamilton (ON): B.C. Decker; 1998.

- This efficient study guide in the "pretty darn quick" series introduces the reader to the world of epidemiology; it covers data-gathering, sampling procedures, study designs, biases, measuring reliability and validity, and much more.

Evidence-based medicine

Godwin M, Hodgetts G. *The Bedford murder: an evidence-based clinical mystery.* Philadelphia (PA): Hanley & Befus; 2003.

- This murder mystery novel reveals clinical pearls and the concepts of evidence-based medicine.

Greenhalgh T. *How to read a paper: the basics of evidence-based medicine.* 3rd ed. Oxford (UK): Blackwell Publishing; 2006.

- One of the best-selling texts on evidence-based medicine, this book is used by health care professionals and medical students worldwide. With chapters on topics such as "statistics for the non-statistician," it serves as a good critical appraisal primer for journal clubs.

McKibbon A, Wilczynski N. *PDQ evidence-based principles and practice.* 2nd ed. Shelton (CT): People's Medical Publishing House; 2009.

- "Provides a plain-language approach to basic principles of evidence generation and application" (Brian Haynes, Chief, Health Information Research Unit at McMaster University). This text has a good section on systematic reviews.

Starting

Riegelman RK. *Studying a study & testing a test: how to read the medical literature*. Boston (MA): Little, Brown and Company; 1981.

- This self-study, active-participation book was written to show clinicians how to read the medical literature thoughtfully and efficiently. It includes a good chapter on diagnostic test statistics, covering sensitivity, specificity and predictive values.

Straus SE, Richardson WS, Glasziou P, Haynes RB. *Evidence-based medicine: how to practice and teach EBM*. 3rd ed. Edinburgh (UK): Elsevier Churchill Livingstone; 1997.

- In the preface to this short and practical text, David Sackett is acknowledged as the senior author of the first edition and mentor to Sharon Straus.

Heath measurement scales

Streiner DL, Norman GR. *Health measurement scales: a practical guide to their development and use*. 2nd ed. Oxford (UK): Oxford University Press; 1995.

- This text enables experienced and novice researchers to develop accurate, sensitive and easy-to-use measurement scales.

Knowledge translation

Straus SE, Tetroe J, Graham ID. *Knowledge translation in health care: moving from evidence to practice*. Oxford (UK): Blackwell Publishing; 2009.

- Insights from Canadian leaders in knowledge translation, especially on approaches for researchers to use to foster the application of their results.

The media

Cohn V, Cope L. *News & numbers: a guide to reporting statistical claims and controversies in health and other fields*. 2nd ed. Ames (IA): Blackwell Publishing Professional; 2001.

- "Victor Cohn of the Washington Post has prepared this manual to help reporters cut through statistical tangles. By such efforts, scientists and writers may gradually upgrade the whole communication system, scientific and journalistic" (Frederick Mosteller, Professor Emeritus of Mathematical Statistics, Harvard University).

Woloshin S, Schwartz LM, Welch HG. *Know your chances: understanding health statistics*. Berkeley (CA): University of California Press; 2008.

- Written by leaders in knowledge translation, particularly in the area of risk management, this book explains how to see through the hype in medical news, ads and public service announcements.

Publishing

Lang TA. *How to write, publish, & present in the health sciences: a guide for clinicians & laboratory researchers*. Philadelphia (PA): American College of Physicians; 2010.

- "Lang's earlier book on how to report medical statistics proved so useful that I bought a second copy to keep in my home office. His new book features the same type of pragmatic advice on the nuts and bolts of scientific writing" (David Grimes, University of North Carolina School of Medicine).

Lang TA, Secic M. *How to report statistics in medicine: annotated guidelines for authors, editors and reviewers*. 2nd ed. Philadelphia (PA): American College of Physicians; 2006.

- This text is an excellent guide to reporting and interpreting statistical presentations.

Research design

Hulley SB, Cummings SR, Browner WS, Grady DG, Newman TB. *Designing clinical research: an epidemiologic approach*. 3rd ed. Philadelphia (PA): Lippincott Williams & Wilkins; 2001.

- This book offers thorough coverage of all elements of designing retrospective, prospective and experimental studies. It addresses sample size estimation with examples for different study designs.

Jadad A. *Randomised controlled trials*. London (UK): BMJ Books; 1998.

- This is a good little text for readers who wish to understand the basic principles of randomized controlled trials and their role in health care decisions.

Pocock SJ. *Clinical trials: a practical approach*. Toronto (ON): John Wiley & Sons; 1983.

- This excellent text contains good chapters on methods of randomization, crossover trials and sample size estimation.

Schultz KF, Grimes DA. *The Lancet handbook of essential concepts in clinical research*. Edinburgh (UK): Elsevier; 2006.

- "Few doctors would quibble with the view that their skills in evaluating clinical research are modest. This book provides a superb and indispensible guide to the interpretation of research for the busy doctor" (Richard Horton, Editor, *The Lancet*). Each chapter represents a peer-reviewed article published in *The Lancet* from 2002 to 2005.

Survey research

Alreck PL, Settle RB. *The survey research handbook*. Boston (MA): Irwin/McGraw-Hill; 1995.

- This handbook covers topics from planning and designing a survey to analyzing the data and has a good chapter on sampling.

Dillman DA, Smyth JD, Christian LM. *Internet, mail and mixed mode surveys: the tailored design method*. 3rd ed. Hoboken (NJ): John Wiley & Sons; 2007.

- This edition emphasizes the use of the Internet in conducting surveys.

Salant P, Dillman DA. 1994. *How to conduct your own survey*. New York (NY): John Wiley & Sons; 1994.

- Start with this book, a step-by-step guide to survey research.

Starting

SUMMARY CHECKLIST

- ❑ Meet with your program director or departmental research coordinator as soon as possible.
- ❑ Look for resources that provide an introduction to the basic concepts of research methodology and critical appraisal.
- ❑ Find a research supervisor.
- ❑ Pose a focused and specific research question.
- ❑ Develop a research outline.
- ❑ Meet with methodological (especially biostatistical) specialists with particular expertise in your area of study.
- ❑ Develop the research protocol.
- ❑ As applicable, obtain institutional and research ethics approval.
- ❑ Seek necessary funding.
- ❑ If you are conducting a clinical trial, ensure that it is registered with ClinicalTrials.gov
- ❑ Collect and analyze the data.
- ❑ Present your findings.
- ❑ Prepare and submit a manuscript describing the study and its results to a suitable journal.
- ❑ If your manuscript is accepted, revise it according to the editors' and reviewers' comments.
- ❑ Celebrate with your coauthors.

2
Research in residency, other health care training, and practice: Why, when and how?

Robert L. Reid, MD, FRCSC

ILLUSTRATIVE CASE

A second-year Obstetrics and Gynecology resident is told by her program director that she must present a research project at the annual resident research day next year. She is swamped with clinical work and is using every spare moment to study for an upcoming departmental exam. The last thing she needs to add to her workload is a research project, and so she asks her director if she can duck the "researcher role" and spend the extra time and energy becoming a better clinician.

■ The CanMEDS 2005 Physician

Competency Framework[1] identifies seven overlapping core competencies as essential in the preparation of physicians to meet the needs of patients in the 21st century. Among these, the Scholar Role serves to anchor contemporary medical practice in continuing professional development, research literacy, critical appraisal skills and the ability to educate others. The best practice is informed by scholarship. A failure to adequately equip graduates with skills in critical appraisal and an understanding of research methodology has been identified as a common deficiency of training programs,[2] and examples of the devastating effects of this scientific illiteracy abound.[3]

To fulfill the Scholar Role, physicians must demonstrate that they:

- maintain and enhance professional activities through ongoing learning;
- critically evaluate information and its sources, and apply this appropriately to practice decisions;
- facilitate the learning of patients, families, students, residents, other health professionals, the public and others, as appropriate; and,
- contribute to the creation, dissemination, application and translation of new medical knowledge and practices.[1]

This guide has been designed to provide a framework to help learners acquire basic skills as researchers, in keeping with the fourth component of the Scholar Role. However, research experience enhances the other competencies of the Scholar by fostering lifelong learning along with skills in critical evaluation and the translation of new knowledge to others. Experience in the conduct of research helps clinicians and other health care practitioners to more capably challenge claims based on faulty research or improper interpretation, and to confidently incorporate into their practice those innovations that have been demonstrated to improve the quality of care.

CHAPTER OBJECTIVES

After reading this chapter, you should be able to:
- describe why scholarly activity, including research, is an essential prerequisite for residents, other health care trainees, and practitioners;
- list the key components of the CanMEDS Scholar Role; and
- highlight the two most critical choices in planning a research project—especially one's first.

Starting

The chapters of this guide provide a road map for the novice health care researcher. They examine what constitutes a scholarly project; emphasize the importance of finding a qualified supervisor or mentor and a working environment that supports research; and explore the fundamentals of conceiving and formulating a research question, conducting literature searches, choosing an appropriate study design, obtaining institutional approval, collecting and analysing the data, and reporting the results. Annotated lists of references and resources are provided to assist in the planning and implementation of a research project. Throughout the guide, the authors—all of whom are experienced investigators—offer practical advice on building a solid foundation for successful health research.

Why me?

No doubt, many resident physicians, other health care trainees and practitioners reading this introduction will think, "That's all fine, but I didn't decide to become a health professional so that I could do scientific research. I'm not looking for a Nobel Prize. I just want to be a competent and caring health care practitioner."

The answer to "Why me?" lies in the many career paths open to graduates of residency and other health care training programs. Graduating practitioners are charged with two responsibilities: (1) to provide the highest possible quality of health care to patients and populations; and (2) to educate the next generations of health care practitioners. Research is essential to evaluating and improving performance in both of these roles.

You may think at the start of your training that a research role would be better left to your colleagues who received Masters or PhD degrees before they entered health practice training. Although it is true that such individuals bring specialized knowledge and research skills to their training, many excellent researchers were not "turned on" to a research career until they encountered a challenging practice-based problem during their residency, other health training, or practice. Moreover, often because of lifestyle factors or the influence of mentors, many health science students and trainees change career course during clinical training, and so it is wise to keep one's options open as long as possible for advanced supplementary training—where research involvement is often expected.

Those who choose to enter practice as soon as they complete their training will need to acquire at least the basics of critical appraisal skills if they hope to elevate discussions with patients above the level of what they hear from popular media. New health care practice subscription services are emerging on the Internet that identify and summarize important discipline- and specialty-specific research findings while providing a short critical appraisal of the quality of the research. Although these services can be extremely helpful to busy health care practitioners, they generally require a basic understanding of key research concepts and sufficient skill in critical appraisal to judge the quality of evidence and facilitate meaningful interpretation and discussion. In addition, practitioners who acquire basic knowledge and skills with regard to health research will be better equipped to contribute to relevant research themselves, such as by identifying patients who meet the enrolment criteria for a clinical trial or even by serving as a study co-investigator.

When can I find time?

The trainee in our case example is no doubt experiencing the same worry about participating in research as many of her peers have before her: she wonders where in the world she will find the time—and the energy—to fit a research project around all of her clinical responsibilities.

Within the time frame of a health care practitioner training program, it is generally unrealistic to expect to have a significant period of protected time in which to conduct research. Exceptions are the Royal College Clinical Investigator Program and a few residency programs that are able to offer a one- or two-year deferral for the completion of a Masters or PhD degree. For most trainees, however, any research project will need to be undertaken simultaneously with training activities. A short elective devoted to the development of a research project can be ideal, although this is not available in all programs. Given the demands of any training program, it is important to plan a research project realistically and at an early stage. Time will be needed to identify and meet with a qualified supervisor or mentor, to develop the research idea, establish necessary collaborations, and prepare the proposal and other documentation for ethics review. Care in the planning stage will pay big dividends later on.

For a first foray into research, it often makes sense to design, in consultation with a supervisor or mentor, a project that examines data retrospectively; examples are a systematic review, survey-based study or chart audit. More ambitious projects that collect data prospectively, as in a clinical study of a new test or treatment or a multi-centre trial, require considerably more preparation and, of course, the requisite funding. It is better, at first, to think small and see a project through than to start an enormous project that falls apart for want of time, funding or subject recruitment, or because of investigator burnout.

Where do study ideas come from?

Dramatic innovations in health and science over the past 60 years have propelled us into the 21st century with a momentum that is already revolutionizing the delivery of health care and the way we live our lives. Did these discoveries happen by accident? Although there are many serendipitous findings in science, discovery and "happy accident" often occur to those who are the most alert and prepared. Many of the most exciting revelations result when discoveries in the basic sciences are brought to bear on pressing clinical problems by those with an open mind and a willingness to critically challenge existing dogma. Witness the discovery by Australian clinician-scientists Robin Warren and Barry Marshall that peptic ulcers are not, in fact, caused by stress or the consumption of alcohol or spicy food, but by infection with the bacterium *Helicobacter pylori*. Marshall and Warren challenged conventional thinking on the subject, "rewrote the book" on peptic ulcer disease, and were awarded the 2005 Nobel Prize for Medicine or Physiology for their insight and efforts.

Those who work in the trenches of health practice face common problems for which there appears to be little progress toward a solution. An unwillingness to explore new strategies is often explained by a shortage of time, which seems to lead to complacency. Unfortunately, many accept what appears to be a suboptimal approach simply because "that's the way it's always been."

Novel ideas arise when old problems are considered from a new perspective. However, new ideas are often dismissed with a quick rebuke: "If the solution were that obvious, someone else would have done it already." Good hunches can be discarded for any number of reasons. Albert Szent-Györgyi, the first scientist to isolate vitamin C, made important discoveries by paying attention to results that another researcher had literally poured down the drain. Not all ideas work out. But, to use a phrase attributed to Nobel Prize winner Linus Pauling, "The best way to have a good idea is to have a lot of ideas." Health care leaders emerge from those who are willing to take the time to pursue a new idea, accept failure if it occurs and move on with other attempts to solve the problem.

"A discovery is said to be an accident meeting a prepared mind."[4]

Albert Szent-Györgyi (1893–1986)
Nobel Prize laureate in 1937

How do I get started?

When you have an idea for a solution or a new approach to a problem, write it down before it vanishes among all the other issues arising from the countless health care concerns you encounter in the course of a day. Then, when you have more time, do a thorough literature search to see whether someone has tested your idea before. Make sure, before you embark on a research project, that you won't end up simply reinventing the wheel.

If, like many health trainees and practitioners, you feel stuck for a clever or feasible research idea, turn to your supervisor or mentor for help. Qualified supervisors and mentors have a track record of productive research. Typically, they have a host of ideas relating to their own research but not enough time to pursue each one. A keen trainee who is willing to tackle one of these projects can forge a long-term collegial relationship that can potentially benefit both parties for years to come.

Conclusion

An understanding of the basics of research methodology and practice are essential for all health trainees and practitioners to allow them to critically evaluate new health science developments. During your health practice training, you will have valuable opportunities to enhance these skills by entering research training programs, studying texts such as this one, participating in activities such as journal clubs and research projects, and interacting with experienced researchers at your university. Taking advantage of these opportunities at an early stage of your career will help you to become a well-rounded practitioner and to develop further the important competencies of the Scholar Role. ∎

Starting

Starting

CASE POSTSCRIPT

Searching her department's website, the resident informed herself about the range of research projects that were in progress within the department and about the research interests and activities of individual staff. She asked senior residents about the quality of supervision, support and mentorship offered by different staff. She then approached a qualified and supportive faculty member to see if he would be willing to serve as her research supervisor. The resident spent a one-month elective later in the year developing a research idea and writing her proposal. This involved several meetings with her faculty supervisor. Her supervisor facilitated a meeting with a statistician during the planning stages to ensure that the study's sample size would be adequate to demonstrate a difference between two labour-induction protocols. Knowing that the project was well planned and adequately powered, the resident and her supervisor submitted the protocol to the university and hospital Research Ethics Boards and received approval. The resident then involved several other residents from the labour and delivery floor in data collection over the next year, and all contributed as co-authors to a prize-winning paper presented at the departmental research day one year later. The resident was also gratified to have her findings published in a leading journal of Obstetrics and Gynecology several months later.

REFERENCES

1. Royal College of Physicians and Surgeons of Canada. *CanMEDS 2005 Physician Competency Framework*. Ottawa: The College; 2005. Available from: http://rcpsc.medical.org/canmeds/CanMEDS2005/index.php

2. Mason AD, Biehler JL, Linares MY, Greenberg B. Perceptions of pediatric emergency medicine fellows and program directors about research education. *Acad Emerg Med*. 1991;6(10):1061–5.

3. Jordan B, Mooney C. Why we need to truly understand the medical literature. *Contraception*. 2007;75(6):405–6.

4. Szent-Györgyi A. Looking back. *Perspect Biol Med*. 1971;15(1):1–5. Available from: http://profiles.nlm.nih.gov/WG/Views/AlphaChron/date/10005/

SUMMARY CHECKLIST

❑ Describe at least three reasons to get involved in the world of research.
❑ Consider, personally and professionally, what you want to get out of being involved in research.
❑ List three people you can talk to about research.
❑ Get started. Let this book be your guide!

3
Finding a research supervisor

Sarah Jane Lusina, MSc
Scott Garrison, MD
Stefan Grzybowski, MD, MCISc, FCFP
Karim Khan, MD, PhD

ILLUSTRATIVE CASE

A family medicine resident is required to complete a research project but isn't sure where to start. Her program director suggests that she start by trying to identify a faculty member to serve as her research project supervisor. Although that seems reasonable, she isn't sure what she should be looking for in a potential faculty supervisor.

■ **You will read about designing,** conducting and interpreting research in other chapters of this guide. Before any of that can begin, however, you will need to find a research supervisor. In this chapter, we will outline various aspects of supervision for you to consider. Specifically, we will highlight the benefits of selecting a supervisor who can provide access to a research team, in contrast to basing that selection solely on what a prospective supervisor can offer individually. This is important because research in the real world is rarely an individual pursuit.

Choosing your topic: What comes first—the project or the process?

The research interests of many health practitioners and trainees are inspired by something they have seen in practice or have experienced. For others, the research component of professional training is merely a hurdle they must clear to meet program requirements. Regardless of which case applies to you, gaining experience in research is an important part of your training and professional development that will enhance your understanding of the health sciences and of the practices you apply every day. Perhaps, if the years of clinical experience ahead of you generate new insights and research questions, you will find yourself continuing to include research as a rewarding dimension of your professional career (see ch. 32).

Before you can seek out a suitable supervisor, you must first evaluate your personal **priorities** and goals. Is it your priority to advance your content knowledge in a particular area (e.g., prevention of *Chlamydia* infection in teenaged snowboarders)? If so, finding a supervisor with expertise in

CHAPTER OBJECTIVES

After reading this chapter, you should be able to:
- describe the issues to consider in the selection of a research supervisor
- discuss the qualities to look for in a research supervisor
- describe the concept of a team approach to research and research supervision

---

KEY TERMS

Authorship	Informal learning	Research environment
Collaborative	Interdisciplinary	Supervisory team
Communication	Norms	Team skills
Conflict resolution	Priorities	
Expectations	RACI management tool	

Starting

that area will be the most important aspect of your search. Or is the research process more important to you, such that, regardless of the topic, you are seeking a supervisor who will provide you with an environment for superior research training? Ideally, you will find a supervisor who can support a research project in an area that you are keenly interested in and offer an effective environment for training in research processes and methods. You may, however, have to choose between the two.

Let's say you choose to pursue the ideal training environment alternative. Fittingly, the first step is to research your options. Scan your department and your wider research and health care network to find out which professors or research groups have a reputation for good supervision and training as well as for producing high-quality research. For example, suppose you discover that a group of renowned clinician-scientists with full professorships are working with a diverse team of researchers to examine the risks of shorter postpartum stays on the maternity ward, but you have limited knowledge of, and have never been particularly interested in, maternity care. Because the training environment is your priority, you pursue this opportunity in view of the benefits of working with this expert team and the exceptional research skills and experience that you will gain in this environment. Of course, this productive and successful team of researchers will be sought after by many trainees, and so you will have to convince them that you are a worthy candidate. This is where your preparation and negotiating skills come into play: Be sure to update your résumé and curriculum vitae before beginning the search for a supervisor, and be prepared to write a cover letter (or equivalent email) to make your request for supervision and to highlight the skills and strengths you can bring to the team.

Whether your approach is process-focused or content-focused, developing an excellent research question should be of paramount priority. Whether you are keenly interested in the topic or not, a good research experience will be facilitated by a thoughtful, well-formed research question. If your goal is to learn how to perform research, to benefit from the guidance of your supervisor, and to produce a publication, a well-formed research question is essential (see ch. 6). Make sure that you review your question with your supervisor and your supervisory team to ensure that you are on track to produce interesting, worthwhile results that will add to the knowledge base of your field.

Selecting supervision and teaming up for success

Finding a supervisor with skills, interests, resources and traits that are matched to your learning needs, expectations and priorities is the key to success. A number of considerations should be taken into a account in the selection of a supervisor: we highlight a few essential factors here.

First, the purpose and responsibility of a supervisor is to provide guidance and support to a research trainee as his or her work progresses. Thus, finding a supervisor who will actually be available and able to perform this oversight over the course of your project is fundamental.

Second, the supervisor needs to have skills and experience in your research area. Ideally, that experience will take many forms: knowledge of the content areas and of research methodology and process, a history of conducting research, and a track record of research success. Your supervisor's job is to ensure that your work is valid, is based on sound ideas and methodology, and advances toward the identified research goal. Also, the ideal supervisor will have experience in supervising trainees, preferably across a broad spectrum of levels from undergraduate students to postdoctoral fellows.

In addition to availability and experience, your supervisor should have access to resources to support your work. These resources can also come in many forms: laboratory or office space, research tools or equipment, access to databases, or access to potential study participants or recruitment possibilities. However, among the most valuable of these resources are networks and teams of skilled experts who can assist with and facilitate your research project.

In our opinion, the ideal supervisor would provide access to a team who can add to the supports your supervisor can offer as an individual: that is, additional guidance, expertise, training in specific research techniques and facilitation of your project's goals. Although individual team members will likely be interested only in certain aspects of a project (e.g., the biostatistical methods) or the application of results (e.g., effective strategies for *Chlamydia* prevention), the team approach harnesses all of these interests to enhance your experience and network of support. Thus, a **collaborative** group with a range of technical and administrative skills can be extremely beneficial to your research experience. Research teams come in many shapes. You may be working in a team comprising other trainees, research assistants or staff. Alternatively, you may find yourself working in a team that includes a few mid-level and senior faculty members. Whatever the team's composition, you will need to function effectively within it, taking advantage of what can be learned from the different members and understanding the unique contributions of each. This also means that you will need to develop the skills to work productively within a team. If it seems difficult at times to work collaboratively, take comfort in knowing that the **team skills** you acquire now will benefit you in your clinical practice, which undoubtedly requires a team approach. The notion of a **supervisory team** is discussed at greater length later in the chapter, but keep it in mind as you read on.

An important trait worth being acutely aware of as you seek a research supervisor is attention to deadlines. A supervisor who is mindful of your timeline will ensure that you stay on track with your desired project milestones and will be receptive to queries and unexpected obstacles that require troubleshooting. A great supervisor will ensure that all members of the team are productive and that they have opportunities not only to use their current skills, but also to develop new ones. Further, a good supervisor will ensure that the team has the capacity to resolve problems as they arise, and that they feel empowered to do so. Lastly, and arguably most importantly, the ideal supervisor will have enthusiasm for the topic and the research process as well as an appreciation for the team approach to research. Clearly, finding a good research supervisor requires a fair bit of research on its own.

In summary, think about what research supervision means to you and where you expect to need the most support. The following checklist outlines some considerations that might help you to find the best person possible to supervise your research project; these apply to both supervisors and supervisory teams.

- ❑ **Other students and trainees.** Talk with other research students or graduate students who have trained with the supervisor you are considering. They are the best source of information on what your experience might be like.
- ❑ **Research process experience.** Does the supervisor you have in mind understand the challenges one faces in research, and can he or she offer practical tips for troubleshooting problems that arise? Current and former students and trainees should be able to provide insight here.
- ❑ **Content expertise.** Does your potential supervisor know the topic area well and its application to and

interconnection with other topic areas? Finding out how long he or she has been active in the area and whether he or she teaches courses on the topic should give you a good sense of this.

- ❑ **Methodological expertise.** Make sure that the supervisor you have in mind is well versed in the approaches that you will need to use for your project, ranging from laboratory techniques to biostatistics.
- ❑ **Management experience.** Does the supervisor you have in mind have a good track record in organizing and managing people, resources, data, space and multiple responsibilities?
- ❑ **Enriching environment.** Will your prospective supervisor be able to enhance your research experience through access to educational workshops and conferences, or key national and international experts?
- ❑ **Matching expectations.** Do your expectations for your research project match those of the supervisor you have in mind? To broach this question, when you meet with a potential supervisor, come prepared with a list of your expectations and offer it as something that you can work on together. This gesture should open up the discussion nicely. Before your meeting, be sure to discuss your expectations with respected colleagues, especially those with research experience, to ensure that they are realistic and appropriate.
- ❑ **Funding track record.** Can your potential supervisor provide the resources to carry out the proposed project? Biographies posed on your department's website can give you a sense of what faculty or staff can offer. You may find curriculum vitae and information on their collaborations, resources and recent grants.
- ❑ **Publication track record and scientific writing skills**. Is your potential supervisor well published? Search literature databases such as PubMed, or the person's own website, if available, for his or her publication record. Is he or she able and willing to coach you through the writing and submission process, and knowledgeable about possible journals that might be interested in publishing your research?

You might think of other items of particular concern to you to add to this list.

Milestones for management, and establishing norms

Starting

For the trainee, a first research project is, among other things, an exercise in independent adult learning, project management and time management. Establishing **norms**—standard, agreed-upon rules for the conduct of the research team—before the work begins can help to ensure that the project runs smoothly.

You may find that the approach to the research component of your training will be different from approaches you have grown accustomed to in your training so far. Your research experience will be greatly enhanced if you quickly become comfortable with the idea that you, for the most part, will be directing the course and pace of your project. Acquiring a certain savvy in project management and time management will help you stay on track (see ch. 23). Set timelines and milestones to keep you on course.

Before the project begins, certain norms should be discussed and agreed on by you, your supervisor and your team. You may find that you have to be the one to bring up the topic of establishing norms, and you should feel empowered to do so. Before you do, though, consider what processes and standards of behaviour you are most comfortable with, what you think is fair, and what you need, considering your skill set. Although it may feel awkward initially, you will be thankful that you initiated the norms conversation at the outset of the project: It will save you some headaches (and potential conflicts) down the road. Also, by doing so, you will demonstrate your conscientiousness, maturity and foresight. Some of the most important norms to discuss include communication, authorship, expectations and conflict resolution, although you and your team may come up with more.

Establishing norms for **communication** is important. Knowing how, in what manner and how frequently (weekly or daily) to communicate is essential to moving your project forward. Does your supervisor prefer face-to-face, phone or email communication? How casual or assertive a communication style is everyone happy with? How long is an appropriate wait time for a reply? Do the team members work over the weekend and into the evenings and expect communication about the project to extend into this time (it may be the best time to get their attention, especially if they are busy during "regular" hours). Explicitly ask your supervisor and team members what the best methods of communication are for each of them. Do they prefer a structured process involving regularly scheduled meetings

to discuss progress, deliverables and timelines? Or do they prefer a more informal working style in which you feel you can "pop in" to ask a quick question and provide "side bar" progress updates?

Authorship is another important expectation to discuss. Before the project commences, identify who will be authors on any publications arising from your project, in addition to any other products that might flow from the work. If you are unsure of what is appropriate, seek out sources that define authorship, such the International Committee of Medical Journal Editors criteria or other standards commonly accepted at biomedical journals.[a] Also, decide collectively the order of authorship on any publications and ensure that everyone understands and is comfortable with the plan. For example, research supervisors are often listed last (but sometimes second), indicating that they are the most senior investigator. Make the topic of authorship a discussion point with colleagues and mentors to learn how they have approached this topic and applied authorship criteria in the past. Be sure to rework the plan if roles change. Research projects are dynamic, and it is highly likely that you will end up being responsible for tasks that you and your team never anticipated.

It is also important to address **expectations** about how the work will get done, by whom, and within what time frame. Be aware of what you would like, and what your supervisor and team can actually provide, so that expectations are aligned. Be prepared: by providing thoughtful background material, clear outlines, and the flexibility to accommodate team member's schedules, you can enhance your chances of success. For example, get a time commitment on deliverables from your supervisor. A promise such as "I will read over your draft of the protocol so you can put it in for ethics review" is meaningless without a date. Encourage follow-through on promises with patience, persistence and smiles: Negativity won't get you anywhere. Set an example by meeting the timelines you proposed and being accountable to your commitments. This also means ensuring that your proposed timelines are realistic. When timelines aren't being met, it will be helpful if you have established a working culture within the team in which checking in and following up are seen as appropriate and, indeed, an essential element of accountability. Of course, this is easier to say than do when the recidivist is the dean of medicine, but the principle is important to keep in mind.

---

a   For the ICMJE criteria, see www.icmje.org/ethical_1author.html

Although the trickiest norms to talk about are likely those concerning **conflict resolution**, they are arguably (pun intended) the most important. You might not be able to predict where conflict will arise, but you can make sure that you have a plan for dealing with it when it does. For example, between you, your supervisor, and your team you might agree that if a disagreement arises the parties involved will first try to sort it out (privately) between themselves. If that turns out to be unsuccessful, a mediator will be sought—ideally, someone who is not tethered to the project or source of conflict. Many student services offices and departments have information on where to find a mediator. If conflict does arise, address it early; otherwise, it could snowball, leaving you in a bit of a predicament.

This brings us to the importance of identifying a supervisor or team of supervisors that you feel comfortable with and with whom you believe you will have a pleasant working relationship. Does the chemistry feel right? If not, you may need to look further. The selection is important. Not only will you learn better in a positive environment where you feel respected and included, but you may find that supervision around a project evolves into important professional and career mentorship. For all of these reasons, it is important to choose well (see also ch. 5).

After the norms conversation, write up what you understand to be the decisions and share them with your supervisor and others who will be involved in your project. Seek confirmation that the norms document represents what they understood to be the agreement; if changes and additions are needed, this is a great time to make them. The norms document will hopefully serve as a compass for your research project that you can refer back to in the event of a misunderstanding.

Parallels between health care practice and the research environment

As in health care practice, achieving high-quality results in research requires a team effort, and thus you shouldn't rely solely on your supervisor. Research is more of a team enterprise than some trainees realize, and supervision and support often come from many people on many different levels. As a health care practitioner, you are accustomed to working in care teams that might include physicians, pharmacists, nurses and physiotherapists. Many of the teamwork skills you have developed in clinical settings will be helpful in the research setting. Of course, you will need to

seek the commitment of an "official" supervisor, but you should also be open to supervision, guidance and mentorship from others.

These days, resident research projects are rarely carried out by one trainee at a bench or computer with support from a single supervisor in an adjacent office. Ideally, you will find a supervisor who works with a variety of experts, to whom you will have access and who may become part of a supervisory team focused, at least in part, on you and your project. Other people might link into your project because of a keen interest in the topic area or the particular methodological approach you plan to use. Embrace and seek out these team opportunities in your research experience. You and your research will certainly benefit from doing so.

As with many of the skills and techniques acquired during a health sciences training program, proficiency in the research process requires specific training. With effective training and experience you can acquire the necessary set of critical thinking skills, analytical approaches and perspectives necessary to conduct high-quality research. Good supervision can facilitate the development of these skills, but the successful heath research trainee will be open to obtaining them from a variety of people and in a range of settings.

In health research, where the question under investigation is complex and multi-faceted, investigators often collaborate across disciplines. For example, a research team interested in preventing falls among seniors through the examination and testing of various exercise training programs could include collaborators with expertise in kinesiology, medicine, physical therapy, epidemiology, biostatistics, health economics and program evaluation. The roles of the team members might range from lead investigators, to masters, doctoral and postdoctoral students, research assistants, data administrators, and you! This **interdisciplinary** approach provides an ideal way to learn about alternative approaches relevant to your research topic. And, because most new researchers have a limited research background and experience working in an interdisciplinary setting, you have the most to learn. So, treat every interaction, whether with an expert investigator in biochemistry or a research assistant charged with data collection, as a valuable learning opportunity.

In addition, when selecting a supervisor you will need to seek a champion who is willing to work with you and to be an advocate for your project. Many supervisors have a

Starting

number of trainees that they are working with and many other diverse responsibilities, so they might not devote as much time and energy as they would like to promoting your work, although they are still proficient in the supervisory role. Consequently, your "champion" might turn out to be your program director, a research mentor, someone with content expertise, someone who can provide practical support with ethics applications and approvals, or someone who can assist with participant recruitment.

Being the small fish in a big and new pond

It is important to realize that much of your research training will take place in informal and unstructured settings: this is where you will learn the most. You will not be called into your supervisor's office or required to sit through long lectures on how to calibrate the data acquisition system to record beat-by-beat blood pressure, or how to systematically write the discussion section of your paper.

It is likely that your supervisor will facilitate group learning activities, such as attending presentations by experts and journal club meetings. A journal club meeting, in which a relevant paper is discussed in detail with particular focus on the methods, can be a fantastic setting for learning. The content might be directly relevant to the work that you need to do, such as estimating the sample size needed for a certain study. Even topics that, on the surface, have no relevance to your current project can spark new ideas for refining your research question or analysing your data. Especially valuable learning venues are research rounds or meetings where team members present data for critical analysis and constructive criticism. These offer a great opportunity to develop critical thinking skills and to practise the evaluation of research results: skills that will certainly come in handy when it is time for you to evaluate your own study and its results, or when you are reviewing published research to inform your clinical practice.

Your supervisor might offer a number of **informal learning** opportunities, such as tutoring you on preparing a research protocol for an ethics application during a lunch break at a research conference. Other informal learning opportunities might arise when you are given a desk in a room with other trainees, where you might find that conversations on data interpretation sprout up from time to time, providing an opportunity to passively and actively gain insights applicable to your own work. Seek out these environments for informal learning and other potential opportunities to engage with other researchers and research trainees: they are among your most valuable classrooms. Make an effort to develop camaraderie with colleagues and to foster peer-learning opportunities. A discussion of how you and your colleagues might network and share competencies stemming from previous work or research experience is beyond the scope of this chapter; see chapter 4 for a discussion of research networks and their benefits.

Practical tips for managing your supervision

Once you have a grasp of your topic area and your research question, have secured a commitment from your research supervisor, and have identified your supervisory team, take some time to consider a little "team theory." Yes, theoretical and practical research literature provides an evidence-informed approach to research and the research team process! The literature on team dynamics and organizational psychology demonstrates the importance of identifying a "compelling goal" for the team as well as clear roles and responsibilities for all involved in the project.[1] To get a project done, those involved need to believe that it is interesting and important and will lead to the achievement of a particular goal or aspiration. As the one with the vested interest in and responsibility for your project, you need to instill in your team members a sense of the importance of the project and its multiple benefits for all involved. It can help to point out the direct benefits of the project to your team and supervisor. However, it is unlikely that you will have any authority over team members and the delivery of their components of the project. This is why establishing explicit roles and responsibilities is important.

Successful research projects take teamwork, and teamwork requires coordination. It will be your responsibility to orchestrate this coordination for your research project. One useful guide from the corporate world is the **RACI management tool**, which can be used to identify, and to prevent confusion about, roles and responsibilities during the course of a project.[2] Where there is no confusion about roles and responsibilities, conflict is less likely. The elements that make up the acronym are:

- **Responsible**. The person who has responsibility for getting the work done or a decision made. Ideally, this responsibility is assigned to one person (e.g., the research trainee).

- **Accountable.** The person who is accountable for the correct and thorough completion of the task. This must be one person (e.g., research supervisor). The "responsible" person is accountable to and has his or her work approved by the person in this role.
- **Consulted.** The people who provide information for the project are often subject experts (e.g., other research project co-supervisors/co-investigators). Here, there is two-way communication.
- **Informed**. These are the people who are affected by the outcome and need to be kept informed about the progress of the project. Here, the communication is one-way.

Thus, applying the RACI framework, you will likely be "responsible" for the entire exercise, your supervisor will likely be "accountable" for the project, and the rest of the supervisory team will provide "consultation." Your program administrators will need to be kept "informed" of your progress and completion of the project. You will also have to "inform" your friends that you can't go out because you are deeply engaged with the literature (or, more likely, are stuck trying to figure out how to get your referencing software to work because no one else on the team knows how to use it).

The RACI tool will become important when you need to make decisions relevant to your research. You will often get conflicting opinions when you ask different people the same question (e.g., should you use the full Mini-Mental State Exam, or the abbreviated version, as a measure of cognitive impairment in your study?). With RACI you can clarify the roles of each team member: some have a consultative role, while others have more leverage in the decisions that will be made. Always make sure that you, your supervisor, and your team members are clear about their roles from the outset of your work together, before any decisions need to be made.

Putting your research into context

It is important to know that the research projects reported in major medical journals, or even the mid-level journals, often have budgets that exceed $1 million. The average 5-year operating grant awarded by CIHR (the Canadian Institutes of Health Research) exceeds $750,000 in total.

This does not count the cost of the investigators' salaries, which are paid through other sources, or the value of "in kind" equipment and infrastructure costs that support many studies. Major multi-centre drug studies powered to obtain statistically significant results for important clinical outcomes may require budgets of over $1 billion. These projects often have a multi-million dollar budget just for their industry sponsors to purchase reprints to distribute to physicians as part of the post-study publicity!

Knowing about the funding structures of a research program is important (see also ch. 19). This information will help you appreciate the resources that your supervisor dedicates to you and your project. Further, it will give you perspective on the demands placed on your supervisor and supervisory team to continue their research work as well as the competitive nature of the **research environment** in the pursuit of funding.

Research is hard work—as with most things, proficiency takes time and practice!

Our expectations invariably colour our experiences. From the outside, research may seem like something you can easily take in stride. The fact that you have made it this far in a professional health sciences training program means that you have had many positive experiences. As a health trainee or practitioner, you may receive positive feedback many times a day. However, be warned: the world of research has many daunting aspects that may come as an unwelcome surprise. Three specific aspects of research should be considered as you contemplate the hard work that goes into research: grants, publications and time frame. First, even the most successful researchers fail in half (or more) of their attempts to obtain competitive grant funding. For example, in 2010–2011, the Canadian Institutes for Health Research funded only 23% of the applications received in the open operating grant competition.[b] Grant applications take a lot of time to put together and, given their low success rate, a great deal of time and effort can be invested in funding proposals before a research project is up and rolling. Second, it's not easy to get published. Journals often reject papers outright, or require many revisions even for preliminary acceptance. It should be noted that researchers who never have their papers rejected are not sending them

b   See www.cihr-irsc.gc.ca/e/42857.html

Starting

to sufficiently competitive journals. Third, at the senior levels, a major study such as a cohort study or a randomized controlled trial often takes five or more years to complete. Thus, health trainees who enter into a relationship with a research supervisor must be prepared for a different pace and a delayed sense of gratification compared with clinical work. Even a health trainee's research project will take months rather than weeks to complete. An excellent draft manuscript will still need dozens of corrections (which can be considered negative feedback by those who are rarely corrected) and may receive no specific plaudits.

In short, research is hard. But our warnings are offered with the best of intentions to improve your research experience. Some senior health practitioners find themselves looking for "quick wins" and "short-cuts" to research success without truly taking time to learn the skills that are required. In *Outliers: The Story of Success*, Malcolm Gladwell highlights research showing that excellence across a range of activities such as music, sport and academics required 10 000 hours of training.[3] This was more important than a myriad of factors such as genetic predisposition and childhood environment. Interestingly, this time requirement can be applied to research as well. And, clearly, you don't have that many hours for your initial research project! Further, some clinicians working in research have not caught on to the importance of teamwork, especially when addressing complex health problems that require interdisciplinary approaches. Consequently, their research endeavours will be limited in scope and application.

Conclusion

So that brings us back to where we began: You need help! Quality supervision, from an individual or team, is a key factor for success. You are unlikely to perform well in research as a soloist. However, we fear that the widely accepted term, *supervisor*, emphasizes the wrong elements of the relationship by stressing "oversight" above assistance, support, guidance, growth, collaboration and teamwork.

We hope that we have provided some insight into the wonderful world of research. The aim of this chapter was to allow you to consider the importance of research supervision and to encourage you to consider your goals for your project and research experience. Further, we wanted to allow you to place your research project in context, thus making realistic choices about how you will pursue your research project. Good luck! ■

CASE POSTSCRIPT

Using what she learned from this chapter and the advice of others, the resident consulted the department website and senior residents to determine which faculty members might be potentially suitable supervisors. After meeting with four promising candidate supervisors, she chose one of them based on his research interests, methodological expertise and success in getting research grants and in being published. Further, feedback from other trainees who had worked with him on other occasions confirmed her impression that his working and interpersonal style would suit hers. Not only was her research project a success, but after her residency program she continued to collaborate with her research supervisor on several successful projects. Now, as a new faculty member, she has the opportunity to serve on a supervisory team for residents as they conduct their first research projects.

REFERENCES

1. Hackman JR. *Leading teams: setting the stage for great performances.* Boston (MA): Harvard Business School Press; 2002.

2. Value Based Management.net. *RACI model.* Available at: www.valuebasedmanagement.net/methods_raci.html

3. Gladwell M. *Outliers: the story of success.* London & New York: Allen Lane; 2008.

Starting

EXERCISES

1. Consider these questions

- What are your priorities for your research project: pursuing a research topic that you are really interested in, or finding a superior research environment where you can gain valuable skills and experience that you can apply to future research endeavours?

- Do you have good knowledge of the work of the research groups within your program, department, faculty and university? Do you have a concept of potential supervisor's approach to research and research supervision? Do you have a network of people who might be able to give you insight into how these groups function and into where, considering your priorities, you might best fit in?

- Do you have the necessary skills to work collaboratively in a research team? Should you seek training to improve your collaborative skills?

2. Seek out one or more of the following through the Faculty of Graduate Studies or Student Development Centre at your university:
   - graduate student supervision guidelines
   - codes of behaviour for trainees and research supervisors
   - technical/scientific writing courses

Starting

SUMMARY CHECKLIST

- ❏ Consider personal priorities: Is it your goal to acquire content knowledge in a particular topic area, or in research skills and methodology?
- ❏ Do some research: Scan your department for a supervisor who fits with your priorities.
- ❏ Ramp up your résumé, curriculum vitae and negotiating skills, as they may be required in your request for supervision.
- ❏ Formulate a manageable and interesting research question.
- ❏ Match your learning needs, expectations and priorities with the skills, interests, resources and traits of your supervisor.
- ❏ Look for a supervisor or supervisory team with content knowledge, experience in specific methodological approaches and the research process, a history of conducting research, a history of successfully supervising students, and a track record of research success.
- ❏ Consider your potential supervisor's access to resources: laboratories, office space, research tools or equipment, data–bases, and study participants/recruitment options.
- ❏ Most importantly, try to seek supervision where you will have access to a diverse team of skilled experts who are interested and able to help you!
- ❏ Find a supervisor/supervisory team who pays attention to deadlines and timelines.
- ❏ Get comfortable with self-managed, self-directed learning: time management and project management skills are key to successful research projects.
- ❏ Establish norms with regard to communication, authorship, expectations and conflict resolution.
- ❏ Look for the parallels in health care practice and the research process.
- ❏ Seek a champion for your project—someone who is willing to put in the time to help it along and to advocate for its importance. This could be almost anyone—from a supervisor or a team member to a manager or fellow trainee.
- ❏ Be open to dynamic learning at every opportunity and from a variety of people.
- ❏ Use the RACI tool to manage supervision and your research project.
- ❏ Take it all in stride and put your research into context. Don't expect to cure cancer overnight and recognize the constraints of time and funding common to research.
- ❏ Remember that failure is part of the research process. You are treading on new territory: embrace setbacks as part of the experience.
- ❏ Have fun!

4
Research teams and networks

Terry P. Klassen, MD, MSc, FRCPC

ILLUSTRATIVE CASE

In anticipation of the Fellows Research Day at the annual meeting of the Pediatric Emergency Research of Canada (PERC) research network, an Emergency Medicine resident is encouraged to present a research idea he has been developing about how the Ottawa Ankle Rules might perform in the context of pediatric care. Although he is rather daunted by the prospect of presenting to a large group of colleagues and research experts an idea that is still at a preliminary stage, he decides to prepare a presentation. He also wonders about the value of joining this research network as a trainee. Specifically, he is unsure whether he is sufficiently qualified to join and whether the required investment of time and effort will pay off.

■ **This chapter will examine the role** of research teams and networks in fostering and promoting research and illustrate how they can provide a fertile environment in which trainees and other novice health researchers can develop knowledge and skills. The last decade has witnessed a blossoming of research networks and teams, enabled in part by national and provincial research bodies that direct funding specifically to team- or network-based research.[1-4] One great advantage of the team-based approach is the capacity it affords to recruit large sample groups over relatively short periods of time, thus achieving the statistical power necessary to confidently address important issues faced by patients and health care providers. Some of these issues are sufficiently complex that only a research team or network will have at its disposal the array of scientific disciplines, perspectives and approaches that are needed to solve the problem. Moreover, firm connections between research networks and health care environments can provide an ideal context for **knowledge translation** (see ch. 30), maximizing the chances that research findings will be applied to health care practice and decision-making.

This chapter will explore these benefits by means of a concrete example, describing how the Pediatric Emergency Research of Canada (PERC) network has advanced the knowledge base for pediatric emergency medicine and has had a positive impact on health outcomes among children in need of emergency care.

CHAPTER OBJECTIVES

After reading this chapter, you should be able to:
- describe research networks and teams and their value in today's research world, using Pediatric Emergency Medicine as an example;
- describe a research network and how it functions, outlining the benefits and challenges it presents; and
- discuss how health care trainees and others new to health research can benefit from working in such an environment.

KEY TERMS

Iterative loop

Knowledge translation

Research disciplines

Research environment

Research training

The PERC network

In Canadian emergency departments in the mid 1990s, there was little clarity with regard to determining which children who presented with a minor head injury involving loss of consciousness should receive a computed tomography (CT) scan of the head. Concerned clinicians and researchers from pediatric emergency departments across the country gathered to discuss approaches to this problem. From this effort arose PERC, whose first study demonstrated that there was substantial variability—as great as four-fold—across nine pediatric emergency departments in the frequency with which CT scans were ordered for children with the same type of minor head injury.[5] Led by Dr. Martin Osmond, and with funding from the Canadian Institutes of Health Research (CIHR), members of the PERC Head Injury Study Group and others developed a decision rule to guide clinicians that was eventually published in 2010.[6]

The theoretical model for this research program is based on the "measurement **iterative loop**" described by Tugwell and colleagues in 1985,[7] which provides a framework for assembling, acting upon and evaluating health information to reduce the burden of illness.[4,8] The logical sequence for research described by the loop includes the following steps:

- quantifying the burden of illness
- identifying causative factors
- identifying gaps in evidence through systematic reviews and evaluating the efficacy of treatment options through randomized controlled trials
- determining treatment effectiveness in the field
- evaluating the cost-effectiveness of interventions
- identifying barriers to transfer and uptake of information by end users
- conducting systematic reviews to identify optimal ways for knowledge translation to reduce the gap between clinical practice and research
- disseminating research findings from clinical and knowledge translation research
- allowing for the natural diffusion of results in the "real world"
- assessing "real world" outcomes

The PERC team modified the original iterative loop into a double loop, highlighting two areas that we believe to be critical to the optimization of health outcomes (Fig. 4.1): clinical research (evaluating therapeutic interventions), and knowledge translation (implementation and uptake of proven interventions).

PERC's work in croup serves to illustrate how this can work. Croup is a relatively common respiratory disease in children, with a peak incidence in 1 to 2 year olds.[9] It is known that most cases are caused by parainfluenza virus and that its incidence peaks in alternate years. The main pathophysiological abnormality is subglottic edema and narrowing of the trachea[10] (steps 1 and 2 in Fig 4.1). Debate raged in the 1970s as to the effectiveness of glucocorticoids in reducing this swelling and achieving a clinical benefit. A meta-analysis by Kairys and colleagues[10] in 1989 demonstrated that, for croup patients admitted to hospital, treatment with glucocorticoids would result in a significant decrease in hospital admissions and reduce the probability of intubation (step 3). This then spurred research in emergency departments to examine the effectiveness of glucocorticoids in this context. A series of randomized controlled trials (RCTs) demonstrated a decrease in hospital admission rates and more rapid clinical improvement with glucocorticoid therapy[11] (step 3). A study of the "real world" effect of glucocorticoids demonstrated a significant decrease in hospital admissions for croup over a 14-year period, which was coincident with the publication of the evidence of the effectiveness of glucocorticoids for croup[12] (step 4). An economic evaluation, included as part of an RCT, demonstrated that cases treated with placebo cost $93, as compared with $72 for those treated with dexamethasone, and had better outcomes with respect to the resolution of croup symptoms and lower rates of hospital admission[13] (step 5). Research is currently under way to examine the knowledge translation portion of the loop[14] (steps 6–10).

To succeed as a network, PERC has had to bring together collaborators from a variety of disciplines. It has also focused on having researchers at all levels participate, from trainees all the way to very senior, accomplished researchers. To be successful in the clinical research loop, it has engaged clinicians, statisticians, epidemiologists and health economists. To be successful in knowledge translation, it has formed a strong partnership with leaders in this field, ensuring that the team includes qualitative researchers, cognitive psychologists and medical sociologists. In our cluster RCT examining three methods for ensuring how croup guidelines are best incorporated into clinical practice, it was noticed that responses varied among the various health care providers in the different hospitals across Alberta with respect to adopting the evidence on treatment for croup (unpublished data). A qualitative researcher, as part of the team, conducted focus groups to elucidate the underlying reasons for the variation in response.

Figure 4.1: **A paradigm for research: the iterative figure-eight.** KT = knowledge translation; SRs = systematic reviews; RCTs = randomized controlled trials. Reproduced from Hartling et al.[4] by permission of John Wiley and Sons.

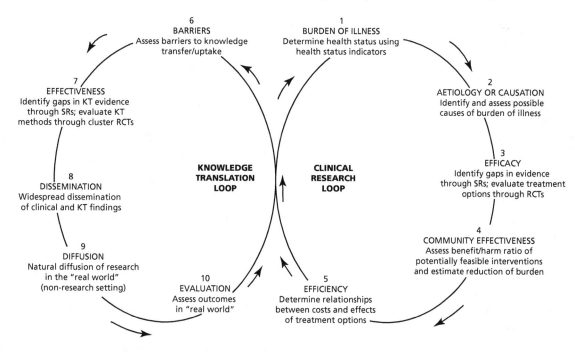

PERC has believed so strongly in creating the next generation of researchers that, from its first formal national meeting, it has held a Fellow's Research Day. Fellows in pediatric emergency medicine from across Canada present their research projects at all stages, from idea-generation to completed projects. In a positive environment, their peers and senior researchers offer constructive feedback to improve their work. With a broad array of disciplinary backgrounds, it offers a very stimulating and supportive environment. The trainees also attend the portion of the annual meeting where staff researchers present their work, giving them a strong sense of the **research environment** and possibilities for the future. Fellows and trainees who have graduated from the program now attend as junior staff members.

Conclusion

This chapter, through the example of the PERC research network, has explored the potential role of research networks and teams in health **research training**. Such networks offer a positive environment in which trainees and others can acquire research skills and observe role models. Research networks provide exposure to a variety of **research disciplines** and methodologies, insight into how networks operate, and practical experience in collaborating with peers and more senior researchers. Additionally, if the resident decides on research as a career option, early experience working with a network provides a valuable foundation, forging links with a community that can play an important part in his or her future development in health research. ■

CASE POSTSCRIPT

The resident's presentation was well-received, and he was encouraged to carry out a systematic review on the pediatric use of the Ottawa Ankle Rules. Being part of a network, he had access to a statistician, an epidemiologist and a librarian, and was able to complete the systematic review and have it published in *Academic Emergency Medicine*.[15] It was also selected as one of the articles relevant to InfoPOEMs (which provides short reviews of articles relevant to primary care) and was rated as very relevant to 89% of those accessing this POEM.[16]

Starting

REFERENCES

1. Babl F, Borland M, Ngo P, Acworth J, Krieser D, Pandit S, et al. Paediatric Research in Emergency Departments International Collaborative (PREDICT): first steps towards the development of an Australian and New Zealand research network. *Emerg Med Australas*. 2006;18(2):143–7.

2. Walker DM, Tolentino VR, Teach SJ. Trends and challenges in international pediatric emergency medicine. *Curr Opin Pediatr.* 2007;19(3):247–52.

3. Pediatric Emergency Care Applied Research Network. The Pediatric Emergency Care Applied Research Network (PECARN): rationale, development, and first steps. *Acad Emerg Med*. 2003;10(6):661–8.

4. Hartling L, Scott-Findlay S, Johnson D, Osmond M, Plint A, Grimshaw J, et al. Bridging the gap between clinical research and knowledge translation in pediatric emergency medicine. *Acad Emerg Med*. 2007;14(11):968–77.

5. Klassen TP, Reed MH, Stiell IG, Nijssen-Jordan C, Tenenbein M, Joubert G, et al. Variation in utilization of computed tomography scanning for the investigation of minor head trauma in children: a Canadian experience. *Acad Emerg Med*. 2000;7(7):739–44.

6. Osmond MH, Klassen TP, Wells GA, Correll R, Jarvis A, Joubert G, et al. CATCH: a clinical decision rule for use of computed tomography in children with mild head injury. *CMAJ*. 2010;182(4):341–8.

7. Tugwell P, Bennett KJ, Sackett DL, Haynes RB. The measurement iterative loop: a framework for the critical appraisal of need, benefits and costs of health interventions. *J Chronic Dis*. 1985;38(4):339–51.

8. Scott S, Hartling L, Grimshaw J, Johnson D, Osmond M, Plint A, et al. Improving outcomes for ill and injured children in emergency departments: protocol for a program in pediatric emergency medicine and knowledge translation science. *Implement Sci*. 2009 Sep 22;4:60.

9. Denny FW, Murphy TF, Clyde WA Jr, Collier AM, Henderson FW. Croup: an 11-year study in a pediatric practice. *Pediatrics*. 1983;71(6):871–6.

10. Kairys SW, Olmstead EM, O'Connor GT. Steroid treatment of laryngotracheitis: a meta-analysis of the evidence from randomized trials. *Pediatrics*. 1989;83(5):683–93.

11. Russell KF, Liang Y, O'Gorman K, Johnson DW, Klassen TP. Glucocorticoids for croup. *Cochrane Database Syst Rev*. 2011;(1):CD001955.

12. Segal AO, Crighton EJ, Moineddin R, Mamdani M, Upshur RE. Croup hospitalizations in Ontario: a 14-year time-series analysis. *Pediatrics*. 2005;116(1):51–5.

13. Bjornson CL, Klassen TP, Williamson J, Brant R, Milton C, Plint A, et al. A randomized trial of a single dose of oral dexamethasone for mild croup. *N Engl J Med*. 2004;351(13):1306–13.

14. Johnson DW, Craig W, Brant R, Mitton C, Svenson L, Klassen TP. A cluster randomized controlled trial comparing three methods of disseminating practice guidelines for children with croup. *Implement Sci*. 2006 Apr 28;1:10.

15. Dowling S, Spooner CH, Liang Y, Dryden DM, Friesen C, Klassen TP, Wright RB. Accuracy of Ottawa Ankle Rules to exclude fractures of the ankle and midfoot in children: a meta-analysis. *Acad Emerg Med*. 2009;16(4):277–7.

16. Canadian Medical Association. Ottawa ankle rules accurate for children aged 6 years and older. *Daily InfoPOEMs*. Available from: www.cma.ca/index.cfm?ci_id=50728&la_id=1&gmAction=/infoPoems/displayPoem.do?poemId=110622.

SUMMARY CHECKLIST

- ❏ Describe how a research network could benefit your research.
- ❏ Describe how a research network could help you develop as a researcher.
- ❏ List potential research networks to join. If you are unsure, find an experienced researcher who can advise you.

5
Looking for an academic mentor

David L. Sackett, OC, MD, FRSC, FRCP

IS THIS YOU?

Although some of your colleagues see the "Resident Research Project" as a hurdle to be jumped (crawled?) over, you see it as a leap into your chosen career of academic clinician-investigator. You'd really like to divide your time and energy between being a master clinician and a groundbreaking researcher. Moreover, although your research supervisor is excellent for your resident research project, you want to link up with someone who would take a long-term interest in you and your career. If this is you, read on. If it isn't, stop reading this chapter and get on with the other bits of this guide that will get you over that "Resident Research Project" hurdle.

◼ What will determine your success

as an academic clinician-investigator? If you want to become a top-flight, study-designing, grant-getting, study-finishing, first-authoring, prematurely promoted, tenure-holding, award-winning, highly respected and widely recruited academic clinician-investigator, you won't get there on your brains, imagination and energy alone. You will need three more things: good academic mentoring,[1,2] effective priority-setting and rigorous time management.

- *Fact:* Previous academic performance accounts for only 6% of the variance in postgraduate medical competency.[3]
- *Fact:* Canadian obstetrics and gynecology fellows with mentors were more than twice as likely to receive academic promotion.[4]
- *Fact:* Graduates of U.S. internal medicine research fellowship programs who had "influential mentors" during their training were 5 times as likely to publish at least one paper and 3 times as likely to be PIs on a funded research grant.[5]
- *Fact:* A full half of U.S. psychiatric residents given mentors, research courses and an academic stipend went on to pursue research careers.[6]
- *Fact:* Although gender-based inequalities exist in running households and raising children, women are as successful as men in having their U.S. National Institutes of Health research grants approved and renewed.[7]

- *Fact:* Burnout affects up to a third of physicians, is more common among women, has a lousy prognosis and is prevented by control over workload, setting limits, having a mentor and having adequate administrative support.[8]
- *Fact:* In a recent survey, 41% of the Canadian residency program directors who responded agreed or strongly agreed that there was a need for more formal mentorship within the training program.[9]

What a good academic mentor provides

For newcomers (such as graduate students, research fellows, or new faculty), academic mentoring provides three things. First, it provides *resources* without obligations. Second, it provides *opportunities* without demands. Third, it provides *advice* and *protection.* I hope it's therefore obvious that an academic mentor is not the same thing as a research supervisor.

By *resources,* I mean that a really good mentor would supplement the resources that might be provided in the short term by your research supervisor and provide you with:

- longer-term space to work;
- productivity-enhancing equipment;
- free photocopy, email and Internet access;
- occasional secretarial support;
- money to go to courses and meetings;
- salary supplements if your fellowship doesn't provide for necessities and simple graces; and
- bridge-funding of your research until you get your first grant.

Starting

In some departments, all or most of these resources are provided by the chair, and in others, none. In either setting, your mentor should "wheel and deal" until the resources are in place. You should be spared both the time and the humiliation of begging for these resources on your own.

By *opportunities* at the beginner's level, I mean the systematic examination of everything that crosses your mentor's desk for its potential contribution to your scientific development and academic advancement.

1. The opportunity to join one of your mentor's ongoing research projects. This can provide more than just "hands-on" practical experience in the application of your graduate course content. You can also learn how to create and function as a member of a collaborative team, and to develop skills in research management.

   Taking on a piece of your mentor's project to run, analyze, present and publish is a two-edged sword. On the one hand, it provides an excellent opportunity to go beyond the classroom and develop your practical skills in data management and analysis. Moreover, it gives you the opportunity to start to learn how to combine "science and showbiz" in presenting your results and writing for publication. Finally, your curriculum vitae (CV) will benefit.

   On the other hand, being given a project by your mentor can be harmful. The greatest risk here is that your mentor might "give" you a pre-designed sub-study or research project and encourage you to use it as your major (e.g., thesis) learning focus. Although often done with the best intention, accepting this "gift" is bad for you. This is because taking on a pre-designed project robs you of the opportunity to develop your most important research skills. First, you'll lose the opportunity to learn how to recognize and define a problem in human biology or clinical care. Second, you'll lose the opportunity of learning how to convert that problem-recognition into a question that is both important and answerable (see ch. 6). Third, you'll lose the opportunity to learn how to select the most appropriate study architecture to answer your question (see ch. 9). Fourth, you'll lose the opportunity to identify and overcome the dozens of "threats to validity" that occur in any study. These

four skills are central to your development as an independent investigator. Without them, you'll master only the methods that are required for your "given" project. Like the kid who received a shiny new birthday hammer, you'll risk spending the rest of your career looking at ever-less-important nails to thump with your same old, limited set of skills.

2. The opportunity to carry out duplicate, blind (and, of course, confidential) refereeing of manuscripts and grants. The comparison of these critiques not only sharpens your critical appraisal skills, but also permits you to see your mentor's refereeing style and forces you to develop your own.

3. The opportunity to accompany your mentor to meetings of ethics and grant review committees to learn first-hand how these groups function.

4. The opportunity, as soon as your competency permits, to join your mentor in responding to their invitations from prominent, refereed journals to write editorials, commentaries or essays. Not only will the joint review and synthesis of the relevant evidence be highly educational. It also provides you the opportunity to learn how to write with clarity and style (see ch. 29). Finally, it adds an important publication to your CV. As soon as your contribution warrants, you should become the lead author of such pieces. The ultimate objective is for you to become the sole author (all the sooner if your mentor casts a wide shadow).

   One note of caution about invited chapters for books: unless the book is a very prestigious one, authoring a chapter in it adds little or no weight to your CV.

5. The opportunity to take over some of your mentor's invitations and learn how to give "boilerplate" lectures (especially at nice venues and for generous honoraria).

6. Your inclusion in the social as well as academic events that comprise the visit of famous colleagues from other institutions should become automatic.

7. The opportunity to go as part of a group to scientific meetings, especially annual gatherings of the research clan. This has several advantages. First, it gives you the chance to meet and hear the old farts in your field. Second, it allows you to meet and debate with the other newcomers who will become your future colleagues. Third, you

can compare your impressions and new ideas with your mentor while they are fresh, in a relaxed and congenial atmosphere.

8.   The opportunity to observe, model and discuss teaching strategies and tactics in both clinical and classroom situations. When you are invited to join your mentor's clinical team, you can study how they employ different teaching strategies and tactics as they move from the post-take/morning report, to the daily review round, to the clinical skills session, to grand rounds. With time, you should take over these sessions and receive feedback about your performance. The same sequence should be followed in teaching courses and leading seminars in research methods.

It is important that these opportunities are offered without coercion and accepted without resentment. Crucially, they must never involve the off-loading of odious tasks with little or no academic content from overburdened mentors to the beholden mentored.

By *advice,* I mean providing frequent, unhurried and safe opportunities for you to think your way through both your academic and social development. Topics here include your choices of graduate courses, the methodological challenges in your research projects, the pros and cons of working with a particular set of collaborators, and how to balance your career with the rest of your life. For example, some mentors refuse to discuss academic issues at such sessions until they have gone through a checklist of items encompassing personal and family health, relationships, finances, and the like. Their advice should take the form of "active listening," should focus on your development as an independent thinker, and should eschew commands and authoritarian pronouncements.

As long as gender-based inequalities exist in running households and raising children, mentors must be knowledgeable and effective in addressing and advising around the special problems that face women in academic careers.[10] Although only 20% of female academics in one study stated that it was important to have a mentor of the same gender, it is imperative that all women pursuing academic careers have easy access to discussing and receiving informed, empathic advice about issues such as timing their pregnancies, parental leave, time-out, part-time appointments, sharing and delegating household tasks, and the like. When the principal mentor is a man, these needs are often best met by specific additional mentoring around these issues from a woman.

When listening to you sort through a job offer, it is important for your mentor to help you recognize the crucial difference between "wanting to be wanted for" and "wanting to do" a prestigious academic post. You'd be crazy not to feel elated at "being wanted for" any prestigious job, regardless of whether it matched your career objectives and academic strengths. However, an "actively listening" mentor can help you decide whether you really "want to do" the work involved in that post. It is here that they may help you realize that the post is ill-matched to your interests, priorities, career stage, competencies, or temperament.

By *protection,* I mean insulating you from needless academic buffeting and from the bad behaviour of other academics. Because science advances though the vigorous debate of ideas, designs, data and conclusions, you should get used to having yours subjected to keen and critical scrutiny. For the same reason, you needn't be tossed in at the deep end. Thus, for example, you should rehearse formal presentations of your research in front of your mentor (and whoever else is around). They can challenge your every statement and slide in a relaxed and supportive setting. As a result (especially in these days of PowerPoint), you can revise your presentation and rehearse your responses to the likely questions that will be asked about it. The objective here is to face the toughest, most critical questions about your work for the first time at a rehearsal among friends, not following its formal presentation among rivals and strangers.

Similarly, your mentor can help you recognize the real objectives of the critical letters to the editor that follow your first publication of your work. Most of them are attempts to show off (the "peacock phenomenon"), to protect turf, and to win at rhetoric, rather than to promote understanding. When serious scientists have questions about a paper, they write to its authors, not to the editor. Your mentors can also help you learn how to write responses that repeat your main message, answer substantive questions (if any), and ignore the tawdry slurs that your detractors attempt to pass off as harmless wit.

Finally, disputes between senior investigators often are fought over the corpses of their graduate students. This means you. Your mentor must intervene swiftly and decisively whenever they detect such attacks on you, including especially those related to your sex, gender, race, handicap, or orientation. The intention of your mentor's

Starting

rapid retaliation needn't be to overcome your attacker's underlying prejudice or jealousy. It should merely make the repercussions of picking on you so unpleasant for him that he never tries it again. If it wasn't already part of your core training, a study of the classic paper on "how to swim with sharks" should be part of this exercise.[11]

How should you find an academic mentor?

In a recent survey of young investigators awarded their first career awards from the Alberta Heritage Foundation for Medical Research,[12] the preferred route was for the host department to provide a list of potential mentors and let the newcomers meet them informally and identify the one that best matched their needs and aspirations. As emphasized earlier, women must have ready access to additional mentoring around the issues of women in academia, from another source if necessary.

What should you look for when picking an academic mentor?

Your academic mentor should possess five crucial prerequisites:

1. Your academic mentor has to be a competent investigator. Although most will be clinicians, this needn't be the case. Some of the most successful academic clinicians I know (including me) were mentored by biostatisticians.

2. Your academic mentor must not only have achieved academic success themselves, but must treat you accordingly. That is, your academic mentor must feel secure enough that they are not only comfortable taking a back seat to you in matters of authorship and recognition. They must actively pursue this secondary role. Everything fails if your academic mentor competes with you for recognition. Unfortunately, such competition is common, and you should seek help from your chair or program director if this happens to you (I devote lots of time to trying to resolve such conflicts before they destroy friendships and damage careers).

3. Your academic mentor should not directly control your academic appointment or base salary. Such controls interfere with the free and open exchange of ideas, priorities, aspirations and criticisms. For example, you may find it difficult to turn down an irrelevant, time-consuming task offered by your academic mentor when they also control your salary.

4. Your academic mentor must like mentoring and be willing to devote the time and energy required to do it well. This includes a willingness to explore and solve both the routine and the extraordinary scientific and personal challenges that arise when they take on this responsibility.

5. Some institutions still lack policies for stopping the tenure clock for childbirth and caring for a young child, or for "re-entry" rights and discounted "résumé gaps." Your academic mentor should be informed about these, and should fight for them when they are lacking.

6. Finally, your academic mentor must periodically seek feedback from you about how well they are performing. They must periodically evaluate their own performance, decide whether they remain the best person to mentor you (and, if not, help you find a more suitable mentor), and identify ways to improve their mentoring skills.

Space does not permit a discussion of priority-setting and time-management, the other main determinants of a successful career in academic medicine, in this chapter. However, I have recently discussed them in the Clinician-Trialist Rounds series in the journal Clinical Trials.[13,14]

Acknowledgement
This chapter draws in part from: Sackett DL. On the determinants of academic success as a clinician-scientist. *Clin Invest Med* 2001;24(2):94–100. The kind permission of the Canadian Society for Clinical Investigation is gratefully acknowledged.

REFERENCES

1. Sambunjak D, Straus SE, Marušić A. Mentoring in academic medicine: a systematic review. *JAMA*. 2006;296(9):1103–15.

2. Sambunjak D. Straus SE. Marušić A. A systematic review of qualitative research of the meaning and characteristics of mentoring in academic medicine. *J Gen Int Med*. 2010;25:72–8.

3. Ferguson E, James D, Madeley L. Factors associated with success in medical school: systematic review of the literature. *BMJ*. 2002; 324(7343):952–7.

4. Wise MR, Shapiro H, Bodley J, Pittini R, McKay D, Willan A, et al. Factors affecting academic promotion in obstetrics and gynaecology in Canada. *J Obstet Gynaecol Can*. 2004;26(2):127–36.

5. Steiner JF, Lanphear BP, Curtis P, Vu KO. Indicators of early research productivity among primary care fellows. *J Gen Intern Med*. 2002;17(11):845–51.

6. Kunik ME, Hudson S, Schubert B, et al. Growing our own: a regional approach to encourage psychiatric residents to enter research. *Acad Psych*. 2008;32:236-40.

7. Ceci SJ, Williams WM. Understanding current causes of women's underrepresentation in science. *Proc Natl Acad Sci*. 2011;108(8):3157–62.

8. Spickard A Jr, Gabbe SG, Christensen JF. Mid-career burnout in generalist and specialist physicians. *JAMA*. 2002;288(12):1447–50.

9. Donovan A, Donovan J. Mentorship in postgraduate training programmes: views of Canadian programme directors. *Med Educ*. 2009;43(2):155–8.

10. Mason MA, Goulden M. Do babies matter: the effect of family formation on the life long careers of women. *Academe*. 2002;88(6):21–7.

11. Johns RJ. How to swim with sharks: the advanced course. *Trans Assoc Am Physicians*. 1975;88:44–54.

12. Straus SE, Chatur F, Taylor M. Issues in the mentor-mentee relationship in academic medicine: a qualitative study. *Acad Med*. 2009;84(1):135–9.

13. Sackett DL. Clinician-trialist rounds: 3. Priority setting for academic success. *Clin Trials*. 2011;8(2):235–7.

14. Sackett DL. Clinician-trialist rounds: 2. Time-management of your clinical practice and teaching. *Clin Trials*. 2011;8(1):112–4.

EXERCISE

Track down the Assistant Professor in your clinical department who is considered their brightest potential star and in whose footsteps you'd most like to tread. Over drinks and dinner (read: beer and pizza—you pay), get their suggestions on the most important stuff you should do right now in preparing for your future academic career.

SUMMARY CHECKLIST

- ❏ List the roles you would like an academic mentor to play for you.
- ❏ List the characteristics you would like to find in an academic mentor.
- ❏ List possible candidates to be your academic mentor.
- ❏ Meet with these candidates. Select one and see if he or she will agree to mentor you.
- ❏ Clarify expectations.

Starting

6
Conceiving and formulating the research question

Christian Vaillancourt, MD, MSc, FRCPC, CSPQ

ILLUSTRATIVE CASE

It is the beginning of a new academic year, and a cohort of Emergency Medicine residents are being welcomed into the program. Their program director discusses the CanMEDS Roles and reviews a list of objectives for the residency program, which include a requirement to complete a research project. One resident has never been involved in a research project before and is quite anxious about finding a topic.

■ **All activities associated with a** project are anchored to a research question. Formulating that question is arguably the most important and the most difficult step in any research project. It can help to begin with a general research idea, but as the project takes shape your initial idea will need to be refined into a specific and clearly defined research question. Research questions are often revised several times during the planning stages of a project as input from the research team is gathered, feasibility assessments are conducted, and the key elements of the study are taken into account. Who is the target population? What is the intervention? How should groups be compared? What outcome measures and what study design should be used? This chapter will help you find a research idea and transform it into a specific and "operational" research question.

Formulating a research idea

Where to start?

■ With a broad topic. We all have a reason for doing what we do in our professional sphere. Whether your training has led you to emergency medicine, surgery, radiology, pediatrics or public health, perhaps something in your life experience has guided your choice. Or perhaps something particular within a field of practice has captured your interest, drawing you to a more specific area such as pre-hospital emergency medical care, traumatology, intervention radiology, neonatal care or the health of seniors. As in health care practice, so in research: it is important to work in an area that you are passionate about. Developing a research project and bringing it to fruition requires a sustained effort and is much easier to accomplish when you are motivated by a keen interest.

What topics are you passionate about?

_____

_____

CHAPTER OBJECTIVES

After reading this chapter, you should be able to:
- develop a strategy to find a research idea
- transform a research idea into a research question
- understand the importance of a properly constructed research question

---

KEY TERMS

Confirmatory study	Knowledge translation	Research idea
FINER criteria	Operational research question	Research question
Hypothesis generation	Parameter estimation	
Hypothesis testing	PICOT question	

Planning

■ With a health condition, procedure, or tool. Not infrequently, we encounter extraordinary patients or circumstances that make an impression on us or spark an interest in finding the best way to approach a problem. You may have been struck by the processes of care involved in attempting to resuscitate a patient in cardiac arrest, or by the insertion of a chest tube using a minimally invasive technique, or by a colleague's suggestion to use ultrasonography to look for a pneumothorax. Many clinical experiences can give rise to questions and a desire to learn more.

What was "cool" about the last interesting patient for whom you provided care?

_____

_____

■ With a research methodology. Sometimes a research interest stems from a desire to learn how to go about addressing questions of a certain kind, in which case the particular research topic might be less important to you than the methodology or study design used to approach it. Perhaps you are interested in working with an experienced investigator to become familiar with a particular research method, or perhaps you have identified a specific research skill that you want to hone for a future research project you have in mind. This interest in method might lead you, for example, to learn how to develop a clinical decision rule, or to perform a good chart review, conduct a survey, or carry out a systematic review.

Is there a specific research method you would like to learn about and apply?

_____

_____

Where to look?

■ Researchers, educators and colleagues. Perhaps the best way to get started is to identify the researchers and educators in your group. Most successful researchers develop a niche or an area of expertise as one research question leads to another. Many researchers have more research questions than time to answer them, and you may find points of intersection between your interests and theirs. Such opportunities might on occasion lead you to a research collaborator, supervisor or mentor outside your own field or discipline.

List the research projects in your field of interest that are in progress in your department and the department faculty members who are most active in research.

_____

_____

■ Reading textbooks and articles. You might be surprised to learn that much of what we practise or take for granted in health care is based on little or no scientific evidence. As you review specific textbook chapters, pay attention to areas of controversy or knowledge gaps noted by the authors. Seek out and read any references cited, but bear in mind that most textbooks are at least five years out of date by the time they are published. Any exploration of a controversial topic will also need to include the most recently published articles available.

Reviewing and discussing recent journal articles with your colleagues can be a great opportunity to generate a research idea. For example, you might find that a particular article raises an interesting idea but uses a flawed method to address it. Another article might describe an exemplary research method that you could apply to a different research question of your own. Many articles generate hypotheses or draw conclusions that should be confirmed in further studies.

List gaps in knowledge or evidence that you have identified in your recent readings.

_____

_____

Planning

■   Meetings and abstracts. There is perhaps no better place to meet researchers and be exposed to the work they do than a scientific meeting. Most research presentations include a rationale and clear objectives for the work reported, and many give a sense of the questions that remain unanswered. If you have not yet had a chance to attend a scientific meeting or are unable to in the near future, you can browse instead through published abstracts in conference proceedings or association journals.

Find out where and when the next national scientific meeting in your area of interest will take place.

_____

_____

■   Granting agencies. If your goal is to obtain funding from a granting agency, carefully review the criteria and requirements of their funding applications. National granting agencies often put funds aside for the study of specific health conditions. Although the topic may be broad (e.g., diabetes in First Nations communities), it encourages researchers to follow a specific line of research.

Are there granting agencies for your field of interest that might be able to provide funding for your project? What are their timelines for funding applications?

_____

_____

Practical considerations

■   Frequency of disease or test use. Because the timeline to complete a research project during a health training program is often very short, it might be wise to choose a research idea that involves a health condition or test that is commonly encountered or used, particularly if you plan to recruit participants prospectively. Common conditions or tests can be identified intuitively from your clinical practice, or by a review of statistics collected by your department.

What conditions or tests do you most commonly see or use in your practice?

_____

_____

Refining your research idea

The answers you have jotted down to the questions above have likely pointed the way to some research possibilities.

Review your answers and write down the first three research ideas that come to mind. You might start with "I wonder if …"

1. _____

2. _____

3. _____

Need help? List at least three researchers you could approach to supervise, mentor or collaborate with you.

1. _____

2. _____

3. _____

A FINER idea

Now it's time to start refining your initial concept. Consider the **FINER criteria**. Your research idea needs to be:

> **F**easible
>
> **I**nteresting
>
> **N**ovel
>
> **E**thical
>
> **R**elevant

It is not always easy for inexperienced researchers to determine whether it is *feasible* to find the answer to a particular research idea. Many things have to be taken into account, including the study design that is best suited to approach the problem, your ability to recruit a sufficient number of participants, how to go about measuring outcomes, the availability of adequate technical expertise, and the time and other resources that you and your research team, if you can join one, will have at your disposal. Input from an experienced research supervisor, mentor or collaborator will be important to assessing and enabling the study's feasibility.

You will be spending a significant amount of time working on your research project. The question you choose to answer has to be *interesting* to your peers and, most importantly, to you!

Please—not another study on the benefits of buffering lidocaine to decrease pain during subcutaneous infiltration! Try to find a *novel* idea. Be imaginative. Will your study confirm or refute previous study findings? Will it extend previous findings to a new population? Will it provide new findings?

Your research project needs to respect the *ethical* concepts of autonomy, integrity, justice, beneficence and non-maleficence. It must not pose unacceptable risks to study participants or invade their privacy (see also ch. 18).

The effect of various diets on the skin tone of worms may be of very little relevance to you, but it is extremely *relevant* to some fishermen. Will the findings of your study add to scientific knowledge? Are they likely to influence clinical practice, health policy, or both? Will they be relevant in guiding future research directions? Not all research ideas will pass the "So what?" test, which is why you were asked to write down three possibilities.

From research idea to research question

If, after this examination of your **research idea**, you still believe it is worth pursuing, then you will need to formulate a specific **research question**. A research idea is your starting point: it is less specific and less operational than a research question. A research question, on the other hand, is relatively narrow and needs to be clearly defined. It is the research question that will enable you to determine what study design to use.

What kind of question is that?

In determining the approach to your research project, it's important to know what kind of question you are asking. As you formulate your question, consider which of the following categories best describes your inquiry.

Parameter estimation for a health condition or diagnostic test. Sometimes we observe that a health condition is present in a given patient population, such as depression among elderly patients seeking care in the emergency department, but we lack good information on its actual prevalence. Or, we might need to determine the diagnostic accuracy or other characteristics of new health technologies, such as the ability of ultrasonography to detect a pneumothorax at the bedside.

Hypothesis generation. There are many disease processes for which our understanding is limited and for which we would like to formulate hypotheses. Studies that look for associations between an exposure variable and an outcome are designed to generate new hypotheses rather than to demonstrate causality. For example, you could explore whether there are any associations between nutritional factors during pregnancy and the incidence of autism in children.

Hypothesis testing. Some research questions are formulated to test a hypothesis as rigorously as is feasible. Studies based on these questions need to have sufficient power (i.e., a sufficient sample size) and an appropriate design to establish causality (e.g., a randomized controlled trial). The example of hypothesis generation given above points to some of the challenges posed by this type of question. How would you test the hypothesis that vitamin D intake in pregnancy influences the incidence of autism? One possible research question might be: "Do children born to women randomly assigned to receive close supervision to

Planning

ensure they consume high doses of vitamin D during pregnancy have a lower incidence of autism compared to those whose mothers are not given specific follow-up regarding vitamin D intake?"

Confirmatory study. You thought you had found the perfect research topic, but when you performed a quick electronic search of the literature you discovered that several papers on your topic had already been published. Don't be discouraged: a study can always be replicated in a bigger or better way! Published studies may have flaws, or may have been conducted with a very different patient population than the one of interest to you. Besides, new knowledge is unlikely to be readily adopted in practice without a number of confirmatory studies. One exception … did I mention the excess of studies on buffered lidocaine?

Knowledge translation. Even if an exposure or intervention has been tested and confirmed in various study populations and in various relevant environments and settings, there are still no guarantees that stakeholders will put this knowledge to use. For example, we know that cardiopulmonary resuscitation (CPR) can achieve a two- or three-fold improvement in survival after out-of-hospital cardiac arrest, yet fewer than 30% of victims receive CPR from a bystander before emergency medical services arrive. Or, to return to our earlier example: Is buffered lidocaine still not being used routinely in your institution, despite all the supporting evidence?

Making your research question operational

Of course, many types of research question are possible, and the categories given above are not exhaustive. The important thing is to understand what *type* of question you are asking and then to make it "operational." An **operational research question** should:

- specify the population to be studied (who?)
- specify the intervention, exposure or behaviour under study (what?)
- specify the timeframe (when?)
- specify the setting (where?)
- reflect a theoretical rationale (why?)
- specify the methodology (how) and primary outcome
- communicate the hypothesis

To get the best answer, formulate the best **PICOT question** you can:

Population (or **P**eople, or **P**atients)
Intervention (if applicable)
Control (or **C**omparison)
Outcome
Timeframe

Here's an example of a bad question: "Is anti-coagulation beneficial in patients with atrial fibrillation?" Here's why. The PICOT ingredients of your research question are the same essential ingredients of a properly designed research protocol. Although these will be covered in detail in chapter 17, you can already appreciate the limitations of the question we just asked: It fails to take the following elements into account.

- What type of anticoagulation?
- What type of benefit?
- In which specific patient population?
- In acute or chronic atrial fibrillation?
- What method will be used to test the hypothesis?
- What is the time frame of interest?

Now compare the previous question with the following one. Which is better? "Do patients over the age of 75 with atrial fibrillation for longer than 48 hours who are randomly assigned to receive coumadin have a lower 1-year risk of embolic cerebrovascular accident compared with those randomly assigned to receive aspirin or placebo?"

Because it is so precise, this question allows you to focus on exactly the information you are trying to obtain and allows others to clearly understand what your research is meant to achieve. Who are these "others"? They are:

- institutional ethics review boards
- funding agencies
- colleagues
- journal editors
- patients and lay people
- consumers of your research results

Now try to formulate you own research question.

Planning

Planning

Use what you think is the FINER of the three research ideas you had earlier. Make sure to include all of the PICOT elements. And remember: Your research question is a work in progress and will likely be modified as you read the other chapters in this guide and meet with your research supervisor.

_____

_____

Conclusion

Formulating a research question can be a daunting task, especially for those new to research. The objective of this chapter was to provide you with a strategy to find and develop a research idea and with the tools to transform that idea into an operational research question. A properly constructed research question will make a world of difference in your ability to design an effective study using the research methodology best suited to your task. ■

CASE POSTSCRIPT

The Emergency Medicine resident was introduced to an excellent, established researcher from the Department of Family Medicine. They both shared an interest in sports medicine, and collaborated on a chart review project evaluating muscle necrosis in patients with acute compartment syndrome. This resident took a liking to research, decided to complete a research fellowship at the end of his residency, and wrote the chapter you just read!

ADDITIONAL RESOURCES

Haynes RB. Forming research questions. In: Haynes RB, Sacket DL, Guyatt GH, Tugwell P, editors. _Clinical epidemiology: How to do clinical practice research_. 3rd ed. Philadelphia, PA: Lippincott Williams & Wilkins; 2006:3–14.

Hulley SB, Cummings SR, Browner WS, Grady DG, Newman TB. _Designing clinical research: an epidemiologic approach_. 3rd ed. Philadelphia: Lippincott Williams & Wilkins; 2007. Chapter 2, Conceiving the research question; p. 17–26.

Smith KM. Building upon existing evidence to shape future research endeavors. _Am J Health Syst Pharm_. 2008;65(18):1767–74.

Stone PW. Popping the (PICO) question in research and evidence-based practice. _Appl Nurs Res_. 2002;15(3):197–8.

Thabane L, Thomas T, Ye C, Paul J. Posing the research question: not so simple. _Can J Anaesth_. 2009;56(1):71– 9.

- The resources listed above can help budding researchers develop comprehensive and well-formulated research questions.

SUMMARY CHECKLIST

- ❑ Off the top of your head, list some problems or areas of interest that you might want to research.
- ❑ List some potential research topics from recent clinical cases or situations.
- ❑ List some researchers or colleagues with whom you might want to work. What are they researching?
- ❑ List some research methods or approaches that interest you.
- ❑ List some potential research ideas from recent texts or papers you have read or presentations you have heard.
- ❑ List any granting agencies that might support work on your topics of potential interest.
- ❑ Looking at your list, select one or two ideas to develop into a question. Refine these using the FINER criteria.
- ❑ Operationalize your question using the PICOT framework.
- ❑ Share your idea with colleagues and your supervisor. Is it ready to use?

7
Searching the literature

Lorie A. Kloda, MLIS, PhD (candidate)

Planning

ILLUSTRATIVE CASE

A resident in Otolaryngology is interested in designing a study to investigate the effectiveness of ventilation tubes in reducing the incidence of recurrent ear infections in young children. In a quick scan of the literature, she locates a systematic review in the Cochrane Library. The review concludes that, although the insertion of ventilation tubes has been shown to be effective in reducing the rate of infections at six months after surgery, many of the studies conducted in this area are flawed and more research is needed. The resident realizes that an overview of the available evidence will be crucial in convincing a granting agency to support her research, but she has never conducted a comprehensive literature search before.

■ **In an age when any health sciences** researcher with an Internet connection can access a wealth of information quickly and freely, the art of searching the literature is often overlooked. A literature search is an important early step in the research process. It enables the researcher to become familiar with the published evidence in an area, to refine his or her research question, and to justify the research project itself by identifying limitations and gaps in the current state of knowledge. Nevertheless, researchers often underestimate the time and thought required to conduct a proper literature search and then create a review to support and justify a research project. The support of a qualified **librarian**—typically, with a master's degree in library and information studies—who has experience searching the biomedical and allied health literature will be essential to the quality and comprehensiveness of your literature search.

The literature search consists of several steps. The first is to identify the information needed, which is often broader than the research topic. In our case example, the research question concerns one type of intervention for otitis media in young children, but the literature search could be expanded to include other approaches, such as antibiotic therapy, or other patient groups, such as older children or even adults. Once the scope of the information being sought is defined, sources where relevant literature can be located are selected and searched, using strategies appropriate to each source. The results of these searches are typically managed using specialized software, and the records are reviewed by the researcher for relevance. The relevant items are then retrieved and integrated into a narrative **literature review** that can be incorporated into a grant proposal or a manuscript.

CHAPTER OBJECTIVES

After reading this chapter, you should be able to:

- describe the various steps involved in conducting a literature search;
- select appropriate sources to search;
- create search strategies for the retrieval of relevant literature;
- save search strategies and results;
- document a literature search; and
- describe the professional librarian's role in supporting literature searches, particularly for systematic reviews.

KEY TERMS

Bibliographic databases	Embase	Literature review	Scopus
BIOSIS	Google Scholar	MEDLINE	Snowball searching
Citation indexes	Grey literature	MeSH	Subject headings
Citation software	Hand searching	Pearl-growing	Web of Science
Cochrane Library	Librarian	PubMed	

41

Planning

Selecting sources

Most medical researchers start their literature searches with **MEDLINE**, the premier biomedical database provided free of charge (through the **PubMed** interface) by the U.S. National Library of Medicine. Although MEDLINE is an excellent source, indexing journal publications back to 1950, it is far from the only one. Several databases should be searched to increase the yield of records retrieved and to reduce geographic bias. Also, because different databases use different indexing practices, searching several will help to compensate for any skewing of results that might be created by a reliance on only one indexing system.

Bibliographic databases

Bibliographic databases contain records of publications such as journal articles, abstracts, conference proceedings, books and book chapters, theses, and other materials. Some databases, such as MEDLINE, are limited to journal articles, while others include all types of publications. The contents of these databases often do not include complete ("full text") articles. The database records contain several fields containing descriptive information about each publication, such as title; authorship; the source journal, book, or conference; and volume, issue number and page range. Bibliographic records also commonly include fields for an abstract and for keywords or subject headings. Fields can be searched separately or in combination.

In addition to MEDLINE, databases to consider searching for biomedical topics include **BIOSIS**, which contains references to biomedical and life sciences research, and **Embase**, which complements MEDLINE through more comprehensive indexing of records published in Europe and Asia. For pharmacology research, Embase is a more detailed and comprehensive index than MEDLINE,[1] and a search of Embase is recommended in any case if the comprehensiveness of a MEDLINE search for a particular topic is in doubt.[2] The MEDLINE, BIOSIS and Embase databases are often available through university libraries.

To locate systematic reviews in health care, DARE (Database of Abstracts of Reviews of Effects), provided free of charge by the Centre for Reviews and Dissemination in the United Kingdom, as well as the **Cochrane Library** are important sources. Searching first for a recent systematic review can provide you with both an overview of your research topic and a useful list of existing publications. Depending on your topic, you may wish to search databases in allied health care fields, such as rehabilitation, nursing

and psychology. A selection of other databases that may be worth considering is provided in Table 7.1.

You might also want to conduct searches in databases outside biomedicine and allied health. For example, management and computer science databases are relevant for informatics-related research, and educational databases are useful for psychosocial research. Many specialized databases are available as well, such as AutismData[a] and POPLINE.[b] Consult a librarian for assistance in selecting and gaining access to appropriate databases. Various vendors offer access to licensed databases, and your institution library's website is an excellent gateway to these resources.

Citation databases

In addition to bibliographic databases, **citation indexes** such as **Web of Science** and SciVerse **Scopus**[c] can be used as part of a complete literature search by helping you to identify journals, books, conference proceedings and other sources where the references of interest to you have already been cited. In this way, starting with one or more key references on a topic, you can enhance your literature review by tracking citations to those references across scientific and academic disciplines, potentially discovering related research in unexpected areas. Web of Science and Scopus are subscription based and should be available through your institution's library. For a more complete picture of citations to a publication of interest, you can also use **Google Scholar**, which is freely available through the Internet.[3]

Designing a search strategy
Subject searching

When you search a bibliographic database, it is important to generate terms that will yield relevant records and to reduce the number of irrelevant records retrieved. The PICOT mnemonic for formulating an "operational" research question, described in chapter 6 of this guide, can also help you frame your literature search.[4] In the case presented, the question "What is the effectiveness of ventilation tubes in reducing the incidence of recurrent ear infections in young children" can be broken down into the following components:

---

a See www.autism.org.uk/autismdata

b See www.popline.org/

c See http://thomsonreuters.com/products_services/science/science_products/a-z/web_of_science/ , www.info.sciverse.com/scopus/ and http://scholar.google.ca/ for Web of Science (Thompson Reuters), Scopus (Elsevier) and Google Scholar, respectively.

- Patient, Problem, Population: middle ear infections in young children
- Intervention: ventilation tubes
- Comparison/Control: antibiotics therapy/no intervention
- Outcome: reduction in recurrence
- Time frame: 6 months after surgery

In your search, select the most important concepts and search these separately. In this case, we can search the concepts middle ear infections (P) and ventilation tubes(I).

Ideally, **subject headings**, if available, can be used to maximize the search results. MEDLINE's extensive list of Medical Subject Headings, known as **MeSH**, is useful for searching. Embase uses its own list of headings, called Emtree. These standardized headings are organized hierarchically and provide the option of including narrower headings in your search by using the "explode" feature. For example, the MeSH for Middle Ear includes several narrower headings:

Ear, Middle
    Ear Ossicles
    Eustachian Tube
    Glomus Tympanicum
    Stapedius
    Tensor Tympani

Searching the "exploded" MeSH "Ear, Middle" will yield records of articles that discuss the middle ear, as well as those that discuss any of the narrower terms (e.g., Eustachian tube). This will increase the number of records retrieved by your search and ensure that relevant items are not inadvertently excluded.

MEDLINE offers other relevant MeSH for the topic, including "Otitis Media" and "Middle Ear Ventilation." Searching these MeSH, and the terms subsumed within them (using the "explode" feature, indicated with the abbreviation "Exp") will retrieve all records in MEDLINE indexed with those terms. As you search for the correct MeSH in MEDLINE, remember that the database offers "scope notes," or definitions of the subject headings. Reading the scope note for a particular MeSH will help you decide whether it is the correct choice and perhaps lead you to an alternative or an appropriate combination of headings.

In addition to searching subject headings, it is also recommended that you search keywords (also called textwords). Searching keywords requires some creativity: because these are the words as they appear in a record's title, abstract and subject heading list, they can take many forms. Brainstorm word variations, alternative spellings and synonyms to increase the potential for a match to be found in your database search. When appropriate, use the truncation feature (typically indicated by an asterisk) to search word stems with various endings or the plural form.

Be sure to combine search terms using logical operators (AND, OR) and to record your search on paper so that you can visualize the relation between terms before they are entered into the database. For example, if you want to design a search strategy in MEDLINE to retrieve as many records as possible that pertain to the use of ventilation tubes for otitis media in children, the following strategy is possible:

Exp Otitis media (MeSH)		Ventilation (MeSH)
OR		OR
Mastoiditis (MeSH)		Tubulation (MeSH)
OR	AND	OR
Tympanitis (MeSH)		Grommet*
OR		OR
Exp Ear, middle (MeSH)		Tympanostom*

AND (infect* OR inflam*)

After this search is conducted, it could be combined with the MeSH Middle ear ventiliation using the logical operator OR.

Once the search terms are selected and run against the database, other options are available for refining the results. These "limits" restrict the search by publication year, language, publication type, study design, age group, sex and many other attributes. The limits that are available vary by database. For our example search, limiting retrievals to publications that discuss infants (aged 12 to 23 months) OR preschool children (2 to 5 years) would be appropriate. Keep in mind that MEDLINE and other databases offer many features that you can take advantage of to increase or reduce the number of records retrieved. To learn about these, consult the user guides available for each database (see Additional Resources).

Planning

■ **Table 7.1: Bibliographic databases relevant to literature searches in the health sciences**

Database	Coverage	Sponsoring agency or owner	Access
AMED (Allied and Complementary Medicine Database)	Over 152 000 records from approximately 600 journals in three separate subject areas, covering 1985 to the present: • professions allied to medicine • complementary medicine • palliative care Many of these journals are not included in other biomedical indexes. Journals are mainly European; most titles are in English. Search terms are based on MeSH. See www.bl.uk/reshelp/findhelpsubject/scitectenv/medicinehealth/amed/amed.html	Health Care Information Service of the British Library	Subscription based; medical and university libraries
BIOSIS	BIOSIS Previews. Indexes life sciences and biomedical research from over 5000 journals as well as non-journal literature; up to 18 million records from 1926 to the present. Biological Abstracts. Index to the international life sciences literature, covering over 4200 journals from 100 countries; contains over 11.3 million records from 1926 to the present. See http://thomsonreuters.com/content/science/pdf/BIOSIS_Factsheet.pdf	Thomson Scientific	Subscription based; medical and university libraries
CINAHL (Cumulative Index to Nursing and Allied Health Literature)	Indexes journals, books, chapter, theses and other publications covering nursing and allied health care disciplines. Uses MeSH as well as CINAHL subject headings. See www.ebscohost.com/cinahl/	EBSCO Publishing	Subscription based; medical and university libraries
Cochrane Library	A collection of six databases indexed using MeSH: • Cochrane Database of Systematic Reviews (Cochrane Reviews) • Cochrane Central Register of Controlled Trials (CENTRAL) • Cochrane Methodology Register • Database of Abstracts of Reviews of Effects (DARE) • Health Technology Assessment Database (HTA) • NSH Economic Evaluation Database (NHS EED) See www.thecochranelibrary.com	John Wiley & Sons, UK Cochrane Reviews, CENTRAL and the Methodology Register are produced by member groups of the international, not-for-profit Cochrane Collaboration. DARE, HTA and NHS EED are maintained by the Centre for Reviews and Dissemination, University of York, UK	Subscription based, but free by arrangement in some countries and Canadian provinces.

Table 7.1 continued

DARE (Database of Abstracts of Review of Effects)	Contains 15 000 abstracts of systematic reviews, including over 6000 quality-assessed reviews and details of all Cochrane reviews and protocols. Focused on effects of health interventions; includes reviews of interventions that are clearly health related; interventions with the potential to affect health; adverse effects; diagnostic and prognostic studies; and individual patient data. See www.crd.york.ac.uk/crdweb/	Centre for Reviews and Dissemination, University of York, UK	Free access through the Internet
Embase	Contains 24 million records, indexing over 7500 journals in biomedicine and pharmacology, including over 2000 biomedical titles not covered in MEDLINE. Also includes conference abstracts. Records are indexed using Emtree subject headings. See http://embase.com/info/what-is-embase	Elsevier	Subscription based; medical and university libraries
HaPI (Health and Psychosocial Instruments)	Contains over 145 000 records from 1985 to the present relating to approximately 15 000 measurement instruments (e.g., questionnaires, tests, checklists, rating scales, etc.) in health and psychosocial sciences. The database does not provide access to the instruments, but rather to information about them.	Behavioral Measurement Database Services, Pittsburgh, PA	Subscription based; medical and university libraries
LILACS (Latin American and Caribbean Literature on Health Sciences Database)	Database with English, Portuguese and Spanish interfaces covering more than 800 medical journals from 19 countries in Latin America and the Caribbean, of which most are not indexed in MEDLINE. Covers human health sciences, including medicine, public health, dentistry, nursing, veterinary medicine, sanitary engineering, pharmacy and chemistry, biology, nutrition, psychology, ecology and the environment. See http://bases.bireme.br/cgi-bin/wxislind.exe/iah/online/?IsisScript=iah/iah.xis&base=LILACS&lang=i&form=F	BIREME (Biblioteca Regional de Medicia) and PAHO (Pan American Health Organization)	Free access through the Internet
MEDLINE	Contains 18 million citations to the life sciences literature from approximately 5400 journals in 39 languages; Records are indexed using MeSH. Of citations added in 2008, 47% were to articles published in the United States and 92% to articles published in English. Focuses on biomedicine and health, encompassing life sciences, behavioural sciences, chemical sciences, and bioengineering relevant to clinicians, health researchers, and those engaged in public health, health policy, or health care education. See www.nlm.nih.gov/pubs/factsheets/medline.html	US National Library of Medicine	Free access throughPubMED at www.ncbi.nlm.nih.gov/pubmed/ or the NLM Gateway at http://gateway.nlm.nih.gov Subscription based though medical and university libraries, as well as the Canadian Medical Association

Planning

Table 7.1 continued			
PsycINFO	Abstracts and citations to the scholarly literature (mainly journals) in the psychological, social, behavioural and health sciences. Coverage is mainly of journals. Approximately 2500 journals, mainly from North America, are represented. Indexed using subject headings from the Thesaurus of Psychological Index Terms. See www.apa.org/pubs/databases/psycinfo/index.aspx	American Psychological Association	Subscription based; medical and university libraries

Pearl-growing

Devising an effective search strategy is a daunting task, and asking for assistance from a librarian is strongly recommended. To get started, however, you can use the **pearl-growing** technique, which is useful for subject searches. For this technique, begin with a known reference and use it to generate more subject headings and keywords. In MEDLINE, you could locate the record for the Cochrane review mentioned in our case, for example, and examine the title, abstract and MeSH terms for possible search terms. These subject headings and keywords can then be used to help devise your own search strategy in the same database. Librarians use this technique especially when their searches retrieve few relevant results.

Storing searches and results

Saving search strategies and creating alerts

Many databases allow the user to save multiple search histories in a personal account. Saving your search strategy so that you can replicate or modify it later is strongly advised. To benefit from this feature of most databases, register for a personal account at the outset and save various iterations of your searches. You can share these later when consulting with a librarian or colleague, and revisit them in cases where a topic is of ongoing interest. MEDLINE, for example, allows you to rerun a saved search to retrieve references that were added to the database since the last time your search was run. An alternative to rerunning a saved search is to set up an alert in order to receive notifications of new database records that match your criteria. Details such as search frequency and email recipients can be entered, and new records matching your search will be sent to you automatically as the database is updated.

Citation software for storing search results

Software such as EndNote or RefWorks is useful for storing, finding, citing and sharing references. Free alternatives to these products are frequently appearing, Zotero and Mendeley[d] being two recent examples. **Citation software** has the capability to find, link to and attach the full-text publication (if it is available online as a PDF [portable document format] file, for example), creating a virtual library or personalized database of literature pertinent to your research interests.

If you don't already use citation software, you should consider several factors in selecting the right one. If you are working as part of a team, determine what others are using, as collaboration will be hindered by incompatible software. Similarly, not all software products are available for all operating systems. Some products exist only in the online environment and may not be compatible with all word processors. You may also want to contact your library and information technology department to determine whether they offer training and support for a particular product.

To support literature searches and the writing of reviews, citation software is used to import references directly from the databases once each search is conducted. After each database has been searched, and the results added to a citation software database, duplicates can automatically be identified and removed. You can sort the references alphabetically or chronologically and review them for relevance directly within the software, rather than online in the database. These personalized databases can be saved and shared with others. For grant proposal and manuscript preparation, collaborators can use citation software to find and cite relevant literature and create reference lists. Citation software is becoming increasingly useful not only for systematic reviews, but also for the management of references relevant to one's research and practice.

d   See www.zotero.org/ and www.mendeley.com/

Documenting the search

When you embark on a new research activity, it's always a good idea to keep track of your work and of all the decisions you make along the way. The literature search is no exception. Whether you are conducting the search yourself, as part of a team, or with the assistance of a librarian, maintain records of the sources selected (and rejected), your search strategies and any supplemental search methods employed. This information will be useful to you and your collaborators during the literature review process and can help to inform your literature searches in the future.

Systematic reviews

If you are conducting a systematic review, you will be required to provide, in the methods section of your published report, extensive details regarding your literature search. As a form of research study, systematic reviews require rigorous methodology (see ch. 15). You will need to become well acquainted with current PRISMA[e] guidelines for documenting and reporting on literature searches for systematic reviews and to enlist the services of a librarian with experience conducting and documenting literature searches for systematic reviews. PRISMA requires the peer review of the search strategy to ensure that it meets strict quality criteria.[5] PRISMA also requires the use of a flow diagram to document the stages of the literature search and the selection of included studies.

Locating relevant literature: supplemental methods

Depending on the scope of your research, you may wish to enhance your literature review by using sources other than databases. For systematic reviews, **hand searching** is often conducted, such that seminal journals and conference proceedings are identified by the research team and their tables of contents screened for relevant references. **Grey literature** searches can be conducted as well. Grey literature includes all forms of literature that fall outside the realm of traditional commercial publishing and are therefore not indexed in databases. Grey literature includes, for instance, government and association reports, websites, brochures and theses. Various resources are available to support searches information in this format (see Additional Resources).

In any literature review, you will likely engage in **snowball searching** (also called reference harvesting). In the case described, the resident would likely use the Cochrane review as a starting point for her literature search and scan its list of references to identify potentially relevant publications. The routine scanning of reference lists is always advised for those conducting systematic reviews, and is helpful for any researcher wanting to gain familiarity with a research area.

The role of the librarian

Throughout this chapter, you have been encouraged to consult or enlist the services of a librarian to support the literature search process. Librarians serve many roles in the research process, including advising and offering training on sources to search and on effective search strategies, and providing access to resources and software. A librarian with experience in the health sciences and training in expert searching can conduct literature searches to meet specific research needs. In our sample case, enlisting a librarian to conduct a thorough search before beginning the clinical trial could prevent potential errors and the needless duplication of research efforts.

For systematic reviews, librarians are typically invited to be members of the research team.[6] They can direct you to validated search strategies, also called "hedges," which are designed to optimize retrieval from certain databases. Hedges exist for all types of study designs, including qualitative approaches,[7] and for several databases, typically MEDLINE, Embase and CINAHL. As a member of the research team, the librarian may also manage other aspects of the literature search, such as overseeing hand searching and grey literature searching, and documenting the search process.

Conclusion

This chapter provided an overview of the steps required to successfully complete a literature search as the foundation of a literature review. Whenever possible, consult a librarian or your library's website for guidance and support in this process. Start by refining your information needs and selecting appropriate sources for searching. Develop search strategies, or use hedges to retrieve relevant records from the databases, and consider citation searching and supplemental strategies. Finally, manage your references and document the literature search process: your present and future research projects will benefit as a result. ■

---

e   The acronym PRISMA stands for Preferred Reporting Items for Systematic Reviews and Meta-Analysis. The most recent PRISMA checklist and explanatory documents can be accessed at www.prisma-statement.org

Planning

CASE POSTSCRIPT

After consulting her librarian, the resident conducts a literature search in several health sciences databases, including MEDLINE, Embase, LILACS and DARE. Using a combination of subject headings and keywords, and limiting her search to research about children, she retrieves many references to relevant studies. In addition, a citation search in Scopus confirms that no important papers were overlooked. The resident keeps a record of her search strategy for each database so that, should her grant application be successful, she will be able to rerun the searches in order to update her literature review in the course of preparing her manuscript.

REFERENCES

1. Brown CM. The benefits of searching EMBASE versus MEDLINE for pharmaceutical information. *Online Inf Rev.* 1998;22(1):3–8.

2. Sampson M, Barrowman NJ, Moher D, Klassen TP, Pham B, Platt R, et al. Should meta-analysts search Embase in addition to Medline? *J Clin Epidemiol.* 2003;56(10):943–55.

3. Kloda LA. Evidence summary: Use Google Scholar, Scopus and Web of Science for comprehensive citation tracking. *Evid Based Libr Inf Pract.* 2007;2(3):87–90.

4. Richardson WS, Wilson MC, Nishikawa J, Hayward RS. The well-built clinical question: a key to evidence-based decisions. *ACP J Club.* 1995;123(3): A12–3.

5. McGowan J, Sampson M, Lefebvre C. An evidence-based checklist for the peer review of electronic search strategies. *Evid Based Libr Inf Pract.* 2010;5(1):149–54.

6. McGowan J, Sampson M. Systematic reviews need systematic searchers. *J Med Libr Assoc.* 2005;93(1):74–80.

7. Grant MJ. How does your searching grow? A survey of search preferences and the use of optimal search strategies in the identification of qualitative research. *Health Inf Libr J.* 2004:21(1):21–32.

ADDITIONAL RESOURCES

Canadian Agency for Drugs and Technologies in Health (CADTH). *Grey matters: a practical search tool for evidence-based medicine.* Ottawa: CADTH; 2009. Available from: www.cadth.ca/media/pdf/Grey-Matters_A-Practical-Search-Tool-for-Evidence-Based-Medicine.doc

- A directory of sources to search for health care literature, including bibliographic databases and an extensive list of online sources for grey literature.

Centre for Reviews and Dissemination. *Finding studies for systematic reviews: a resource list for researchers.* York (UK): University of York; 2010. Available from: www.york.ac.uk/inst/crd/pdf/Finding_studies_for_systematic_reviews.pdf

- A directory of sources to search for studies to support systematic reviews.

———. *The InterTASC Information Specialists' Sub-Group Search Filter Resource.* York (UK): University of York; n.d. Available from: www.york.ac.uk/inst/crd/intertasc/index.htm

- This resource organizes research on optimal search strategies (hedges) by study design and other topics, linking directly to original publications measuring the sensitivity and specificity of these.

———. *Systematic reviews: CRD's guidance for undertaking reviews in health care.* York (UK): University of York; 2009. Available from: www.york.ac.uk/inst/crd/index_guidance.htm

- This online manual describes the process of creating a systematic review, giving step-by-step instructions.

PubMed Online Training. Available from: www.nlm.nih.gov/bsd/disted/pubmed.html

- This site links to the full PubMed tutorial as well as to quick tours that demonstrate how to search using MeSH, save searches, and export search results to citation software.

EXERCISES

- Identify one or two key articles relevant to your research question, either by asking knowledgeable colleagues or by doing a PubMed search. Look at the subject headings assigned to the article(s) and read the abstract(s) to identify potential keywords. Use these terms to develop a search strategy that will retrieve relevant literature.

- Brainstorm databases that may contain relevant references. Look at library websites for subject guides or contact a health sciences librarian for suggestions. Run a brief test search using a few keywords in each database to determine whether it contains relevant references.

- Conduct a citation search starting with a key publication related to your research topic in all three citation databases, if your institution provides access: Web of Science, Scopus, and Google Scholar. Compare the retrieval from the three databases. Which one provided the most useful results, and why?

Planning

SUMMARY CHECKLIST

- ❑ Describe the information you need to search for. Write it down.
- ❑ Select the sources you will use for your search.
- ❑ Create an effective search strategy.
- ❑ Select a high-value reference that you have found, and use its terms to refine your search strategy.
- ❑ Discuss your search with a professional librarian or information specialist. Refine your strategy again.
- ❑ Save your search appropriately.
- ❑ Create alerts for your topics of interest.
- ❑ If desired, supplement your strategy with hand searches and grey literature. Contact knowledgeable authors in the field for their recommendations.

Planning

8
Data: Variables and levels of measurement

Bart J. Harvey, MD, PhD, MEd, FACPM, FRCPC

ILLUSTRATIVE CASE

A nurse practitioner student completing a placement at a Community Health Centre wants to determine what proportion of people served by the centre received the recommended preventive services during the previous 2 years. After speaking to his field supervisor and deciding to carry out a review using the centre's electronic health record (EHR) database, he realizes he will need to determine which EHR data elements will be needed for the study.

■ Health information about people

and conditions is often ascertained by counting, making observations, and taking measurements. These collected values form a set of data that can be quite varied, as the following examples demonstrate:

- In preparation for a strategic planning retreat, the executive director of a local community health centre determines the country of birth and language spoken at home for each patient seen at the centre during the previous 2 years. She finds the most frequent to be China and Mandarin, respectively.
- A woman with a 2-year history of high blood pressure uses her home blood pressure cuff to learn that her blood pressure is 150/90 mm Hg.
- On his first visit to a primary care centre, a man reports that he has 3 adult children.
- As part of a hospital self-evaluation, a health services researcher develops and administers a questionnaire that includes an item asking each of 500 randomly selected respondents to use a five-point scale, ranging from "poor" to "excellent," to rate their last clinical visit at the hospital.

- A genetic assessment determines that a woman carries the *BRCA1* gene.

When these counts, observations and measurements differ from person to person or from time to time, they are referred to as **variables.** Variables are the building blocks of many research studies, especially those that use quantitative methods. Statistical tools, described and discussed in chapters 24 and 25, help us better understand and make sense of the data collected with respect to these variables. However, the choice of statistical techniques or tests used to describe and analyze variables will depend on the type of data being examined. In preparation for the later discus-

CHAPTER OBJECTIVES

After reading this chapter, you should be able to:
- define **data variable** and **level of measurement;**
- list, describe and recognize the three roles that data variables play in research studies; and
- list, describe and recognize the five common levels of measurement used in research studies.

KEY TERMS

Categorical data	Dichotomous (binary) data	Interval data	Quantitative data
Continuous data	Discrete data	Level of measurement	Ratio data
Co-variable	Explanatory variable	Nominal data	Response variable
Data	Exposure variable	Outcome variable	True zero point
Data variable	Independent variable	Ordinal data	Variables
Dependent variable	Indicator variable	Predictor variable	

Planning

sions in this guide on specific research approaches and methodologies (ch. 9), the collection and management of data (ch. 22), and techniques for analyzing data (chs 24 & 25), this chapter discusses the three kinds of data variables used in research studies as well as the five levels of measurement (also called types of data). This chapter, however, does not apply to the kinds of data that arise from qualitative research studies, which are addressed in chapter 16.

Types of data variables

Three types of variables are used in research studies: outcome variables, predictor variables and co-variables. Each type has a specific purpose.

Outcome variables

An **outcome variable** serves as an endpoint of interest. Also referred to as the **response** or, more traditionally, the **dependent variable,** the value of an outcome variable is one that is believed to be affected by the potential causes (measured by predictor variables, defined and discussed below) being investigated in the research. An example of an outcome variable is the diagnosis of lung cancer among participants in a study examining the risk factors for this disease.

Predictor variables

A **predictor variable** is one that is being measured to determine whether it affects the outcome of interest. Also known as **independent, exposure, indicator** or **explanatory variables,** these may be measured before the study begins (e.g., age, body mass index, sex) or may be assigned as part of the study (e.g., to receive the intervention or placebo in a randomized clinical trial). An example of a predictor variable is the reported level of physical activity in a study examining risk factors for ischemic heart disease.

Co-variables

Co-variables are additional variables collected because they are known or hypothesized to be relevant to the study. These usually include characteristics that are or could be related to the predictor and/or outcome variables being studied, and are therefore often of interest to assess and, when necessary, control for in the data analysis. Examples of co-variables include factors such as age and sex as well as potential competing risk factors such as physical inactivity, smoking history or past occupational exposures.

Whether a variable serves as an outcome variable, predictor variable or co-variable depends on the question that is being asked. For example, in a study examining the possible effect of serum cholesterol on heart disease, cholesterol level is the predictor/exposure variable and heart disease is the outcome variable. However, in a study examining the potential effect of dietary fat on cholesterol level, dietary fat is the predictor/exposure variable and cholesterol level is the outcome variable.

Levels of measurement (types of data)

Data are generally either **categorical** or **quantitative**. **Categorical data**, as the name suggests, are observations or variables that are classified or categorized by means of labels or other descriptive terms. In the examples listed above, country of birth, language spoken at home, presence of the *BRCA1* gene, and the 5-point scale (ranging from "poor" to "excellent") are categorical measures. **Quantitative data** are observations, counts and measures made by determining quantities or assigning numeric values to the data. In the examples above, the blood pressure of 150/90 mm Hg and the number of children are quantitative measures.

More detailed descriptions of categorical and quantitative levels of measurement are presented below.

Categorical data

Categorical data are data that fall into specified categories. At a categorical level of measurement, some particular quality of the observation is used to classify it into one and only one of a series of categories. Categorical data should satisfy two conditions: (1) the categories must be mutually exclusive (a quality should fall into only one category); and (2) the categories must be collectively exhaustive (all possible responses can be classified). There are three specific types of categorical data: **nominal, dichotomous** (a special kind of nominal data) and **ordinal**.

Nominal data fall into categories that have no inherent order (i.e., the categories simply serve as names). Examples of such categories are occupation, country of birth, language spoken at home, diagnosis and blood type.

Dichotomous (or binary) data are a special kind of nominal data that are frequently used in health research and fall into one of only two possible categories. Examples of the categories used to describe dichotomous data are female/male, treatment/control, diseased/not diseased and alive/dead.

Ordinal data. Like other kinds of qualitative data, ordinal data fall into categories. Unlike the categories used to describe nominal data, those used to describe ordinal data exhibit an inherent ranking (e.g., from lowest to highest). Some examples are the following:

- levels of care: primary, secondary, tertiary, quaternary
- amount of pain: none, mild, moderate, severe, excruciating
- level of health: excellent, very good, good, fair, poor

The differences or "distances" between adjoining points on an ordinal scale are often either unknown or indeterminate. For example, we do not know how much better "excellent health" is than "very good health." Furthermore, the differences between the various points on an ordinal scale are usually not equal; for example, the difference between "moderate pain" and "severe pain" may be greater or smaller than the difference between "mild pain" and "moderate pain."

Although numbers are sometimes used to identify ordinal categories (e.g., cancer stages, the New York Heart Association Functional Classification), these numbers are simply ranked labels, and the difference between each category is usually unequal or unknown. This fact, however, does not stop researchers from performing mathematical operations on ordinal data. Even for a small number of categories, some researchers will compute means and standard deviations or add and subtract the values of categories. This practice is rarely justified and is generally discouraged. However, it is common and appropriate for the frequency of each nominal and ordinal category to be counted and for the applicable percentages to be calculated and reported.

Quantitative data

Quantitative data are those that can be described by numerical quantities; they are observations based on counts or measurements. Two types of quantitative data will be presented in further detail: **discrete data** and **continuous data.**

Discrete data are whole numbers; their values are presented only as integers (i.e., they do not include fractions).

Such data are often collected by counting, as in determining the number of teeth with cavities, the number of pregnancies, and the number of children in a family. Although these data, like ordinal data, can be rank-ordered, the relation between values can be readily determined. For example, a family with 2 children has exactly half as many as another that has 4 children.

Continuous data, as the name suggests, include a full range of evenly spaced and possible fractional values: that is, no matter how close any two values are to one another, other values always exist between them. Of course, whether values close to one another can actually be individually detected usually depends on the precision of the measuring technique being used. However, the measurement and recording of continuous variables may, in practice, be confined to a limited number of points (often integers) on the continuum if greater detail is not warranted by the precision or use (or both) of the measurement. For example, although a particular blood pressure reading may in fact be 154.768923/90.325146 mmHg, it would usually be reported simply as 155/90 mmHg. Other examples of continuous data include blood glucose (mg/100 mL), height (in inches or centimetres), temperature (usually in degrees Fahrenheit or Celsius) and age (which can be measured on any of several possible scales: in hours, days, weeks, months or years).

For continuous data, the absolute difference between values can always be determined by subtraction. However, relative measures involving multiplication and division (e.g., x is twice as big as y) can be performed only with continuous data that have a **true zero point.** For example, because age has a true zero point (i.e., birth), we can determine that a person who is 40 years of age is twice as old as a 20-year-old. In contrast, temperature measured in degrees Fahrenheit or Celsius does not have a true zero point, so it would be inaccurate to state that 50°F is twice as hot as 25°F. However, the Kelvin temperature scale does have a true zero point. Continuous data with a true zero point are called **ratio data,** whereas those without a true zero point are called **interval data.**

Some variables can be reported using more than one level of measurement, depending on the preference of the researcher. For example, a researcher could report a patient's actual blood pressure (continuous), categorize it as low, normal or high (ordinal), or label it simply as normal or abnormal (dichotomous).

Planning

Planning

Conclusion

Data are the building blocks of health research. The level of measurement (i.e., type) of the data collected during the course of a study determines the type of statistical analysis that should be performed on those data. When data, collected as counts, observations and measurements, differ from person to person or from time to time, they are referred to as variables. Variables play three distinct roles in research studies: as outcome variables, predictor variables or co-variables. Later chapters of this guide discuss how data variables are employed in various research methods (ch. 9), in the collection and management of data (ch. 22), and in the selection and conduct of applicable statistical tools to summarize, describe and better understand study data (chs 24 & 25). ∎

Acknowledgement

The development of this chapter was informed by Harvey BJ, Ancker JS, Bairnsfather S, Bukowski JA, Hudson S, Lang TA, et al. *Statistics for medical writers and editors*. Rockville (MD): American Medical Writers Association; 2009. Chapter 2, Types of data; p. 5–11.

EXERCISES

(Answers are given on the following page.)

1. What level of measurement involves only two categories?
2. What level of measurement involves whole-number counts?
3. What level of measurement involves a set of category names with no inherent ordering?
4. What level of measurement includes a full range of possible fractional values?
5. What level of measurement involves a set of inherently ordered categories?
6. In a study of the association between physical activity and mental health, women were asked how many children they had. What level of measurement is "number of children"? What types of variables are "number of children," "physical activity" and "mental health"?
7. Survey respondents were asked to rate their current health on a 5-point scale ranging from "excellent" to "poor." What level of measurement best describes this measure?
8. In the Women's Health Initiative Trial, women who were randomly assigned to receive hormone replacement therapy (HRT) had heart disease more frequently than women who did not receive HRT. What level of measurement is the variable "had heart disease"? What types of variables are "hormone replacement therapy" and "heart disease"?
9. A study was conducted to assess the association between age and the occurrence of osteoporosis. What level of data measurement is "age"? What types of variables are "osteoporosis" and "age"?
10. A study was conducted to assess the association between serum cholesterol concentration (in mg/dL) and systolic blood pressure (in mm Hg). What levels of measurement are "systolic blood pressure" and "cholesterol concentration"?
11. Researchers extracted data from hospital records to explore whether the number of surgical procedures ever completed by each surgeon is associated with the surgeon's rate of surgical complications. What level of measurement is "number of surgical procedures ever completed"? What types of variables are "surgical complications" and "number of surgical procedures"?
12. Researchers conducted a study to assess the effect of radiation exposure (in mSv) on the risk of lung cancer among a group of uranium miners. What level of measurement best describes "lung cancer"? What types of variables are "radiation exposure" and "lung cancer"?

Planning

ANSWERS

1. Dichotomous (binary) data
2. Discrete data
3. Nominal data
4. Continuous data
5. Ordinal data
6. Discrete data; co-variable (number of children), predictor variable (physical activity) and outcome variable (mental health)
7. Ordinal data
8. Dichotomous; exposure variable (hormone replacement therapy) and outcome variable (heart disease)
9. Continuous data; predictor variable (age) and outcome variable (osteoporosis)
10. Continuous (both)
11. Discrete data; predictor variable (number of surgical procedures) and outcome variable (surgical complications)
12. Dichotomous data; predictor variable (radiation exposure) and outcome variable (lung cancer)

SUMMARY CHECKLIST

- ❑ Thinking about your research project, list the types of variables involved.
- ❑ List the kinds of data (i.e., levels of measurement) involved in your research project.

Planning

9

Research methods and design: Bringing the research question to life

Bart J. Harvey, MD, PhD, MEd, FACPM, FRCPC

Designing

ILLUSTRATIVE CASE

Motivated by the recent experience of one of her patients, a Family Medicine resident wants to study the outcomes and experiences, such as death, metastases, incontinence and impotence, of men diagnosed with favourable-risk prostate cancer (i.e., low-grade, localized tumours with a low PSA level) who are managed with active surveillance versus those who are treated by radical prostatectomy. She arranges a meeting with the hospital's chief of Urology to discuss the possibility of designing and carrying out a randomized trial or some other kind of study to address this question.

■ **This chapter builds on the preceding** three chapters—on developing a research question (ch. 6), conducting a literature review (ch. 7) and applying identifying data variables (ch. 8)—each of which lays important groundwork to help you select a research design suitable for your study. To choose the best design for the purpose, you will need to be familiar with the options available and consider the advantages and disadvantages of each. It is important to realize that no single design can answer all types of questions, and so your choice will depend on, among other things, the nature of your research question.

This chapter examines this array of potential study designs in detail, focusing on quantitative designs: that is, those that involve counting, taking measurements and/or categorizing observations. The methods and conduct of qualitative research are discussed in chapter 16. In addition, the research methods used to design and conduct systematic reviews will not be discussed in this chapter, but are presented in chapter 15.

The research question

As discussed in chapter 6, a well-formed research question shapes several components of the anticipated research project, which are often summarized using the PICOT mnemonic: the Population, people and/or patients of interest to be studied; any Intervention that is being assessed; any Comparison that will be made against the intervention; the

applicable primary Outcome to be assessed (and, if applicable, any secondary outcomes); and, finally, any applicable Time frames, such as the period of follow-up. Each of the components specified in the research question should be taken into account as you consider potential research designs.

The Family Medicine resident in our illustrative case will need to choose a research design that enables her to identify and/or recruit a sufficient number of men diagnosed with favourable-risk prostate cancer (patient population), some of whom will be treated with radical prostatectomy (intervention) while others are managed with "watchful waiting"

CHAPTER OBJECTIVES

After reading this chapter, you should be able to:
- discuss the purpose, advantages and disadvantages of descriptive, cross-sectional, case-control, cohort and experimental study designs;
- discuss selection bias, information bias and confounding; how they can affect a research study's results; and how they can be addressed in the study's design, conduct and/or analysis;
- choose an appropriate research design, given a research question and context; and
- argue the relevance and importance of your proposed research project (i.e., answer the questions "So what?" and "Who will care?").

Designing

KEY TERMS

Allocation	Ecologic studies	Non-differential misclassification
Allocation concealment	Effect modification	Observational studies
Before-after (pre-post) studies	Effect modifier	Odds ratio
Bias	Experimental studies	Placebo
Blinded, blinding	External validity	Placebo effect
Case	Generalizability	Prevalence studies
Case-control studies	Historic (retrospective) cohort studies	Quasi-experimental studies
Case reports	Incidence/surveillance studies	Randomization
Case series	Information bias	Random error/variation
Cohort studies	Interaction	Randomized controlled trial (RCT)
Confounding	Internal validity	Relative risk
Control	Interrupted time series analysis	Risk difference
Cross-over studies	Longitudinal surveys	Selection bias
Cross-sectional studies	Masked, masking	Stepped wedge design
Descriptive studies	Matching	Stratified randomization
Differential misclassification	Natural experiments	Two-by-two (four-fold) table
Ecologic fallacy	N-of-1 studies	

(comparison). Each group will be followed for a sufficient period of time (time frame) to determine each participant's health outcomes of interest (e.g., survival in good health, development of progressive prostate cancer, development of treatment complications, death as a result of prostate cancer, or death from another cause).

Research designs

Potential research designs range from relatively simple and straightforward descriptive or cross-sectional studies to complex experimental studies.[1] Research examining a given health issue often progresses from description, to explanation, to prediction, to control.

Descriptive studies

The most straightforward research design is the **descriptive study**, which, as the name suggests, enables investigators to describe various aspects of a phenomenon.[1,2] Features such as who is affected, where they live, when they were affected, and any other characteristics of interest can be determined and summarized. Individual (i.e., univariate) variables are usually summarized using various descriptive statistics (see ch. 24), such as mean, median, percentage, range, standard deviation and interquartile range. Descriptive studies often enable a preliminary analysis of the relationship between variables to be conducted using techniques such as stratified tables and calculations such as ratio of proportions, difference of means and correlation.

The insights gained through descriptive studies may also identify possible causative agents—for example, the role of chimney dust in the development of scrotal cancer.[3] Descriptive studies can also be conducted to gain an initial understanding of observed occurrences, thus helping to identify possible explanations that can be tested using more analytic, comparative, study designs. An initial report of young men diagnosed with Kaposi's sarcoma and *Pneumocystis* pneumonia in the early 1980s is an example of a descriptive study.[4] As is well known, this and other early descriptive studies led to further studies that ultimately resulted in the identification of HIV and AIDS.

There are several types of descriptive studies.[2] **Case reports** and **case series** describe the first instance or instances of a novel illness (e.g., AIDS, SARS), test (e.g., computed tomography, magnetic resonance imaging) or treatment (e.g., laparoscopic surgery). **Incidence/surveillance** studies measure the occurrence of diseases in a defined population (e.g., communicable diseases in Canada). **Prevalence studies** measure the presence of health indicators (e.g., exposures, behaviours, diseases) in a defined population (e.g., people who report being physically active, people with diabetes in a Canadian province or territory).

Cross-sectional studies

Cross-sectional studies use data gathered at one point in time to measure potential exposures, outcomes and other variables of interest together. These studies can be conducted in various ways, such as through phone surveys, self-administered questionnaires or the examination of existing databases. However, because potential exposures and outcomes are measured at the same time, cross-sectional studies are well suited for establishing prevalence (of outcomes and risk factors) but poorly suited for the identification of potential cause-and-effect relationships. Like descriptive studies, they are useful in the formulation of hypotheses that can be tested in more rigorous, analytic, studies.

In cross-sectional studies, individual variables are usually summarized using various descriptive statistics (see ch. 24), such as mean, median, percentage, range, standard deviation and interquartile range. In addition, the relationship between variables can be determined using stratified tables or calculations such as the ratio of proportions, difference of means, and correlations.

Some cross-sectional studies are carried out using population averages rather than data about individual people (e.g., amount of alcohol sold each year in each Canadian province, annual provincial rates of liver cirrhosis). These are called **ecologic studies**. Although this type of study is useful for suggesting hypotheses to be tested in rigorous analytic studies, ecologic studies cannot be used to draw causal conclusions. This is because they do not make clear whether the individual people who developed the outcome of interest were those who were actually exposed to the reported variable (i.e., they do not provide direct cause-and-effect information). For example, the fact that a certain geographic area has both high levels of environmental toxins and high rates of cancer is not sufficient to demonstrate that the toxins are the cause of the cancers. This type of inference is referred to as the **ecologic fallacy**.

Because cross-sectional and descriptive studies can usually be completed relatively quickly and inexpensively, and sometimes with data that are already available, these approaches are often the first to be used to gather initial insights and to determine whether more rigorous, analytic, studies are warranted.

Canada is internationally renowned for its **longitudinal surveys**, such as the National Longitudinal Survey of Children and Youth (NLSCY), the National Population Health Survey (NPHS) and the Canadian Community Health Survey (CCHS). The data collected in these studies are often available to researchers. For example, Naiman and colleagues used data from the CCHS to examine the impact of public smoking bans on self-reported smoking status and exposure to second-hand smoke.[5]

Case-control studies

The **case-control study** design is almost as efficient as descriptive and cross-sectional designs, while providing a more rigorous way to assess potential cause-and-effect relationships.[1,6] The case-control design is one of three "analytic" or "comparative" research approaches in which two or more groups are formally compared to determine whether there is evidence of an association between the outcome (or outcomes) of interest (e.g., occurrence of, or death resulting from, cancer) and the exposure (or exposures) under study (e.g., toxin exposure, level of physical activity, screening mammogram). The other two analytic approaches—cohort studies and experimental studies—will be discussed later.

The first step in designing a case-control study is to identify a group of individuals (**cases**) who have the outcome of interest and a comparison (**control**) group selected to provide an estimate of the frequency of the exposure in the population from which the cases are drawn. In a case-control study, an *outcome* refers to a pre-existing condition or outcome in the case group, such as (1) having being diagnosed with the disease under study, (2) having developed a complication of a certain disease (e.g., metastatic spread of a cancer), or (3) having died from a cause under study (e.g., in a motor vehicle crash, due to a cancer, etc.) As such, the controls should be as similar as possible to the cases, aside from not having the outcome of interest. Although the number of controls is often quite similar to the number of cases being studied, if only a limited number of cases are available the power of a case-control study can be enhanced by selecting multiple controls per case. (However, selecting more than 10 controls per case provides only marginal added benefit.) Once the cases and controls have been identified, information about each group is sought, especially concerning the potential exposure or exposures of interest (e.g., past immunizations, history of smoking). This past-exposure information can come from a variety of possible sources, including health records, other records (e.g., cell phone records, for a study on brain cancers or motor vehicle collisions associated with cell phone use; employment, for a study on the health risks associated with certain occupational exposures), participant self-reports and even reports

Designing

by spouses, other family members or friends. If the exposure is truly associated with the outcome of interest, then the frequency of that exposure should be found to differ significantly between the groups being studied (e.g., a history of smoking being more frequent among those with lung cancer cases than among the controls, a record of influenza immunization being less frequent among those who contracted influenza).

The association between the occurrence of the exposure and case-control status (i.e., in those with and without the outcome of interest) is often summarized with a **two-by-two table** (also known as a **four-fold table**) and quantified using an **odds ratio**—the ratio of the frequency of exposure versus non-exposure among cases and the frequency of exposure versus non-exposure among controls (i.e., A/C ÷ B/D or AD/BC).

	Cases	Controls
Exposed	A	B
Not exposed	C	D

For example, a case-control study of 100 people with lung cancer (the cases) and 100 people without lung cancer (the controls) found the following results:

	Cases	Controls
Smokers	80	20
Non-smokers	20	80

The resulting odds ratio would be 16 (i.e., 80/20 ÷ 20/80 or 80 x 80/20 x 20). Case-control studies can often be analyzed using logistic regression, which readily provides an odds ratio adjusted for any other variables of interest that were also studied (e.g., age, sex).

It should be evident, and will be discussed further below, that the accuracy of case-control studies is highly dependent on two factors. The first is that the cases and controls are as comparable as possible (except, of course, that one group has the disease/outcome of interest while the other does not).[6,7] Controls can be identified by methods such as random selection from the same neighbourhood as the case, or by random-digit dialing in the same telephone exchange, or from the examination of records in the same health system. Although hospital controls are often considered and sometimes used, because individuals in hospitals have associated health issues they generally poorly reflect the characteristics of the underlying population; for this reason, drawing controls from this patient group can lead to biased results.

One strategy that is often used to enhance the comparability of cases and controls is **matching** the selected controls to the cases on the basis of factors that are thought to be important, such as age, sex, socioeconomic status, etc. One of the shortcomings of matching is that, if too many factors are chosen, it might not be possible to find suitable controls for some of the cases, who then cannot be included in the study. Another disadvantage is that the role played by the matching factors in causing the outcome of interest cannot be explored because, by design, these factors do not differ between the case and control groups.

The second key factor affecting the accuracy of a case-control study is the determination of past exposure(s): this must be done as precisely as possible and, in particular, in a manner that is comparable between the case and control groups. The recall of past information by study participants is a common source of systematic error (**bias**) in case-control studies. For example, it has often been demonstrated that people with an illness, or who have a child born with congenital abnormalities, recall past exposures to putative causal agents more accurately than unaffected (control) participants.

To the degree that case-control comparability and the accurate determination of past exposures are not achieved, any observed differences between cases and controls may be biased and, as a result, fail to reflect real differences.

Because the outcomes of interest have already occurred when a case-control study is initiated, these studies can usually be completed relatively quickly and inexpensively, requiring a relatively modest number of study participants. They are particularly well suited for the study of rare diseases (i.e., when the outcome of interest is expected to be infrequent) and for formulating hypotheses that can be tested in further studies using more rigorous analytic designs.

Cohort studies

Whereas case-control studies sample people on the basis of the outcome, **cohort studies** sample people on the basis of their exposure to some putative causal agent, such as smoking or asbestos. By their nature, cohort studies minimize one of the shortcomings of case-control studies.[1,8] Specifically, to reduce the potential risk of the exposure(s) of interest being measured differentially between cases and

Designing

controls, they are designed to determined such exposures prospectively, before the occurrence of the outcome of interest. However, this generally results in cohort studies taking much longer to complete, and therefore being much more expensive, than case-control studies, since more time is required for an adequate number of the participants to develop and be diagnosed with the outcome or outcomes of interest. **Historic (retrospective) cohort studies**, however, are an exception to this, and are possible only when detailed, historical exposure records are available for a well-defined population, such as employees in a specific workplace. However, both prospective and retrospective cohort studies almost always require sample sizes much larger than those needed for case-control studies to ensure that a sufficient number of participants will ultimately develop and be diagnosed with the outcome of interest.

Although case-control studies, by definition, address only those instances in which the outcome of interest is dichotomous (i.e., individuals either do or do not have the outcome of interest), cohort studies can be used to examine a wider range of outcome measures, such as continuous, discrete and ordinal values (e.g., mean serum cholesterol concentrations following a dietary program). Like case-control studies, the association between the exposure and a dichotomous outcome of interest in a cohort study is often summarized with a two-by-two table. However, because a cohort study includes an entire study population, thus enabling incidence rates to be determined (which is not possible in case-control studies), the association between the outcome of interest and any exposures of interest can be quantified by the relative risk or the risk difference. The **relative risk** is the ratio of the frequency (or "incidence") of the outcome among those exposed and the frequency among the non-exposed (i.e., $A/A+B \div C/C+D$). The **risk difference** is a measure of the excess frequency of the outcome of interest attributed to the exposure (i.e., $[A/A+B] - [C/C+D]$).

	Outcomes	No outcomes
Exposed	A	B
Not exposed	C	D

For example, a cohort study of 34 440 British doctors was conducted by Doll and Peto[9] to determine the health effects of cigarette smoking. After 20 years of follow-up, 10 072 of the study participants had died. Deaths were distributed among smokers and non-smokers as follows:

	Died	Alive	Total
Smokers	9132	19 453	28 585
Non-smokers	940	4915	5855
Total	10 072	24 368	34 440

The observed risk of death was 319.5 per 1000 among the smokers and 160.5 per 1000 among the non-smokers. As a result, the relative risk of death among smokers compared with non-smokers during that 20-year period was 1.99 (319.5/160.5). In other words, the study's results suggested that smoking doubled the risk of dying. The risk difference was 159.0 per 1000 (319.5–160.5), suggesting that smoking is responsible for an excess of 159 deaths per 1000 among smokers compared with non-smokers.

Despite their improved measurement of the exposure(s) of interest, cohort studies share with case-control studies the challenge of the potential non-comparability of the groups being studied. Like all of the study designs discussed so far, cohort studies simply examine the potential results of "naturally occurring" decisions (e.g., a person decides to smoke, a health care provider prescribes a treatment). This is why cohort, case-control, cross-sectional and descriptive studies are collectively referred to as **observational studies**: the researcher is simply observing decisions and outcomes determined outside of his or her control. The observational nature of cohort studies means that the groups being compared (e.g., those who smoke, those who are physically active) will likely differ with respect to many other characteristics beyond those being studied. As will be discussed in further detail below, this means that any observed difference in an outcome of interest (e.g., the occurrence of heart attacks) may also be the result of these other, differing, "exposure" factors—both those that are known and measurable as well as those that are currently unknown and therefore cannot be measured. In an effort to account for potential differences between the study groups, researchers often use techniques such as stratification and regression analysis, which enable study results to be calculated in a manner that adjusts for any potential differences. Of course, including any potentially differing factor in such an analysis requires that the factor in question has been measured for all study participants. However, even after adjusting for any known and measured factors, the groups may still differ because of other factors that are either unknown or were not measured.

Designing

The next section will discuss experimental studies, which use research designs that are better able to ensure the comparability of the groups being studied.

Experimental studies

Unlike in observational studies, in which participant or health provider decisions and choices determine the studied exposure, in **experimental studies** each participant's exposure of interest is assigned according to the research protocol specified by the researcher, thus enhancing the comparability of the groups being studied.[1] In both experimental and observational studies, the groups being compared should, ideally, differ from one another only with respect to the exposure of interest—and, the more that this can be achieved, the stronger the evidence will be of any relationship between the studied exposure and outcome. The comparability of study groups is important because it better enables any observed difference in the outcome measure to be attributed to the exposure under study. In contrast, the degree to which the study groups otherwise differ permits alternative potential explanations for any observed differences. In reality, the comparability of study groups can be achieved only through a randomized experimental study design in which participants are randomly assigned to the study groups (e.g., a **randomized controlled trial**). With this design each group (if sufficiently large) will, on average, have a similar distribution of all factors, measured and unmeasured, associated with the outcome of interest. Because of the resulting comparability of the study groups, any between-group difference in the occurrence of the outcome can be more confidently attributed to the exposure (e.g., treatment) being studied.

As a result, experimental studies that use non-random approaches to assign participants to study groups are, like observational studies, at risk of assembling groups that differ from one another with respect to factors other than the exposure under study. It should also be noted that, even with the use of rigorous **randomization** techniques (and, especially, in relatively small clinical trials), study groups can differ from one another simply by chance. As a result, investigators often use **stratified randomization**, so that participants are evenly allocated to the study groups, thus ensuring that they do not differ according to any important co-factors.

However, this comparability is best achieved when participants are randomly assigned[10] to study groups, when the sequence of group **allocation** can be successfully concealed from those involved in the study[11] and, where feasible and applicable, when the participants and those providing care

and making participant assessments are unaware of which study group each participant is in (referred to as **blinding** or **masking**). **Allocation concealment** is used during the assignment of participants to study groups to ensure that the assignment is not manipulated, whereas blinding occurs after group assignment to reduce the risk that those involved in the study will know which study group participants are in, ideally to ensure that all participants are treated in a comparable fashion. Blinding is often applied, where possible, to those in the comparison group receiving a **placebo** intervention, which should be as similar as possible (e.g., pills that look and taste the same) to the intervention under study. In this way, it should be impossible to determine whether a participant is in the study group or the comparison group until the secured allocation information is accessed to "break the code." If this level of blinding of all those involved in the study can be accomplished, then each participant will be treated in a similar fashion (i.e., each will receive the usual standard of care, while one group also receives the intervention under study and the other receives the placebo). Although the phrase "double blinding" is often used, those who are blinded (e.g., participants, those providing care, those making assessments) should be explicitly identified in the study protocol and resulting report.

The association between the exposure and outcome of interest in an experimental study such as a randomized controlled trial (RCT) is summarized and quantified in exactly the same manner as in a cohort study. This should make sense, given that RCTs are cohort studies with the unique feature of the exposure/intervention being determined according to the researcher's study protocol.

Recently, investigators have begun to use a **stepped wedge design** in which the intervention is rolled out in a staged fashion to all participants, such that those receiving the intervention in later stages serve as the comparison for those who began to receive it in earlier stages.[12-14] The implementation of the intervention is often carried out in "clusters" of participants, in which case the order in which each cluster receives the intervention is often determined by a randomization process.

Other research designs

Although the research designs discussed above (and summarized in Table 9.1) represent those that are frequently used in health studies, many other designs can be, and have been, used. Although it is beyond the scope of this chapter to discuss all possible designs, a few are mentioned briefly here to help you determine whether they might be applicable to your research project and warrant further exploration.

Quasi-experiments

In some circumstances, alternative experimental study approaches have been used. These include **quasi-experimental studies** in which participants are allocated to the study groups using non-random methods (e.g., according to birth date or hospital number) or the group assignment is simply alternated as each participant is recruited. (Even worse, in some instances, is the practice of assembling study groups as "grab" or "convenience" samples.) However, because these methods do not assign individuals to study groups in a truly random fashion, the comparability of the resulting groups may be compromised.[15–17]

Natural experiments

Another variant is a **natural experiment** in which naturally occurring circumstances result in one group of individuals being exposed while others are not.[18,19] This design is probably more accurately considered a cohort study in which "nature" has determined exposure. However, because the exposure is naturally determined, the groups being compared may be more comparable than is usually the case in cohort studies.

Before-after studies (also known as pre-post studies)

As the name suggests, in **before-after** studies measures are made of research participants before and after some intervention or event (e.g., level of physical fitness level before and after participation in a physical activity program).[20] Because the participants serve as their own controls, many other relevant factors remain constant, and so the study's ability to detect an effect is strengthened. However, it has been shown that simply being included in a research study can change people's behaviour, and so it is not always clear whether any observed change is due to the intervention under study or to some other change motivated consciously or unconsciously among study participants. Also, it is also possible for participants to experience a **placebo effect** simply because they have been started on a treatment, even if that treatment has no efficacy. As a result, many researchers will also include a parallel comparison study group that receives an "inert" control intervention (e.g., a series of educational sessions, weekly newsletters or a placebo treatment) to help assess what role, if any, the experience of being studied might have played in the observed results.

N-of-1 studies[21–23] are a special kind of before-after study in two ways: (1) only a single individual is studied and (2) that individual serves as his or her own control. These studies are often used to help guide treatment decisions by comparing the effects experienced by a patient when he or she receives, in a randomized fashion, the active treatment or the placebo. Of course, such studies are possible only under specific circumstances, such as recurrent illness (e.g., asthma, headaches) and when the active treatment given will "wash out" over a reasonably short period after it is stopped. Authors have also considered the feasibility of combining the results of multiple N-of-1 trials.[24] Although these studies are largely focused on informing treatment decisions, they also provide a valuable introduction to many of the methods necessary for research.

Interrupted time series analyses

Although similar in approach to before-after studies, **interrupted time series analyses** usually involve multiple measures both before and after the intervention being assessed.[25] These multiple data points provide a much more complete understanding of any temporal changes leading up to and following the intervention of interest. Although these studies can be used to collect data concerning individual people, they are often used to assess the effects of population-wide policies and practice, such as the application of clinical guidelines,[26] the enactment of anti-smoking laws[5,27] or seat belt legislation,[28] and the impact of published research on prescribing patterns.[29]

Cross-over studies

As in before-after studies, participants in **cross-over studies** also serve as their own controls.[30–34] However, in cross-over studies it is also possible for the intervention to be administered to participants more than once and for those administrations to be determined in a blinded fashion and using random allocation. This design is often used to assess the efficacy of drugs. Of course, this design requires an intervention whose effects readily subside during a "wash-out" period before the cross-over, and that the health issue being studied will recur after that period. It would therefore be inappropriate to use this design to study an intervention, such as an educational program, that is expected to have long-lasting effects. A cross-over design would be suitable, for example, to assess the efficacy of a new drug for the treatment of tension headaches.

Designing

Designing

■ **Table 9.1 A comparison of study designs**

Study design	Characteristics	Advantages	Disadvantages
Descriptive	Enables the characteristics of a group to be summarized	Usually efficient (quick and small) Data may be readily available and plentiful Provides initial insights	Provides description only Unable to determine causal relationships
Cross-sectional	"Survey" of a single "population" Data from a single point in time	Usually efficient (quick and small) Data may be readily available Provides population prevalence estimates	Unable to determine causal relationships Exposure and outcomes measured at same time
Case-control	Comparison of two groups (according to outcome status) Exposure occurs "naturally"	Usually efficient (quick and small and retrospecive (i.e., the outcomes of interest have already occurred)	Potential for biased exposure measurment Potential confounding as a result of group diffrences Weak design for determniing causal relationships
Cohort	Comparison of two or more groups (according to outcome status) Exposure occurs "naturally"	Exposure measured prior to outcome Moderately stong design to detemine causal relationship	Usually large and lengthy Costly Potential confounding and biases as a result of group differences
Experimental	Comparison of two or more groups (according to intervention assignment)	Most rigorous research design Comparability of study groups Strongest design for determining causal relationships	Usually large and lengthy Costly

Other study factors

Several general design issues apply to all research studies. These include the context within which the study is carried out and potential factors that can compromise the accuracy of a study's results. These factors are discussed briefly below.

Study context and generalizability

As you design your study, consider those to whom the results will apply. Research studies are almost always carried out to gain insights and draw conclusions that are applicable beyond the individuals who participate in the study. The study population indicated in the research question defines the broader context of your research: this is the population from which your study sample should be drawn, and to which your results should be applicable. For practical and ethical reasons, only a limited number of partici-pants can and should be included in any given study; however, the selection of this group will dictate the degree to which the study and its results might be generalized. (This is also referred to as the **external validity** of the study.) For example, if a researcher wishes to determine the proportion of patients with diabetes who have had an ophthalmologic examination in the previous 24 months, the choice of how participants are identified and recruited—whether from a diabetes specialty clinic, a primary care practice or a province-wide diabetes registry—will dictate the applicability—that is, the **generalizability**—of the study's results.

Study error and internal validity

When a research study is carried out, it is hoped that its results will reflect the "truth," such that the observed effects are "real." However, the results of a given study can sometimes be explained by factors other than truth. The first of these is **random error/variation**. This arises when, by chance, the individuals selected for the study are not representative of the group being studied. As a result, the study's results do not reflect the truth, but differ because a non-representative group of participants was selected by chance. It should be noted, however, that chance can affect a study's results in either direction, being equally likely to lead to overestimation or to underestimation. As discussed in chapter 25, statistical tests and techniques are used to determine the probability that random variation (i.e., bad luck) might be responsible for the observed study results.

As suggested above, factors such as non-comparable study groups and inaccurate measures of exposures and/or outcomes can alter a study's results so that they do not reflect the true relationship between the exposure(s) and outcome(s) being studied. These are examples of other factors, such as bias and confounding,[33] that can distort a study's results. The potential for bias and other errors should be taken into account as you select a study design, for each approach differs in its susceptibility to these problems. In addition, unlike the random effects of chance, bias and confounding are systematic errors and, as such, can arise because of weaknesses in a study's design and/or conduct, resulting in a predictable over- or underestimation of the effect being assessed. **Internal validity** is the term used to describe the soundness or rigour with which a study is designed and conducted. It is also an indicator of the accuracy of the study's results (i.e., how well they approximate the "truth").

There is often a trade-off between internal and external validity. The more tightly controlled the selection of participants for a study (e.g., with long lists of inclusion and exclusion criteria) and the delivery of the intervention, the greater the internal validity will be, but at the cost of the generalizability of the results (external validity).

Study biases

Biases are factors that, arising from the design and/or conduct of a study, cause the results to diverge from the truth. Although many different types of bias have been described,[34,35] they generally fall into two main categories: selection bias and information bias.

Selection bias arises when the groups being compared differ as a result of how study participants are chosen. As discussed above, in observational studies this can arise when the groups being studied are selected in a way that fails to ensure that they are comparable. This poses a particular challenge in case-control studies, where, ideally, one strives to select the control group from the same population in which cases occur.[6,7] Although the selection of controls is straightforward in some circumstances, it is not always clear what kind of controls should be used: neighbourhood, friend, associate, relative or hospital. However, without the selection of a suitably comparable control group, the study's results will be systematically biased and provide an inaccurate estimate of the true relationship between the exposure(s) and outcome(s) being studied. In fact, as discussed above, even experimental study designs can be affected by selection bias, particularly if the methods used for randomization[10] and allocation concealment[11] are not sound. Of course, as discussed earlier, even when an appropriate randomization technique is used, groups are still at risk of differing sizably from one another simply by chance. Selection bias also comes into play in determining who gets into a study. Those who volunteer (in some studies, this can be as few as 20% of those approached) differ from the general population, jeopardizing to some degree the external validity of the study. This is a problem for all research designs that enrol participants.

Information bias arises as a result of how information is collected about the participants in a study. This can occur at any juncture from initial recruitment to final follow-up where the measurement of the study groups might differ, but it is particularly likely when the exposure and/or outcome of interest are measured. For example, **differential misclassification**/information can result when a questionnaire does not accurately collect sought-after information or when study participants are not followed for a sufficiently long period for the outcomes of interest to be observed. It can also arise if those who are providing and/or collecting participant information are aware of which group a participant is in. As discussed above, one way to reduce this risk is to mask (blind) any applicable individuals (e.g., the participants themselves, practitioners providing care, those making the measurements or adjudicating outcomes). If blinding is accomplished successfully, then the measurement of information should be achieved in a comparable manner, independent of which group a participant is in.[36]

Selection and information biases are of particular concern in comparative studies: if the groups are affected differentially, their comparison can potentially be distorted. Further, the groups compared in non-randomized experimental and observational studies may differ from one another with respect to factors other than the exposure (e.g., treatment) being studied. As a result, special care must be taken in the design, conduct, analysis and interpretation

Designing

of these kinds of studies. However, it should be noted that, even if the measurements are made comparably among the study groups, there might still be some level of inaccuracy. Although such **non-differential misclassifications**/measurements will not result in a favouring of one group over the other, they do bias the study's result toward the null. That is, the resulting "random error" causes the result observed by the study to underestimate the "true" result.

Confounding

Confounding occurs when the apparent effect of the exposure under study is the result of its association with another causative (confounding) factor. To be a confounder, a factor must be associated with the exposure, must be an independent determinant of the outcome, and must not be an intermediate step in the causal pathway. For example, although a study might find an increased risk of ischemic heart disease associated with coffee drinking, it is possible that this apparent association is confounded by some other risk factor for ischemic heart disease, such as smoking, which is also associated with coffee drinking. The presence and effect of potential confounders can be determined by assessing the level of risk of the exposure under study while controlling for any potential confounding factor. This is accomplished by carrying out a stratified analysis that adjusts for the amount of such a confounding variable (smoking), which enables the effect of the other variable (coffee drinking) to be determined independently of the potential confounder's effect. If confounding is present, the level of risk associated with the exposure under study will be reduced (i.e., the amount of risk attributable to the confounding factor has been removed/controlled for). On the other hand, if confounding is not present, then the level of risk will remain unchanged when the potential confounder is controlled for.

Effect modification

Stratified analyses are also used to explore whether a factor might be an **effect modifier**. As the name suggests, such a factor modifies the effect of another factor. For example, studies have shown that the effect of asbestos exposure is magnified in those who also smoke. This is why the risk of developing mesothelioma, a cancer uniquely associated with asbestos exposure, is markedly greater among those with a history of smoking. This would become apparent in an analysis stratified by smoking because the level of risk (e.g., odds ratio or relative risk) of mesothelioma would be greater in the smoking as compared with the non-smoking subgroup. Effect modification is sometimes referred to as **interaction**, meaning that factors interact with one another to create a greater effect than either would cause on its own.

Conclusion

A wide range of approaches is available for you to choose from as you design your research study. However, your choice of study design should be guided by how much is known about the subject being studied and by the advantages and disadvantages associated with each possible design. Although this chapter has provided a general overview of the various issues that should be considered in choosing a study design, the seven chapters that follow each address a particular type of study in further detail. ∎

CASE POSTSCRIPT

Although the resident and her supervisor recognize that several research designs, including a randomized clinical trial, could be used to address her research question, to better inform their planning they choose to begin with a preliminary descriptive study to better understand the characteristics and experiences of men diagnosed with favourable-risk prostate cancer who are managed at their medical centre. The findings of this descriptive study allow them to better determine the quality of the data available from the hospital's electronic health records database. Guided by these preliminary results, they then design and complete a retrospective cohort study comparing the outcomes of the men managed with active surveillance versus those attained by men treated with radical prostatectomy.

Designing

REFERENCES

1. Grimes DA, Schulz KF. An overview of clinical research: the lay of the land. *Lancet*. 2002;359(9300):57–61.

2. Grimes DA, Schulz KF. Descriptive studies: what they can and cannot do. *Lancet*. 2002;359(9301):145–9.

3. Waldron HA. A brief history of scrotal cancer. *Br J Ind Med*. 1983;40(4):390–401.

4. Centers for Disease Control. Kaposi's sarcoma and Pneumocystis pneumonia among homosexual men—New York City and California. *MMWR Morb Mortal Wkly Rep*. 1981;30(25):305–8.

5. Naiman AB, Glazier RH, Moineddin R. Is there an impact of public smoking bans on self-reported smoking status and exposure to secondhand smoke? *BMC Public Health*. 2011 Mar 3; 11:146.

6. Schulz KF, Grimes DA. Case-control studies: research in reverse. *Lancet*. 2002;359(9304):431–4.

7. Grimes DA, Schulz KF. Compared to what? Finding controls for case-control studies. *Lancet*. 2005;365(9468):1429–33.

8. Grimes DA, Schulz KF. Cohort studies: marching towards outcomes. *Lancet*. 2002;359(9303):341–5.

9. Doll R, Peto R. Mortality in relation to smoking: 20 years' observations on male British doctors. *Br Med J*. 1976;2(6051):1525–36.

10. Schulz KF, Grimes DA. Generation of allocation sequences in randomized trials: chance, not choice. *Lancet*. 2002;359(9305):515–9.

11. Schulz KF, Grimes DA. Allocation concealment in randomised trials: defending against deciphering. *Lancet*. 2002;359(9306):614–8.

12. Mdege ND, Man MS, Taylor Nee Brown CA, Torgerson DJ. Systematic review of stepped wedge cluster randomized trials shows that design is particularly used to evaluate interventions during routine implementation. *J Clin Epidemiol*. 2011 Mar 15. [Epub ahead of print].

13. Brown CA, Lilford RJ. The stepped wedge trial design: a systematic review. *BMC Med Res Methodol*. 2006 Nov 8;6:54.

14. Hussey MA, Hughes JP. Design and analysis of stepped wedge cluster randomized trials. *Contemp Clin Trials*. 2007;28(2):182–91.

15. Morgan GA, Gliner JA, Harmon RJ. Quasi-experimental designs. *J Am Acad Child Adolesc Psychiatry*. 2000;39(6):794–6.

16. Johnston MV, Ottenbacher KJ, Reichardt CS. Strong quasi-experimental designs for research on the effectiveness of rehabilitation. *Am J Phys Med Rehabil*. 1995;74(5):383–92.

17. Shadish WR, Cook TD, Campbell DT. *Experimental and Quasi-Experimental Designs for Generalized Causal Inference*. Boston (MA): Houghton Mifflin Company; 2002.

18. Petticrew M. Commentary: Sinners, preachers and natural experiments. *Int J Epidemiol*. 2011;40(2):454–6.

19. Petticrew M, Cummins S, Ferrell C, Findlay A, Higgins C, Hoy C, et al. Natural experiments: an underused tool for public health? *Public Health*. 2005;119(9):751–7.

20. Anonymous. A primer on before-after studies: evaluating a report of a "successful" intervention. *Eff Clin Pract*. 2002;5(2):100–1.

21. Jaeschke R, Cook D, Sackett DL. The potential role of single-patient randomized controlled trials (N-of-1 RCTs) in clinical practice. *J Am Board Fam Pract*. 1992;5(2):227–9.

22. Guyatt GH, Heyting A, Jaeschke R, Keller J, Adachi JD, Roberts RS. N of 1 randomized trials for investigating new drugs. *Control Clin Trials*. 1990;11(2):88–100.

23. Guyatt GH, Keller JL, Jaeschke R, Rosenbloom D, Adachi JD, Newhouse MT. The n-of-1 randomized controlled trial: clinical usefulness. Our three-year experience. *Ann Intern Med*. 1990;112(4):293–9.

24. Zucker DR, Ruthazer R, Schmid CH. Individual (N-of-1) trials can be combined to give population comparative treatment effect estimates: methodologic considerations. *J Clin Epidemiol*. 2010;63(12):1312–23.

25. Matowe LK, Leister CA, Crivera C, Korth-Bradley JM. Interrupted time series analysis in clinical research. *Ann Pharmacother*. 2003;37(7–8):1110–6.

26. England E. How interrupted time series analysis can evaluate guideline implementation. *Pharm J*. 2005;275:344–7.

27. Naiman A, Glazier RH, Moineddin R. Association of anti-smoking legislation with rates of hospital admission for cardiovascular and respiratory conditions. *CMAJ*. 2010;182(8):761–7.

28. Masten S. The effects of changing to primary enforcement on daytime and nighttime seatbelt use. *Traffic Safety Facts: Research Note*, DOT HS 810 743. Washington (DC): National Highway Traffic Safety Adminitration; March 2007. Available from: www.nhtsa.gov/people/injury/research/TSF/HS810743/810743.html

Designing

29. Tu K, Mamdani MM, Jacka RM, Forde NJ, Rothwell DM, Tu JV. The striking effect of the Heart Outcomes Prevention Evaluation (HOPE) on ramipril prescribing in Ontario. *CMAJ*. 2003;168(5):553–7.

30. Jackson PR, Yeo WW. Cross-over trials–a commentary. *Eur J Clin Pharmacol*. 1997;52(2):155–8.

31. Jackson PR, Yeo WW. Cross over trials. *Br J Clin Pharmacol*. 1996;42(3):401–3.

32. Jones B, Donev AN. Modelling and design of cross-over trials. *Stat Med*. 1996;15(13):1435–46.

33. Grimes DA, Schulz KF. Bias and causal associations in observational research. *Lancet*. 2002;359(9302):248–52.

34. Sackett DL. Bias in analytic research. *J Chronic Dis*. 1979;32(1–2):51–63.

35. Lang TA, Secic M. In: Lang TA, Secic M. *How to report statistics in medicine: annotated guidelines for authors, editors and reviewers*. 2nd ed. Philadelphia (PA): American College of Physicians; 2006. Appendix 5: Sources of error, confounding, and bias in biomedical research; p. 449–57.

36. Schulz KF, Grimes DA. Blinding in randomised trials: hiding who got what. *Lancet*. 2002;359(9307):696–700.

ADDITIONAL RESOURCES

Dennis ML, Perl HI, Huebner RB, McLellan AT. Twenty-five strategies for improving the design, implementation and analysis of health services research related to alcohol and other drug abuse treatment. *Addiction*. 2000;95 Suppl 3:S281–308.

- An interesting and reasonably extensive discussion of issues to consider to strengthen the design and conduct of health research.

Fletcher RH, Fletcher SW. *Clinical epidemiology: the essentials*. 4th ed. New York: Lippincott Williams & Wilkins; 2005.

- A very readable and informative text describing the various aspects of clinical epidemiology and research.

Hulley SB, Cummings SR, Browner WS, Grady DG, Newman TB. *Designing clinical research: an epidemiologic approach*. 3rd ed. Philadelphia: Lippincott Williams & Wilkins; 2007.

- A readable and informative text discussing the various steps in designing and conducting clinical research.

Streiner DL, Norman GR. *PDQ epidemiology*. 3rd ed. Shelton (CT): People's Medical Publishing House; 2009.

- A concise, informative and very readable "classic" text providing an overview of epidemiology principles and methods from the "Pretty Darn Quick" series.

Grimes and Schulz *Lancet* series

- This is a multi-article series published in *The Lancet*. Each article provides an informative overview of an aspect of clinical research and research design.

Grimes DA, Schulz KF. An overview of clinical research: the lay of the land. *Lancet*. 2002;359(9300):57–61.

Grimes DA, Schulz KF. Descriptive studies: what they can and cannot do. *Lancet*. 2002;359(9301):145–9.

Grimes DA, Schulz KF. Bias and causal associations in observational research. *Lancet*. 2002;359(9302):248–52.

Grimes DA, Schulz KF. Cohort studies: marching towards outcomes. *Lancet*. 2002;359(9303):341–5.

Schulz KF, Grimes DA. Case-control studies: research in reverse. *Lancet*. 2002;359(9304):431–4.

Designing

Schulz KF, Grimes DA. Generation of allocation sequences in randomized trials: chance, not choice. *Lancet*. 2002;359(9305):515–19.

Schulz KF, Grimes DA. Allocation concealment in randomised trials: defending against deciphering. *Lancet*. 2002;359(9306):614–8.

Schulz KF, Grimes DA. Blinding in randomised trials: hiding who got what. *Lancet*. 2002;359(9307):696–700.

Schulz KF, Grimes DA. Sample size slippages in randomised trials: exclusions and the lost and wayward. *Lancet*. 2002;359(9308):781–5.

Schulz KF, Grimes DA. Unequal group sizes in randomised trials: guarding against guessing. *Lancet*. 2002;359(9310):966–70.

Grimes DA. Uncertainty. *Lancet*. 2002;360(9341):1242.

Schulz KF, Grimes DA. Sample size calculations in randomised trials: mandatory and mystical. *Lancet*. 2005;365(9467):1348–53.

Grimes DA, Schulz KF. Compared to what? Finding controls for case-control studies. *Lancet*. 2005;365(9468):1429–33.

Grimes DA, Schulz KF. Refining clinical diagnosis with likelihood ratios. *Lancet*. 2005;365(9469):1500–5.

Schulz KF, Grimes DA. Multiplicity in randomised trials I: endpoints and treatments. *Lancet*. 2005;365(9470):1591–95.

Schulz KF, Grimes DA. Multiplicity in randomised trials II: subgroup and interim analyses. *Lancet*. 2005;365(9471):1657–61.

Grimes DA, Hubacher D, Nanda K, Schulz KF, Moher D, Altman DG. The Good Clinical Practice guideline: a bronze standard for clinical research. *Lancet*. 2005;366(9480):172–4.

Grimes DA, Schulz KF. Uses and abuses of screening tests. *Lancet*. 2002;359(9309):881–84. Erratum in: *Lancet*. 2008;371(9629):1998.

Designing

SUMMARY CHECKLIST

- ❑ Consider your research question and the methods found in this chapter. Which design or designs would be best to choose for your study?
- ❑ Reviewing your design, consider how you will address generalizability and internal validity. Consider potential sources of error and bias. Refine your design.
- ❑ Discuss your selection with your research supervisor(s) and/or a methodologist. Refine your design.

Designing

10
Developing and assessing health measurement items and scales

David L. Streiner, PhD, CPsych

ILLUSTRATIVE CASE

A resident in pediatrics is working in a pediatric epilepsy clinic and realizes that effective management of these patients and their families involves more than simply controlling seizures, because the impact of epilepsy on quality of life must also be taken into account. He does a literature search and finds several scales that try to measure quality of life, but he is not sure how to choose among them. He'd like to know what features he should look for in deciding which, if any, of these instruments to select.

Designing

■ **This chapter outlines what you** should know about evaluating scales used to assess various aspects of health and behaviour, such as quality of life, mood and pain. It is aimed both at people who need to select an instrument to use in a research project, and at consumers of research who want to know whether a scale used to gather data is a good one. The chapter will review how scale items are developed and how to determine whether a scale as a whole is reliable and valid for the use to which it is put. The chapter also provides a launching point for those who want to collaborate with others in developing new scales.

It is relatively easy to measure physical attributes, such as height, blood pressure, creatinine levels, and so forth. After all, if we stand a person on a scale there is no doubt that we are measuring his or her weight, and the company that manufactures a triglyceride test guarantees that triglyceride levels are in fact what their test measures, and not something else. What we require of these measurements is that they be accurate, reproducible and feasible. However,

things becomes more complicated when we try to assess attributes such as moods, feelings, attitudes, beliefs or other internal states that we can't observe directly. How can we be sure that a scale is really measuring a person's quality of life, rather than, say, depression or pain, or that a test of a patient's knowledge about the management of his condition is in fact an accurate reflection of what he needs to know?

These types of attributes, which are not directly observable, are generally referred to as **hypothetical constructs**[1] (or **latent variables**). That is, we do not *see* anxiety or intelligence per se; all we can observe are their outward manifes-

CHAPTER OBJECTIVES

After reading this chapter, you should be able to:
- describe how scales are constructed;
- discuss the properties of a scale, such as reliability and validity; and
- evaluate existing scales.

KEY TERMS

Construct validity	Inter-rater reliability	Psychometrics
Criterion validation	Intra-class correlation coefficient	Reliability
Cronbach's α	Latent variables	"Satisficing"
End-aversion bias	Negative predictive value	Social desirability bias
Hypothetical constructs	Pearson correlation coefficient	Test-retest reliability
Internal consistency	Positive predictive value	Validity

---

tations. For example, if we see that a patient is pessimistic about the future, that her sleep is disturbed, that she has lost interest in doing things that she used to enjoy, has decreased libido, and has been having thoughts of suicide, we hypothesize that all of these are related and arise from an underlying state, or construct, we call *depression*. Similarly, we view a large vocabulary, knowledge about areas outside one's specialty, skill at problem-solving, and speed in solving puzzles as reflections of something we call *intelligence*. Again, note that we do not see the depression or intelligence directly, but only phenomena that they are hypothesized to affect. Many areas that we want to measure in health—pain, quality of life, mood, satisfaction with care, activities of daily living, caregiver burden, and so on—are in fact hypothetical constructs.

Over the past century, researchers primarily in the fields of psychology and education have developed an array of techniques that allow us to develop scales to tap—that is, measure or assess—these constructs relatively accurately. To appreciate these methods, though, requires certain skills along with a particular vocabulary. In this chapter, we will review those techniques, albeit in a non-technical way. By the end, you should be able to critique articles that present new scales. However, just as you wouldn't perform an appendectomy until you've had proper training and have had an expert looking over your shoulder for a sufficient number of cases, developing a new scale is not something you should try on your own. With that said, let's go through the steps required to bring a new scale to life so that you'll know what to look for.

Developing the items

The fact that hypothetical constructs are not directly observable has implications for what items do or do not appear on a scale. It's obvious that a pain scale, for example, should measure intensity, duration and frequency, but what else can and should it cover? Should a pain scale also tap the degree to which the pain interferes with work or leisure activities? Similarly, should a scale of aggressive behaviour in patients with dementia tap only episodes of a patient striking someone else, or should it be broadened to include verbal outbursts, spitting, and so on? To use a phrase that will recur often in this chapter, it all depends. What it depends on is the test developer's theory or understanding of the construct. If "pain," to the scale's author, refers only to the subjective experience—the sensation of

pain—then the effects of pain on the patient's life would not be covered. Conversely, if the developer sees pain in a more holistic way and believes that its effects colour most aspects of daily life, then questions about its impact on normal activities would be included.

For you, as a reader, user or developer of a scale, this matter of defining the construct has three implications. First, it means that you must have a clear idea of the construct in mind before you begin. In your conceptualization of the construct, what should and should not be included? It will be of great help to you later on if you pause to write down these areas for inclusion and exclusion, and in as much detail as possible.

The second implication is that the scale's author should do the same thing in the article that introduces the tool to the world. The result of these two steps—having a clear idea of the construct as it applies to your research or clinical purposes, and understanding how the construct is applied in a given scale—might immediately eliminate some scales from your consideration. For example, if your model holds that quality of life is a purely subjective phenomenon, and that people who are severely impaired can still enjoy a high quality of life,[2] then you would not consider using a proxy scale, such as the EQ-5D,[3] which rates only what people do or seem to experience.

The third implication is that, if you are contemplating developing your own scale, then an explicit statement of what should be included and excluded is mandatory and should be reported in your first paper about your new scale.

After you have a model, either explicitly (ideal) or implicitly (less than ideal), it's time to begin drafting items for the scale. In reality, few scales are developed *de novo*; they borrow from existing scales to varying degrees. It's not easy to write good items, and there are a limited number of ways to ask if a person is feeling sad, for instance, or experiencing pain. So, "borrowing" items from a number of scales to construct a new one is quite common.

At times, however, one must start from scratch because no adequate instrument exists. One example is the CHEQOL-25,[4] which assesses, from their own perspective, the quality of life of children with epilepsy. We began with various qualitative research methods, such as focus groups with the children and their parents, to elicit what the children thought was important,[5] and, based on typed transcripts of the numerous sessions, extracted five or six broad domains (the number varied between the child's and parent's version). The team then wrote a number of items that we felt tapped each domain—far more than we would eventually use, for reasons we'll discuss below—and went back to the original participants to ask: (1) Do the items seem to tap the domains? (2) Do any items appear irrelevant? (3) Did we miss any important ones? and (4) Does the wording seem appropriate?

Checking the items

Whenever you write new items, or use a scale in a population in which it hasn't been tried before, it is important to do some "cognitive interviewing"[6 (p 127–9)] with a sample of respondents. Anywhere from 5 to 10 people are asked, with respect to a given item, "Tell me how you arrived at your answer," or "Rephrase the item in your own words." The answers may alert the developer to difficulties that respondents might have in understanding the wording or intent of the item. Experts in the field are also asked to rate the relevance of each item to the construct, and those items deemed to have low relevance are eliminated. Finally, it's very useful to construct a matrix, assigning a row to each item and a column to each theme you identified earlier as important. You should then be able to match each item with one of the themes, and every theme should have a number of items associated with it.[6] If you can't, then you should either reject the scale (if you were thinking of using it) or go back to the drawing board (if you are developing a scale).

Not every scale that has been developed has been developed well. So, whether you are planning to use someone else's scale or to write your own, you must be aware of what makes an item good or bad. Beware the "double-barrelled" item that rolls two questions into one. For example, an item on a scale of satisfaction with care may be written as, "My doctor was prompt and courteous." The "and" in the sentence is a dead give-away that this is a double-barrelled question. How should the patient answer if the doctor was prompt but rude, or courteous but late? The problem is that different people will arrive at an answer differently: some will answer "False" because both parts aren't true, while others will answer "True" because at least one part is, and you'll never know which respondents favoured which logic. Other double-barrelled questions are more subtly so, especially in scales of health-related quality of life. Take the item, "My arthritis gets in the way of my enjoyment of sports." Does "False" mean that the arthritis doesn't get in the way, or that the person never enjoyed sports to begin with, and so the arthritis has no effect? Again, you'll have no idea.

The many kinds of bias that can influence how a person answers an item are far too numerous for all to be mentioned here, but a more complete list is provided by Streiner and Norman.[6] The most common biases are **social desirability bias, end-aversion bias** and "**satisficing.**" People want others to think well of them, and often give responses that are socially desirable—"I floss my teeth three times a day," "I never drink to excess," or "I always take all of my medications"—sometimes knowing that they are distorting the truth a bit, and sometime unaware that they are doing so. In either case, you can't trust the responses to be accurate reflections of the person's actual behaviour. As the name implies, end-aversion bias refers to people's tendency to avoid the extremes of scales (usually labelled "Always," "Never," "Extremely," and so on) because they can think of an exception. The effect of this is to reduce the number of response options that are actually used, which makes the test less reliable (more about reliability later). "Satisficing" means giving an answer that satisfies the minimum demands of the question—giving a response—but one that isn't the best reflection of the person's attitude or state, or that isn't even accurate. This often happens when the scale is too long, or the person finds the item too difficult to understand and opts for the first or last response alternative in a list or finds some other easy way out.

Once items have been screened with these biases in mind, the test developer should be left with far more items than are necessary or feasible to include. The next task is to weed out items that are redundant, don't perform adequately, or don't fit nicely into one of the domains that were postulated at the outset. Whether you're evaluating how the test developers did this or, more crucially, thinking of developing a scale yourself, the best advice is, "Don't try this at home." You can read more about the techniques that are used for these purposes, such as factor analysis[7] and item response theory,[6] but these are jobs for experts in the fields of statistics and, especially, **psychometrics**.

Reliability

Once the items have been chosen and a scoring scheme developed, it's time to determine whether the scale as a whole performs properly. This "proper performance" has two components: reliability and validity. Over the years, a number of other terms have crept into the literature (especially in medicine) as supposed synonyms of reliability and validity, such as "reproducibility," "precision," "accuracy,"

Designing

"stability," and so on. Later, we'll see why none of these is satisfactory;[8] for now, suffice it to say that you should stick with the original terms, "reliability" and "validity." We'll discuss reliability in this section, and validity in the next.

At the simplest level, **reliability** refers to the stability of a scale's scores. This can—and should—be assessed in a number of ways. If the scale is self-administered (i.e., the person fills it in himself or herself), then we are interested in **test-retest reliability**. That is, if the person completes the scale in one way today, will he or she complete it the same way at a later time (assuming that whatever it is we're measuring hasn't changed)? The rationale is that, if the respondent hasn't changed but his or her score on the scale does, then we can't be confident that we're getting accurate results either time; this would be akin to trying to measure a piece of wood with a rubber ruler—we'd always get a different answer. Usually, the interval between the first and second administrations of the scale is 10 to 15 days. If it were any shorter, then we'd have to be concerned that the person is simply recalling what he or she put down the first time and is repeating it, rather than responding to the questions again; if the interval were too much longer, then the probability would increase that the attribute itself will have changed. Needless to say, the nature of what the scale is measuring affects the interval. Some constructs, such as pain, may change over shorter periods of time; others, like introversion, change slowly if at all, and so the test-retest interval can be adjusted to account for this.

Some scales are filled out not by the person being assessed but by someone else. For example, supervisors evaluate their students; parents act as surrogates for young children; older children are often surrogates for elderly, cognitively impaired parents; psychiatrists or nurses may assess the mood or the thought processes of patients who do not appear to be able to accurately evaluate their own status; and so on. Here, we are interested in the agreement between two or more raters, or the **inter-rater reliability.** Again, the rationale is fairly self-evident: if two observers don't agree about what they've seen, then we likely can't trust either of them. Inter-rater reliability is relatively easy to evaluate in research settings, where both observers can be trained, if necessary, to use the scale, and both have equivalent information about the person being assessed. However, inter-rater reliability can be difficult to achieve in practice. If a mother and father don't fill out a scale about their child in a similar way, does that mean that the scale is unreliable, or that, for example, each parent sees the child in different circumstances? Similarly, if two supervisors disagree about a student, it may be that one has interacted with the student more than the other, or in a different setting. Thus, it can be difficult to differentiate unreliability from unique knowledge. But, even when the latter is at play, it imposes limitations on how a scale can be used and who can complete it. For instance, if parents' reports differ from those of teachers, then either one or the other must be used exclusively; or, if both are used, the study must recognize that they reflect different—and complementary—views of the child.

The most common way to measure test-retest and inter-rater reliability is to correlate two sets of scores with a **Pearson correlation coefficient**.[7] However, a better statistic to use is the **intra-class correlation coefficient** (ICC),[6] because the latter "penalizes" the raters if one is consistently higher (or lower) than the other, or if they systematically report higher (or lower) scores the second time they rate a scale. For example, if rater A consistently evaluated residents one point higher than did rater B, the Pearson correlation would be 1.0, and the ICC would be somewhat lower. Both the Pearson correlation and the ICC can range from 0 to 1, with 0 reflecting no reliability and 1 showing perfect reliability. A rough rule of thumb is that correlations below 0.70 are unacceptable, while those in the 0.70s are fine for the early stages of research, those in the 0.80s are acceptable for more mature research areas, and correlations over 0.90 are required for scales used for clinical or decision-making purposes about individuals.[9]

A third index of reliability is somewhat different from these two and looks at the **internal consistency** of the scale—that is, the degree to which the items are correlated with one another. The rationale is that most scales are designed to tap one attribute, such as depression, pain, attitudes toward end-of-life care, and so forth. Consequently, all of the items should relate to this one construct: that is, the scale should be unidimensional. If the items aren't correlated (i.e., if internal consistency is low), then we can't be sure exactly what the scale is measuring, because it's likely tapping a number of different areas. Some scales are designed to be multifactorial—that is, to tap different aspects of a person or an attribute. For example, a "satisfaction with care" scale may be subdivided to measure satisfaction with physicians and the nurses (who are usually rated quite positively), wait times (always too long), the food (always bad), and the facility (parking spots are always too few and too expensive). In this case, we would be interested in the internal consistency of each of the individual subscales, rather than of the scale as a whole.

Designing

Even so, the notion that a scale should be unidimensional is a bit slippery, because some constructs are more homogeneous than others, and that homogeneity depends on how finely grained we want the scale to be. For instance, if we want a scale to simply detect whether a patient in a family physician's office is depressed, it is sufficient to think of depression as a single, unitary construct and to use a scale that gives us one total score. However, if we were working in a clinic that specializes in depression, we may want a scale that looks at different aspects of depression: the affective component, the behavioural component, the cognitive component, and so forth. In this case, we would want the internal consistency of the entire scale to be lower than for the family doctor's screening tool.

Also be aware that some scales are not meant to be internally consistent, much like checklists of signs or symptoms that may or may not occur together.[10] A prime example of this is the five-item Apgar scale,[11] where it is quite conceivable for a neonate to score low on one item (e.g., muscle tone) but not on the other four. In this case, we would not bother to look at internal consistency. In medical circles, developing this type of scale is sometimes referred to as "clinimetrics,"[12] but, for a number of reasons, I recommend avoiding this term.[13,14]

The most widely used statistic for measuring internal consistency is **Cronbach's** α (alpha),[15] whose value, like that of the Pearson correlation and the ICC, can range from 0 to 1. Cronbach's α is probably the most widely used index of reliability, because the scale needs to be given only once to calculate it, as opposed to two or more times, as in the case of inter-rater or test-retest reliability. Unfortunately, the popularity of this test is not matched by its usefulness. The major problem is that two factors influence the magnitude of α: the internal consistency of the scale (which is good), and the number of items (which is bad). What this means is that if a scale has more than 15 or so items, α is guaranteed to be high even if the items are not internally consistent.[16] So, don't believe that a long scale (> 15 items) is reliable if the only evidence reported is coefficient α; rely on other forms of reliability, or other indices of internal consistency, such as the average item-total correlation (how much each item correlates with the total score) and the average inter-item correlation (how much the items correlate with each other).

If this were the extent of reliability, then terms such as "reproducibility" and "consistency" would seem to be legitimate synonyms insofar as they capture the degree to which scores are replicable across time or raters. But there's another component to reliability, and that is the degree to which the scale can spread people out on a continuum. Despite Thomas Jefferson's declaration that "All men are created equal," scales are based on a different premise, which is that no two people are equal, and it's the job of the scale to differentiate among them. This simple statement leads to some seemingly counter-intuitive conclusions. Imagine that we are evaluating 20 trainees using a typical three-point scale of Unsatisfactory / Satisfactory / Superior. Now, when's the last time you heard of anyone rating a trainee as "Unsatisfactory"? (Even Jack the Ripper would likely get a Satisfactory for technical skills.) In customary practice it's not an option, which means that "Satisfactory" is now the signal to the trainee that he or she had better watch out— and even *this* is rarely used. Thus, virtually everybody is rated as "Superior." So, if I rated all the trainees as Superior and so did you, our inter-rater *agreement* would be 100%. Similarly, if we rated them again two weeks later, we'd likely give the trainees equally high marks, and the test-retest agreement would therefore be 100%. However, the *reliability* of our scale would be 0, because there is no variability among the people we're rating! Consequently, terms such as "agreement" and "reproducibility" are misleading because they do not capture this aspect of reliability: the ability of the scale to repeatedly discriminate among people.

The fact that the variability of scores affects reliability has a second implication, which is that *reliability is not a fixed property of a test.* That is, it's wrong to talk about *the* reliability of a test, as if it were a fixed and immutable quantity. (Indeed, many journals in the field of psychometrics— scale development—automatically reject any article submission that refers to reliability as a property of the test.) Rather, reliability is an interaction among the scale *and* the group being assessed *and* the circumstances. An instrument that may be reliable when used with one group of people may be much less reliable when used with a group of people who have a much smaller range of scores. What this means for you as a user of scales (or of research papers that report data gathered by means of scales) is that you should never accept at face value the author's statement that "the scale has been shown to be reliable." You have to ask whether the variability in scores that you expect to see in *your* patient population is the same as that of the author's group. If you expect that the variability will be less (because, for instance, you're dealing with inpatients or outpatients only, rather than with both, as in the paper), then the reliability in your group may be lower—even much lower— than in the original article.

Designing

Validity

Assuming that the scale has shown adequate reliability with a group of people similar to the one you intend to study, we are ready for the next step in determining whether the scale is performing properly: that is, to assess its **validity.** The conceptualization of validity has changed over the past few decades. If you read a textbook from the 1960s (or recent articles by people who haven't kept up with the field), you'll find definitions along these lines: "Validity tells us if the scale is measuring what we think it is." That is, validity (like reliability) was seen as a property of the instrument that, once established, was established for good. These days, validity is defined as "the degree of confidence we can place on the inferences we make about people based on their scores from that scale."[6] (p 251) In other words, the focus is not on the scale per se, but rather on the scores produced by the scale. This is not simply a semantic difference. Rather, it emphasizes the fact that, again in parallel to the conceptualization of reliability, validity is an interaction among the scale, the people completing it, and the circumstances under which it is filled out. Let's look at some examples of how validity is context-dependent.

Many personality assessment tools, such as the Minnesota Multiphasic Personality Inventory–2 (MMPI-2),[17] have sub-scales that determine respondents' "test-taking attitude": were they under- or overstating the extent of their difficulties; were they being defensive about admitting faults; were they presenting themselves in an unrealistically positive light; and so forth. Few people would endorse an item such as, "I have never told a lie," for example, unless they were trying to create a positive image of themselves. When used to assess hospital inpatients or those seeking help from a health care provider, elevations on these sub-scales are seen as pathological and as reflecting attitudes that can get in the way of successful treatment. However, to take one example, when the MMPI-2 is administered to people who are in the midst of custody and access disputes with an ex-spouse, high scores are interpreted in a much more positive light: the person should be trying to minimize his or her faults, and attempting to portray him- or himself as psychologically healthy. Indeed, if the person's score were not elevated, we'd be concerned about his or her appreciation of social norms and mores.

A second example is the well-known fact that the ability of diagnostic tests to rule in or rule out disorders is dependent on the prevalence of the disorder in the population being tested.[18] Diagnostic tests can (and always do) make two types of errors: they can miss true cases, and they can wrongly identify a healthy person as being ill. Consequently, we are interested in two properties of diagnostic tests: the **positive predictive value** (PPV), which is the proportion of positive test results that are actually from people who have the disorder being tested for; and the **negative predictive value** (NPV), which is the ability of the test to rule out a disorder when it is absent. When the prevalence of the disorder is high, the PPV is often very good while the NPV is poor. Conversely, when the prevalence is low (which is the more common situation), the NPV is usually quite excellent while the PPV is poor, resulting in a high proportion of false positives.[19]

In both of these examples, it is not the test that is valid or invalid, but the use to which it is put, which depends on the circumstances (example 1) and the population (example 2). As with reliability, the leading psychometric journals will reject any article whose authors claim, without making any such qualification, that they have established *the* validity of a test.

There's a second way in which the conceptualization of validity has changed over the years. Older textbooks (and, again, recent articles by people oblivious to developments now over 40 years old) spoke of different types of validity. More specifically, they referred to the "three Cs" of *content, criterion* and *construct* validity. Each of these was often broken down into subtypes, and battles raged as to whether to call a given study an example of, say, "discriminant validity" or "concurrent criterion validity." Now, though, because validity is concerned with the interpretation and meaning of test scores, everything is seen as a form of construct validity. We can talk about **criterion validation** (this is one method of establishing **construct validity**), but not criterion validity, as if it were a different animal from other types of validity testing.

So, what do we mean by construct validity? Let's go back to the beginning: most of what we are trying to measure are hypothetical constructs, or "constructs" for short. Not only do we hypothesize that the construct exists, but we also have theories about the construct itself. These needn't be grand theories that rival those of evolution or relativity in their scope and level of development, but rather a series of hypotheses about what might influence the construct, and how the construct relates to other phenomena. For example, our "theory" about pain would lead to hypotheses such as: (A) patients in an arthritis clinic should score higher on a pain scale than those attending a clinic for dermatitis; (B) scores on a pain scale should decrease after an analgesic is administered; (C) patients who report chronic pain should also score higher on a depression scale than people who are not in chronic pain; and (D) scores on a pain scale should be unrelated to intelligence.

None of these hypotheses is world-shattering or would lead to a Nobel prize in physiology or medicine, but they do point to ways to determine whether the scale is performing as it should. It's worth noting that studies of validity are much more variable in terms of their design and analysis than are reliability studies. For reliability, we simply administer the scale once (for internal consistency) or twice (for inter-rater and test-retest reliability), and calculate the appropriate statistic. The design and analysis of validity studies, on the other hand, are dictated by the question. For hypothesis A, for example, we would give the scale to two groups of people—those in an arthritis clinic and those in a dermatology clinic—and compare the scores using a *t* test. With the second hypothesis, we would administer the scale to the same people, before and after analgesic medication, and use a paired *t* test (or, if we were being fancy, we would have a placebo group, and then use a "group by time" analysis of variance). Hypotheses (C) and (D) are correlational in nature, and so we would have the participants fill out two questionnaires. We hypothesize *a priori* in (C) that there should be a moderate correlation between pain and depression, and in (D) that there should be no correlation between pain and intelligence.

If the results obtained are as hypothesized, then we will know that our theory is valid and that the scale has been validated to some degree *in this population*. However, if the results are not as we expected, then (1) the theory is right but the scale isn't working as expected; (2) the scale is fine but the theory is wrong; or (3) both the theory and the scale are flawed. The problem in this latter situation is that we won't know which of the three explanations is the right one.

You should also note that there is no end to the hypotheses that can be generated and tested using a given scale. In this regard, validity testing is never finished. Another factor that contributes to the never-ending task of validation is that, even when a scale is developed for one group or with one purpose in mind, researchers will always be interested in expanding its reach, so that it can be used with different patient groups or under different circumstances. Because, as we've said, validity is not an inherent property of a scale, but rather depends on the scale *and* the target group *and* the assessment situation, we have to re-evaluate validity whenever any of these factors change.

As mentioned at the beginning of this chapter, the constructs that these scales are trying to measure cannot be seen

directly. Consequently, unlike lab tests or rulers, there is no perfect gold standard against which we can evaluate them. For this reason, terms like "precision" or "accuracy" should be reserved for lab tests, and are imprecise and inaccurate when used with the types of scales we've been discussing. Use "validity."[8]

Utility

The final attribute you should be interested in is the utility, or usability, of the scale: that is, how feasible is it for you to use in your setting? The first consideration is copyright. There are many scales floating around in hospital and university settings that really shouldn't be. If a scale is to be used for research purposes, you can often get permission from the developer to use it free of charge, although some authors request that you let them know of any publications that emanate from the research (a reasonable request). When it is to be used for clinical purposes, though, it is neither ethical nor legal to simply photocopy the scale for your own use.

The next aspect to look at is how the scale is to be completed. Self-administered scales require, in most instances, a Grade 6 reading level in English (the level of the average high school graduate; a sad commentary on our educational system), and so might not be practical to use in certain groups, such as recent immigrants. Nor would a self-administered test be practical in a fracture clinic, where many patients have their arms in a cast. Other aspects to consider: Is the scale self-explanatory, or will the respondent need to be told how to complete it; if the latter, are there staff available to do this? If people are to fill it out while waiting for their appointment, where exactly will this be done? Is there space available? Is there a place where they can write? Is it quiet and free from distractions? These seemingly small things can pose important obstacles in the real world.

If the scale is to be used by one person to rate another, somewhat different questions need to be answered. In many cases, those administering a scale will need some degree of training to know what the response options mean; if this is the case, it will require resources in the form of someone who knows the scale and can do the training, time for the raters to receive the training, possibly someone to act out different behaviours to check on the raters' reliability, and so on.

The next consideration is time. You should allow at least 30 seconds per item, and so even a 20-item scale can take some respondents about 10 minutes to complete. This is rarely an issue in a research context, where participants

Designing

come in just for the study. But, if you are using patients and asking them to complete other scales for a validity study, the battery of tests can seem to them to be an assault and battery.

Finally, how is the scale scored? For most, this is simply a matter of adding up the number of items that have been endorsed, or the scores for each option. Other scales, primarily those used in personality assessment, may have complicated scoring algorithms and can be scored only by computer. This can limit their practicability, depending on the resources available for your research.

Finding and evaluating scales

Fortunately, it's not necessary to dig into the often arcane literature to find out if a scale is ready for prime time. Two excellent compendia of scales are listed in the Additional Resources section at the end of this chapter. They reproduce many frequently used scales (but see the caveat in the preceding section before you blithely photocopy the pages) and, more importantly, critique their psychometric properties and utility. One of the appendices in *Health Measurement Scales* (also listed in Additional Resources) directs you to other, less widely used scales and, in some cases, to their

evaluation. In 2010, the *Journal of Psychosomatic Research* began a series of articles devoted to critiquing scales in a number of areas such as depression, anxiety, quality of life and apathy.[20] If the scale you want to use is not in any of those resources, the Summary Checklist at the end of the chapter will guide you through the process of evaluation.

Conclusion

Once we leave the realm of direct physical measurement and try to measure phenomena such as attitudes, behaviours, feeling states and quality of life, we must use scales that tap these constructs. Developing a good scale—one in which the items are clear, unambiguous and free from bias, and that as a whole is reliable and valid for the population under study—is a time-consuming task. Reliability implies that, if the person hasn't changed, we will get the same response under various circumstances (different time, different raters) and that the scale is measuring only one construct. Validity implies that we can place some meaning on the score and use it to tell us something about the respondent. Finally, to be useful, any scale must be feasible to use within the constraints of the assessment situation. ∎

REFERENCES

1. Cronbach LJ, Meehl PE. Construct validity in psychological tests. *Psychol Bull*. 1955;52(4):281–302.

2. Albrecht GL, Devlieger PJ. The disability paradox: high quality of life against all odds. *Soc Sci Med*. 1999;48:977–88.

3. Tamim H, McCusker J, Dendukuri N. Proxy reporting of quality of life using the EQ-5D. *Med Care*. 2002;40:(12):1186–95.

4. Ronen GM, Streiner DL, Rosenbaum P; Canadian Pediatric Epilepsy Network. Health-related quality of life in children with epilepsy: development and validation of self-report and parent-proxy measures. *Epilepsia*. 2003;44(4):598–612.

5. Ronen GM, Rosenbaum P, Law M, Streiner DL. Health-related quality of life in childhood disorders: a modified focus group technique to involve children. *Qual Life Res*. 2001;10(1)71–9.

6. Streiner DL, Norman GR. *Health measurement scales: a practical guide to their development and use*. 4th ed. Oxford: Oxford University Press; 2008.

7. Norman GR, Streiner DL. *Biostatistics: the bare essentials*. 3rd ed. Shelton (CT): BC Decker; 2007.

8. Streiner DL, Norman GR. "Precision" and "accuracy": two terms that are neither. *J Clin Epidemiol*. 2006;59(4):327–30.

9. Nunnally JC, Bernstein IH. *Psychometric theory*. 3rd ed. New York: McGraw-Hill; 1994.

10. Streiner DL. Being inconsistent about consistency: when coefficient alpha does and doesn't matter. *J Pers Assess*. 2003;80(3):217–22.

11. Apgar V. A proposal for a new method of evaluation of the newborn infant. *Curr Res Anesth Analg*. 1953;32(4):260–7.

12. Feinstein AR. *Clinimetrics*. New Haven (CT): Yale University Press; 1987.

13. Streiner DL. Clinimetrics vs. psychometrics: an unnecessary distinction. *J Clin Epidemiol*. 2003;56(12):1142–45.

14. Streiner DL. Test development: two-sided coin or one-sided Möbius strip? *J Clin Epidemiol*. 2003;56(12): 1148–9.

15. Cronbach LJ. Coefficient alpha and the internal structure of tests. *Psychometrika*. 1951;16(3):297–334.

16. Cortina JM. What is coefficient alpha? an examination of theory and applications. *J Appl Psychol*. 1993;78(1):98–104.

17. Butcher JN, Dahlstrom WG, Graham JR, Tellegen A, Kaemmer B. *The Minnesota Multiphasic Personality Inventory-2 (MMPI-2): manual for administration and scoring.* Minneapolis (MN): University of Minnesota Press; 1989.

18. Meehl PE, Rosen A. Antecedent probability and the efficiency of psychometric signs, patterns, or cutting scores. *Psychol Bull*. 1955;52(3):194–216.

19. Streiner DL. Diagnosing tests: using and misusing diagnostic screening tests. *J Pers Assess*. 2003;81(3):209–19.

20. Keszei AP, Novak M, Streiner DL. Introduction to health measurement scales. *J Psychosom Res*. 2010;68(4):319–23.

ADDITIONAL RESOURCES

Fischer J, Corcoran K. *Measures for clinical practice and research: A sourcebook. Vol. 1. Couples, families and children*. 4th ed. New York: Oxford University Press, 2006.

——— *Measures for clinical practice and research: A sourcebook. Vol. 2. Adults*. 4th ed. New York: Oxford University Press, 2006.

- These two volumes are similar to McDowell's book but cover a much wider scope, including marital functioning, mood and development.

McDowell I. *Measuring health: A guide to rating scales and questionnaires*. 3rd ed. Oxford: Oxford University Press; 2006.

- An excellent compendium of existing scales in areas such as physical disability and handicap, social health and anxiety. The actual scales are presented and critiqued.

Streiner DL. A checklist for evaluating the usefulness of rating scales. *Can J Psychiatry*. 1993;38(2):140–8.

- This article provides a brief "cheat sheet" for evaluating existing scales without going into all of the messy details.

Streiner DL, Norman GR. *Health measurement scales: a practical guide to their development and use*. 4th ed. Oxford: Oxford University Press; 2008.

- This book, as the subtitle states, guides the reader through the steps necessary to develop a scale. It can also be used by people who are interested in appraising scales developed by others and defines the terms necessary to understand articles that describe scales. One appendix tells readers where they can find existing scales in a wide variety of areas.

Designing

SUMMARY CHECKLIST

1. Background

❑ Do the authors explain the theoretical rationale for the scale?
❑ Do they state how this scale differs from other scales tapping the same or similar constructs?

2. The items

❑ Do all of the items seem to relate to the construct?
❑ Are there aspects of the construct that aren't tapped?
❑ Do any of the items seem vague or ambiguous?
❑ Are technical terms used (e.g., "shock," "myocardium")?
❑ Are any items double-barrelled? (Look for "ANDs" and "ORs.")
❑ Is the reading level appropriate for your study population?

3. Reliability

❑ Is the internal consistency > .80?
❑ Does the test-retest reliability meet commonly accepted norms (> .70 for research in new areas; > .80 for research in established areas; > .90 for clinical use)?
❑ If appropriate, does the inter-rater reliability meet these same standards (> .70 for new research areas; > .80 for established research areas; > .90 for clinical use)?
❑ Have these been established in a population similar to the one you are studying?

4. Validity

❑ Have enough validity studies been done so that you're confident about what the scores reflect?
❑ Has validity been established in a population similar to one you are studying?

5. Utility

❑ Is the test copyrighted? If so, do you have permission to use it?
❑ How long does it take to complete?
❑ Are instructions or training required and, if so, do you have the resources for this?
❑ How easy is it to score?

Designing

11
Surveys

Susan J. Bondy, BA, MSc, PhD, FACE

ILLUSTRATIVE CASE 1

An Endrocrinology resident is interested in the experiences of primary care physicians in managing older patients with diabetes. She obtains a mailing list from the College of Family Physicians of Canada from which to draw a simple random sample of physicians and designs a survey following the method of a popular guidebook.

ILLUSTRATIVE CASE 2

An Obstetrics and Gynecology resident wishes to determine and describe the rates of adverse outcomes of labour and delivery in all five of the health region's labour and delivery centres, which vary somewhat in the volume of deliveries they manage. Here the population of interest is composed not of people but of episodes of care. Because the resident had planned in advance to report data for each hospital, she oversamples from the smallest hospital to achieve a minimum sample size that will be useful. All deliveries that occur during a defined period are eligible for the study. At each hospital, a random sample of 500 deliveries is drawn, and the charts are reviewed for the outcomes of interest. Outcome rates are reported for each hospital separately and are presented for the whole region using sampling weights to account for the oversampling in the smaller centres.

■ **The term "survey" is used in many ways**. In the context of research, some people use the word whenever a questionnaire is involved, although this is not necessarily accurate. Not all research that uses questionnaires requires a representative sample, as surveys do, and not all surveys involve questionnaires. Moreover, as the second case example illustrates, not all surveys are surveys of *people*. Representative surveys can be used to describe any population of people or other entities, such as cases or procedures.

It is important also to distinguish between surveys and other forms of cross-sectional research. **Representative surveys** are often done to estimate the prevalence of disease or other characteristics in a population. Many researchers also use **cross-sectional data** (including existing survey data) to test hypotheses about, for example, differences between groups, or the relationship between an exposure and an outcome of interest; these data can be derived from pre-existing large health surveys or gathered by other

CHAPTER OBJECTIVES

After reading this chapter, you should be able to:

- discuss the design elements that characterize survey studies
- describe the importance of correct population sampling methods in survey research
- locate additional resources to guide the development of a survey project
- describe the implications of different sampling methods for the analysis of survey data
- better understand how to use and interpret existing survey-based research

KEY TERMS

Clustered sampling	Finite population correction	Random sampling	Sampling weights
Complex samples	Generalizability	Representative surveys	Simple random sample
Confidence intervals	Margin of error	Representativity	Statistical precision
Cross-sectional data	Measurement errors	Response rate	Stratified sampling
Design effect	Minimizing error and bias	Sample size	Survey data analysis
Estimates	Point estimate	Sampling errors	Survey mode
External validity	Precision of the estimate	Sampling frame	Variance

specifically designed means. Studies such as these, whose primary objective is to test a hypothesis, are more correctly described as cross-sectional analytic studies, or case-control studies in some instances. The sampling design that is most cost-effective in testing a hypothesis is usually very different from the design that would be used to describe a naturally occurring population, as in a representative survey. For the purposes of this chapter, then, a "survey" involves:

- the unbiased selection of individuals to study from a defined population of like individuals;
- the measurement of one or more characteristics or attributes for each member of the sample (e.g., the presence or absence of a particular condition); and
- data analysis to estimate the distribution of that characteristic in the population of interest (i.e., the population from which the sample is drawn).

What makes a survey valid?

The methodological strength of a survey is determined by the degree to which it minimizes error and bias and achieves statistical precision.

Minimizing error and bias means providing statistical estimates that authentically describe the population of interest. To achieve this aim, the researcher must avoid both sampling errors and measurement errors, as follows:

- **Sampling errors** are minimized by ensuring that the sample obtained is truly representative of the population being described. Surveys are held to a higher standard for population representativeness than are most other research designs. For example, in a clinical efficacy trial, external generalizability can be achieved by using explicit and quite narrow inclusion criteria, and random sampling is rarely used to select eligible patients. The findings are generalizable, but only to patients with those same characteristics. In contrast, the people in the population being described in a survey may be quite heterogeneous (e.g., young and old, sick and well). If the survey sample is representative, then the sample should include the same *mix* of characteristics as the underlying population, and in the same proportions (a property called **representivity**). **Random sampling** is an important means to obtain this representativity. **Sample size** is also important. The larger a random sample is, the better the odds that it will be representative.

- Minimizing **measurement errors** requires the use of reliable and valid measures. For guidance on developing measurement scales and questionnaire items, see chapter 10.

Statistical precision is an important attribute in any study design. In surveys, the **precision of the estimate**—or, in other words, the degree of confidence one may have in the estimate obtained—is usually reported using **confidence intervals** or by presenting each statistic along with its **margin of error**. A 95% confidence interval, for example, is a range of values that has a 95% likelihood of containing the true value of the variable that has been estimated (see also chs 24 & 25). Margin of error is reported as a value following a ± sign. For example, for a finding such as "40% of respondents agreed," one could report a 95% confidence interval of, say, 37% to 43% or, equivalently, state that the 40% estimate was accurate to within ± 3%, 19 times out of 20. The statistical methods used to calculate confidence intervals and margins of error for survey results are somewhat different from those used for other research designs discussed in this guide. Different methods and software may be required; these are introduced briefly later in this chapter.

Designing a relatively simple survey

1. Defining who (or what) you want to describe. The first, crucial step in designing a survey is to define the population you wish to study. In doing so, consider your survey's anticipated **generalizability** (or **external validity**): that is, the future and distant populations to whom you expect your results to be applicable. This should underpin the survey's inclusion and exclusion criteria, which define the people or things that make up that wider population. The researcher in our first case example is interested in diabetes care. In formulating her research question (see ch. 6), she decided that she wanted to study the physicians who provided this care. Her design would have been very different had she wanted to study the experiences of diabetic patients regardless of who cared for them. In the second case example, "deliveries" were sampled, which is not the same as sampling individual mothers (who might have more than one delivery within a study period) or individual babies. The sample that is used, and the method to obtain it, must be matched to the target population exactly as defined in the research question.

The second case also illustrates that one study can address multiple, related populations simultaneously (one for each of the five hospitals). Researchers often plan in advance to report statistics for multiple subgroups. We will return to this case example later with respect to the implications for sample size and the approach to data analysis presented by the use of oversampling and stratification. However, we might pause here to note a different but related problem presented by this case. Although multiple births (e.g., twins, triplets) are less common than singleton births, their high complication rates can greatly influence reported outcome rates for the entire study sample. Thus, although including some multiple births would be essential to make the survey generalizable to *all* deliveries, a simple random sample (see step 5, below) of all deliveries would include relatively few multiple births and would therefore have little statistical precision in describing these births separately. A report specific to multiples would have to wait for a separate or much larger study. It is also important to note that collecting data on exceptional cases that do not meet a survey's inclusion criteria and will not be used in the analysis is both costly and unethical.

2. Defining what you want to measure. Many good handbooks on survey design recommend that surveys be constructed on the basis of a breakdown of the specific types of information that you want to be able to report. Ideally, this would involve mapping out detailed mock results tables that show every population-based **point estimate** to be presented (e.g., means, proportions) overall and for each planned subgroup. You will need to define how every statistic will be calculated and who will be included in it. For example, in our survey of physicians, one question might ask about their satisfaction with certain services to which they can refer patients. Some respondents will say this question is "not applicable" because they do not use these services; you will have to decide how to handle these responses, which will have the effect of reducing the sample size for specific questions and statistical measures.

3. Selecting sampling frames and survey modes. A **sampling frame** provides a means to enumerate a population and draw a random sample from it. Sampling frames are often lists, but they can be any means to create a census or register of the individuals in your population of interest. This can include creating maps of where people are found and methods to keep future patients in sequence and draw a fair sample of them. For scientific rigour, all potential

sampling frames should be evaluated for coverage gaps (who is left out) and other errors (e.g., old addresses). Problems with your sampling frame can result in biased samples that do not represent the intended target population well. For one example, in trying to survey a specific professional group, one might have to rely on lists from professional organizations with voluntary membership. This can result in a biased sample, because those who are willing to join (and to pay the membership dues) may be systematically different from those who are not. Old address lists may systematically exclude new graduates and new practices. To give another example, having to rely on sampling based on telephone numbers may include too few young people who use only cellphones or others who have joined no-call lists. These factors can create some bias in the demographic characteristics of the sample.

The term **survey mode** refers to the method by which recruitment and data collection are conducted. Modes with the longest history and the best-developed literature are face-to-face household surveys, telephone surveys and mail surveys. The mode will be determined by considerations such as the contact information available to the researcher (e.g., mailing addresses) and the measures that need to be taken to obtain the relevant information (e.g., blood work cannot be obtained by telephone, although recruitment by telephone might be used). The cheapest mode is rarely the best. For example, Internet surveys have proliferated even though they are frequently ignored by potential respondents. Simple-to-follow but well-researched guides exist for all these modes (see Additional Resources). These guides explain how to recruit participants, maximize response rates, track samples and present data. Household, telephone and large clinical surveys are all best carried out by academically oriented professional services on contract.

However, surveys conducted in health care settings are not addressed in most general survey books, and they present a number of concerns and challenges unique to their setting. Many clinician researchers have tried to conduct a survey alongside the provision of routine care, using existing staff, only to find that the response rates they obtain are very low and that the resulting sample is flawed by selection bias. For example, clinical staff conducting a survey might be more likely to approach patients they know are affected by the problem being studied, or those they perceive to be most likely to participate. A rigorous study plan should be developed, and staff dedicated to the study should be employed.

Designing

Detailed records must be kept of those who were eligible for the survey, were approached, and participated,[1,2] all of which requires a lot of effort. The research plan should be reviewed for scientific merit (by someone with survey expertise, and not only clinical knowledge in the area), and approval should be sought from the appropriate Research Ethics Board.

Patients must feel free to decline to participate in a survey. Approaching a patient with a request to participate in research can be inadvertently coercive if the patient fears that non-participation might jeopardize his or her care. Poor response rates or unreliable responses, on the other hand, can result if patients lack confidence that the information they provide will be held securely and in confidence. A good practice to facilitate informed consent for participation in a survey is to give advance notice of an upcoming survey by phone or mail, and by someone who is not a health care provider. Again, contracting a professional service to do or supervise the work can head off patients' concerns about the impact of survey participation or non-participation on their care.

Anonymous drop-box surveys are often used in patient waiting-rooms using self-explanatory consent materials and questionnaires. Such materials should, of course, have Research Ethics Board approval. However, with respect to representativeness, anonymous drop-box questionnaires are a very weak survey design. Response rates are low and, worse, their response rates are often impossible to estimate because the total number of eligible individuals (i.e., the denominator) cannot be defined. Nor can the researcher be certain who filled out the questionnaires (or, for that matter, who might have done so repeatedly). Such convenience samples rarely result in generalizable or publishable results, although their findings can be of local interest.

For externally funded research, convenience samples are rarely defensible, although there are circumstances for which no sampling frame exists, such as research involving homeless, displaced or hard-to-identify populations. Sampling methods for such populations, such as "snowball" sampling and sampling based on location, are described in the literature (see Additional Resources).

4. Translating the survey objectives into a questionnaire or interview. This aspect of survey design is outlined in chapter 10 and is described in detail in various specialized texts listed under Additional Resources. Such texts provide examples of good and bad questions and describe how to lay out questionnaires as a whole and to pre-test them. In brief, the detailed analysis plan described in steps 1 to 3 is used to generate a list of key measures to be addressed by the survey items. Always start by establishing a clear definition of each concept you want to report on, and review the methodological literature regarding how each of these is best measured. Cherry-picking interesting questions from other people's work can be a dangerous exercise. First, it can lead you off-track and make your questionnaire long and burdensome. Previously used questions should be examined critically, to see whether their reliability and validity were previously assessed. It is common for bad questions to be used again and again, even in major public health surveys. Bad questions include those that are confusing, leading (that is, suggest an answer), impossible to answer within the contraints of the questionnaire (e.g., they require a qualifier such as "it depends"), or are difficult to analyze (e.g., in the case of questions that ask the respondent to provide a ranking order for a set of choices).[2–4] If you need to create new questions, such as new measures for attitudes (or perceived "importance"), seek out expert tips on designing questions and response options from the literature. Writing good questions for surveys is a specialized skill.

Guidebooks and expert consultants also provide useful advice on optimal lengths for survey instruments, with respect to both time required and number of items. In general, surveys are best kept short. However, if the survey is of direct interest to the respondents (e.g., asking patients about their specific condition, or physicians about issues that are important to them), they will usually stay motivated for a longer time. The same guidebooks on survey design also provide tips on making the questionnaire (or web-based forms, etc.) as appealing as possible. These guides can include very specific advice on considerations such as the choice of colour, paper quality, typefaces and the use of graphics.

Ideally, full-scale pre-testing (see ch. 21) will include practice statistical analysis and presentation of results. Many problems can be avoided by pilot-testing a survey design in this way.

5. Creating the sampling design. The most basic survey design is the **simple random sample** (SRS). This design requires:

- that all members of the source population can be identified and have an equal chance of being selected, and that oversampling is not used;

- that elements[a] are sampled independently (e.g., not in clusters); and
- the assumption that one is sampling with replacement[b] from a very large target population and that no finite population correction (FPC) will be used. (The concept of the FPC is described later, under Determining the Sample Size).

In medium- to large-scale surveys, SRS designs, strictly defined, are rare. **Complex samples** are used to accommodate subgroup comparisons and multiple research goals and can make the overall project far more cost-effective. Complex samples can involve any of the following elements:

- **stratified sampling**, in which random samples are drawn separately from each subgroup of interest (e.g., each hospital in our second case example). Oversampling from smaller groups is often necessary to achieve a minimum sample size per group. However, unequal probabilities of selection for different subgroups can make the overall sample non-representative;
- **sampling weights**, which are developed to compensate for oversampling and instances of non-response and are applied to the analysis to restore representativeness;
- **clustered sampling**, by which people are sampled in groups (e.g., one samples students by drawing a large random sample of whole classes, or samples patients by selecting at random a large number of clinics) as a way to reduce field costs.

Novice researchers need to be aware of the implications of all of these design features, each of which will complicate the analysis. For example, the researcher in our second case example draws a random sample stratified by hospital. Estimates describing the entire health region (i.e., across all hospitals) will thus need to be based on stratified and weighted calculations, as opposed to simple ones. Stratified

or clustered sampling and weighting will also affect the margin of error of the calculated estimates. Unless these aspects of the survey design are taken into account in the statistical analyses, the resulting estimates may be biased and the confidence intervals or margins of error will be reported as narrower than they should be.

Clustered sampling, in particular, can easily be misapplied. One mistake is to analyze clustered data as though people had been sampled individually and, as a result, to report an incorrect margin of error. In designing a survey with clusters (or *primary sampling units*, PSUs, in survey methods jargon), two common mistakes should be avoided. The first is to use what amounts to a convenience sample of groups (for practical reasons), and the second is to include too few groups. Just as no study of 3 to 10 people, chosen non-randomly, could provide a reliable estimate of the source population, no sample of 10 families, or 3 treatment centres, chosen by convenience could make for a representative survey sample. Even when the selection of groups is random, it is common to underestimate the number of groups required. Standardized methods for surveys in public health recommend that no fewer than 30 to 50 PSUs be sampled at random from a population set of PSUs many times larger.[3–6] People doing small surveys might stick to an SRS design, or else sample everyone and treat this as an SRS. For any other design, an experienced statistician should be enlisted to assist in creating the sampling design and analysis plan. Again, the need for statistical assistance would include even the fairly simple design described in the second case example, which would require weighted and stratified analyses for the region as a whole, necessitating the use of specialized software (see Additional Resources).

6. Determining the sample size for a simple survey. Your determination of the sample size for your survey will start with the plan you devised in step 1. The minimum sample size needed to achieve the desired level of precision (for each estimate) can be obtained using various sample-size calculators, including some that are available free online.[c] If you are planning to conduct secondary analyses and hypothesis tests, you will need to calculate the minimum sample size to obtain appropriate statistical power for each of these tests or comparisons.

Designing

---

a   In survey jargon, *elements* are the individuals of interest, the single unit of analysis for the study.

b   In sampling with replacement, individuals that are sampled are "returned" to the original sample, such that the sample size and the probability for each individual of being sampled remain constant throughout the sampling process. This means that individuals have some chance of being sampled more than once in the same study. This is rarely done in health surveys, but the assumption is considered to be met where the target population is very large (such as a million or more).

---

c   For an example, see www.OpenEpi.com

Designing

Note that the required sample size refers to the final number of *complete* responses used to calculate each statistic of interest. This is *not* the number of questionnaires mailed, or even all of the completed interviews before subgroups are considered. To determine the size of the initial sample or mailing, and the required budget, the target sample size is multiplied by inflation factors that account for errors in the sampling frame and the expected non-response rate. One should even estimate the percentages of "not applicable" and "don't know" responses for each question. For example, one might ask how satisfied a patient was with a specific service, but perhaps only 40% of the sample have used that service and are thus able to contribute data on satisfaction. Spreadsheets are usually used to estimate how a simple random sample will be naturally distributed over subgroups of interest. For example, if you hope to report pregnancy outcomes by age group of the mother, you will need to guess the percentage of teen mothers that you will have in your sample. This process of determining how large a sample will need to be to adequately represent all subgroups usually increases the sample size targets, and cost, or else suppresses the researcher's appetite for subgroup analyses.

Finally, if you are planning to use a complex sampling design, you will need to inflate the target sample size to correct for the impact that your sampling design will have on the margin of error of estimates. The degree to which statistical precision would be decreased (or the required sample size increased) is referred to as the **design effect** and can be difficult to estimate without the guidance of a statistician.

Comments on small samples from small target populations

It is not unusual in health research to find that the total population of interest is small, comprising just a few hundred patients or an even smaller number of health professionals. In such cases, the best approach is generally to do no sampling and ask everyone to take part, treating the resulting sample as an SRS. The **finite population correction** (FPC) should *not* be used with samples of this kind. The FPC is an advanced concept, but an important one to raise even in this introductory guide. The FPC reflects the fact that the results from a sample of, say, 90 out of 100 potential participants are not likely to be much different from the results from all 100. Because the use of the FPC correction in estimating sample sizes or calculating *P* values and confidence intervals is very rarely appropriate in health research,[d] you will need

to know to turn off this option in the software you are using. (It is common for the FPC to be a default setting.) Using the FPC can result in falsely narrow confidence intervals and findings of statistical significance where none exists. Most peer reviewers will reject the use of the FPC in health research. The bottom line is that small samples produce wide margins of error. There is no quick fix.

Conducting the survey

Developing the field methods for the conduct of your survey is as important as any other aspect of the design. Step-by-step advice on survey recruitment and fieldwork is available for mail, telephone and other kinds of surveys (see Additional Resources). Major considerations in planning the fieldwork methods are: (1) creating interest in the study to maximize participation rates; and (2) quality assurance.

Dillman's social exchange theory[7] provides a basis for the methods he outlines to motivate people to participate in surveys. How the survey is advertised in advance and first presented to potential respondents can influence participation rates. Advance announcements can generate interest and help convince people that the survey is important and legitimate (and not, say, unsolicited marketing). Cover letters and announcements should be pilot-tested to ensure that the language is effective in communicating the value of the research. With respect to approaching people, the best advice is to personalize communications as much as possible, for example by using personally addressed envelopes, real stamps and real ink signatures on cover letters. Professional looking, appealing and easy-to-complete materials increase response rates, too.

Follow-up reminders are essential to achieve a reasonable response rate, although more than 3 to 4 follow-ups will rarely result in much additional return. Again, handbooks on survey research give advice on how many follow-ups to use and at what intervals. Keeping the reminders fresh, appealing and personal is good advice. Research has also shown that small monetary incentives increase response rates by a small but important amount.[2-4]

Even for small surveys, your fieldwork will require very careful record-keeping to manage mailing lists, ensure that people who have already participated are thanked and are not sent further reminders, and to ensure proper handling of informed consent and the appropriate storage of completed questionnaires and data files

---

d Using the FPC can make sense in circumstances such as quality-assurance

audits, which are used only within an organization and whose results would never be applied to any external group or place.

containing personal and health information. Every person in the initial sample must be tracked and given a final determination with respect to who participated, who refused, and who turned out to be ineligible. There are detailed standard definitions for all of these outcomes, and these numbers are used to estimate the response rate in ways that are scientifically acceptable.[2] Depending on the scale and complexity of the study, training and supervision of staff and monitoring of data quality need to be considered. This can include data quality checks, repeating a sample of interviews, and other methods for quality assurance.

Survey data analysis

The analysis of survey data has three main components: reporting a correct **response rate**; calculating the **estimates** without bias; and calculating the margin of error or **variance**, as appropriate to the sampling design.

Response-rate definitions and formulae are given in most survey guides and statements of standard survey practices (see Additional Resources). To report response rates correctly, you will need the detailed notes you kept while you were administering the survey on the number of people who were approached, refused, participated, and turned out to be ineligible.

Point estimates (the actual means or proportions) are often corrected for the bias created by complex sampling designs using sampling weights. Some researchers apply additional corrections for non-response patterns and known differences between the sample and the actual population.

As soon as weighting or clustered sampling is involved, special software is needed to calculate the correct confidence intervals (and any P values calculated for subgroup comparisons and other tests). Many statistical packages now include procedures designed specifically for complex samples; examples include Epi Info, Stata, SAS, the SPSS Complex Samples module, SUUDAN and Wesvar. Within the multi-purpose statistics packages (Epi Info, SPSS, SAS and Stata), only the commands explicitly intended for complex samples should be used. Again, surveys using small samples present a challenge, as the methods that are easiest to use assume large samples. The analysis plan should be considered at the design stage, and always in consultation with a suitably experienced statistician.

The final and important step in doing a survey is to evaluate the net impact of selection and measurement errors. A too-easy marker for potential selection bias is a low response rate. In reality, low response rates (often below 50%) are, with rare exceptions, to be expected, even when best practices to maximize response rates have been followed.[7] There is simply no hard and fast rule as to what response rate is acceptable, as opposed to being too low for the survey results to be valid. An acceptable response rate depends on how much the sample remains representative of the target population specifically with respect to the behaviours or characteristics being reported on, and this will vary from study to study. The statistical issues of selection bias (missing people) and response bias (missing and wrong answers) are discussed in detail in rigorous survey methods books (see Additional Resources). At a minimum, most researchers will describe the demographic and other characteristics of the sample and compare these with the corresponding characteristics in the population they want to describe.

Where to get more information

Many books and guides have been published on survey methods, and it is important to select those that are appropriate to health research and focus on methodological rigour. Among resources aimed at non-experts, some have thorough and easy-to-follow discussions on questionnaire design and data collection. The *Total Survey Design* and *Tailored Survey Design* series by Don Dillman, for example, are well-researched, step-by-step guides to the most common survey modes. Health professionals should choose from the more academic variants of such guides.[3,7,8] At the other end of the spectrum are texts that provide detailed, technical presentations of the statistical aspects of survey design and analysis. These are important resources for people working with data from existing large surveys, or planning a large survey, but their statistical content can be challenging and they do not always apply to smaller studies or clinical research specifically.

The ideal resources are those written for health professionals and the staff of government health agencies. They use language targeted to non-statisticians, but include the level of detail needed for rigorous research, along with material on ethical considerations, privacy and confidentiality. Examples ranging from brief guides to full texts appropriate for public health staff and other health care professionals interested in conducting surveys are listed among the intermediate-level texts in the Additional Resources section.

Designing

Conclusion

Representative sample surveys can be a powerful tool when used to describe actual health-related outcomes and experiences in a known population and to introduce statistical estimates to this evidence. Surveys are a popular research method, and the estimates they produce are of interest to a wide variety of audiences. Surveys also have distinct requirements for methodological rigour and require close attention to many technical considerations, including the principles of sampling and selection bias, measurement theory and statistics, and require support from a biostatistician well versed in survey methodology. Involvement in a large- or small-scale survey project offers a valuable opportunity and challenge for a research trainee. ∎

Designing

REFERENCES

1. Altman DG, Schulz KF, Moher D, Egger M, Davidoff F, Elbourne D, et al. The revised CONSORT statement for reporting randomized trials: explanation and elaboration. *Ann Intern Med.* 2001;134(8):663–94.

2. American Association for Public Opinion Research (AAPOR). *Standard definitions: final dispositions of case codes and outcome rates for surveys.* Lenexa (KS): AAPOR, 2006. Available from: www.aapor.org/Standard_Definitions/3049.htm

3. Statistics Canada. *Survey methods and practices.* Cat. no. 12-587-X. Ottawa: Statistics Canada; 2003. Available from: www.statcan.gc.ca/pub/12-587-x/12-587-x2003001-eng.pdf

4. United Nations. Department of Economics and Social Affairs, Statistics Division. *Designing household survey samples: practical guidelines.* Studies in Methods Series F, no. 98. New York: United Nations; 2008.

5. Hoshaw-Woodward S. *Description and comparison of the methods of cluster sampling and lot quality assurance sampling to assess immunization coverage.* Geneva: World Health Organization; 2001. Available from: www.who.int/vaccines-documents/DocsPDF01/www592.pdf

6. Frerichs RR, Shaheen MA. Small-community-based surveys. *Annu Rev Public Health.* 2001;22:231–47.

7. Dillman DA, Smyth JD, Melani Christian L. *Internet, mail and mixed-mode surveys: the tailored design method.* 3rd ed. Hoboken (NJ): John Wiley; 2009.

8. Aday LA, Cornelius LJ. *Designing and conducting health surveys: a comprehensive guide.* 3rd ed. New York: Jossey-Bass; 2006.

ADDITIONAL RESOURCES

Brief guides to the basics of survey research for health researchers

Abramson J, Abramson ZH. *Research methods in community medicine: surveys, epidemiological research, programme evaluation, clinical trials.* 6th ed. Hoboken (NJ): John Wiley, 2008.

- This popular book is useful with respect to the goals of a community health survey, but provides little information on sampling methods.

Salant P, Dillman DA. *How to conduct your own survey.* Hoboken (NJ): John Wiley; 1994.

- This concise paperback guide contains easy-to-follow discussions of questionnaire design and data collection but does not address proper sampling methods.

University of North Carolina Center for Public Health Preparedness. A guide to sampling for community health assessments and other projects. Chapel Hill (NC): The Center; n.d. Available from: http://cphp.sph.unc.edu/PHRST5/

—— *Two-stage cluster sampling: general guidance for use in public health assessments.* Chapel Hill (NC): The Center; n.d. Available from: http://cphp.sph.unc.edu/PHRST5/

- The above brief guides provide advice on the development of community samples in the form of easy-to-read newsletters.

Intermediate to advanced resources on surveys and secondary analysis of existing surveys for health researchers

Aday LA, Cornelius LJ. *Designing and conducting health surveys: a comprehensive guide*. 3rd ed. New York: Jossey-Bass; 2006.

- This popular textbook for first-level courses on surveys in public health and other disciplines provides a broad introduction to all key topics of survey planning, conduct and analysis and does not require advanced statistical knowledge.

Dillman DA, Smyth JD, Melani Christian L. *Internet, mail and mixed-mode surveys: the tailored design method*. 3rd ed. Hoboken (NJ): John Wiley; 2009.

- This textbook provides a broad introduction to all key topics of survey planning, conduct and analysis, with specific detail on several survey modes. It does not require advanced statistical knowledge.

Groves RM, Fowler FJ Jr, Couper MP, Lepkowski JM, Singer E, Tourangeau R. *Survey methodology*. 2nd ed. Hoboken (NJ): John Wiley; 2009.

- This textbook provides a broad introduction to all key topics of survey planning, conduct and analysis and does not require advanced statistical knowledge.

Statistics Canada. *Survey methods and practices*. Cat. no. 12-587-X. Ottawa: Statistics Canada; 2003. Available from: www.statcan.gc.ca/pub/12-587-x/12-587-x2003001-eng.pdf.

United Nations. Department of Economics and Social Affairs, Statistics Division. *Designing household survey samples: practical guidelines*. Studies in Methods Series F, no. 98. New York: United Nations; 2005. Available from: http://unstats.un.org/unsd/demographic/sources/surveys/Handbook23June05.pdf

United Nations. Department of Economics and Social Affairs, Statistics Division. *Household sample surveys in developing and transition countries*. Studies in Methods Series F, no. 96. New York: United Nations; 2005. Available from: http://unstats.un.org/unsd/hhsurveys/pdf/Household_surveys.pdf

- These classic overall guidebooks are written for applied health researchers and government employees who use survey research. The United Nations volumes are the ultimate guidebooks for population surveys in public and global health. The chapters on methods and sampling are excellent guides to learning about intermediate and advanced aspects of sampling design without advanced statistics training. The Statistics Canada book has good material on questionnaire design and fieldwork and is also exceptionally good for its relevance to the Canadian context, including with respect to information on ethics and confidentiality.

Specialized resources

American Association for Public Opinion Research (AAPOR). *Standard definitions: final dispositions of case codes and outcome rates for surveys*. Lenexa (KS): AAPOR; 2006. Available: www.aapor.org/Standard_Definitions/3049.htm

- This technical reference describes professional standards for survey methods. These standards are widely are used in the private sector as well as by major government and university-based survey research institutes.

Brackertz N. *Who is hard to reach and why*? ISR Working Paper. Melbourne, Australia: Swinburne University of Technology Institute for Social Research 2007. Available from: www.sisr.net/publications/0701brackertz.pdf

Faugier J, Sargeant M. Sampling hard to reach populations. *J Adv Nurs*. 1997;26(4):790–7.

- These resources provide advice on special methods to survey hard-to-reach populations, such as "snowball" sampling and sampling based on location.

McDowell I, Newell C. *Measuring health: a guide to rating scales and questionnaires*. 2nd ed. Oxford: Oxford University Press; 2006.

- This book focuses on the development of self-report measures related to health for use in surveys and any research using self-report measures.

Designing

Texts on technical and statistical aspects of survey design and secondary analysis of surveys

Groves RM, Dillman DA, Eltinge JL, Little RJA. *Survey nonresponse*. New York: John Wiley; 2002.

Korn EL, Graubard BI. *Analysis of health surveys*. Hoboken (NJ): John Wiley; 1999.

Levy PS, Lemeshow S. *Sampling of populations: methods and applications*. New York: Wiley; 2010.

Lohr SL. *Sampling: design and analysis*. 2nd ed. New York: Cengage Learning, 2009.

Lehtonen R, Pahkinen E. *Practical methods for design and analysis of complex surveys*. 2nd ed. Hoboken (NJ): John Wiley; 2004.

Designing

SUMMARY CHECKLIST

For planning a survey:

- ❑ Define the population you want to describe in formal terms.
- ❑ Define the key measures of your survey and review how each is best measured.
- ❑ Design and pre-test your questionnaire (or data collection materials).
- ❑ Identify and critique possible survey sampling frames and data collection modes.
- ❑ Design field-test methods, including quality control measures.
- ❑ Determine what margin of error is acceptable for each estimate.
- ❑ Define random sampling procedures.
- ❑ Determine sample size needed and the budget this will require.

For conducting a survey:

- ❑ Obtain ethical approvals (including for pre-testing, if required).
- ❑ Hire and train staff as required.
- ❑ Announce and promote the survey.
- ❑ Conduct random sampling as per plan.
- ❑ Invite participants and record the outcome of all invitations.
- ❑ Obtain informed consent.
- ❑ Complete data collection according to the study plan.
- ❑ Prepare statistical analyses that describe the population of interest, with honest margins of error, and that reflect the complexity of the sampling design.

12
Medical record review studies

Andrew Worster, MD, MSc, CCFP(EM), FCFP

ILLUSTRATIVE CASE

A second-year resident in Emergency Medicine sees a patient with a swollen and tender lower leg. The patient had been seen in the emergency department just two days before for the same problem. At that time, the patient had a D-dimer test to look for evidence of deep venous thrombosis (DVT). The result was negative, and the patient was discharged. The resident is aware that this test can be used to rule out DVT in patients with a low likelihood — i.e., a low pretest probability (PTP) — of the disease. There is no record of venous thromboembolism (VTE) risk factors or a formal PTP calculation on the patient's chart from his previous visit. The resident wonders if the PTP was taken into consideration before the D-dimer test was ordered and, more generally, how often PTP is documented. The answer to this question may have significant implications regarding the quality of care provided by emergency physicians to patients with suspected VTE. The resident decides to conduct a study to answer her research question: "Is PTP assessment of patients who present to the emergency department with suspected VTE routinely documented before D-dimer testing?"

■ **This chapter provides an introduction** to medical record review (MRR) studies, outlining how they are conducted, and why. Like all research methods, MRR studies serve a particular purpose, allowing the researcher to obtain data to answer certain types of questions. In our case example, the resident discusses with her supervisor the possible study designs she could use to answer her research question. One method that they consider is a survey of emergency department physicians and residents. Both the resident and her supervisor recognize that results from such a survey would be subject to professional desirability bias (i.e., respondents providing answers that they think would make them look good, rather than describing what actually occurs). Another method they consider is a prospective cohort study, in which the resident would observe staff physicians and fellow residents in the emergency department and question them each time they

order a D-dimer test. However, this is not feasible from a resource perspective and would be subject to the Hawthorne effect: that is, once study participants realize they are being observed, they will likely change their behaviour. Instead, the resident and her supervisor decide that the best way to approach her research question is through a review

---

CHAPTER OBJECTIVES

After reading this chapter, you should be able to:
- list the advantages and limitations of medical record review studies
- describe how cases are selected
- discuss how the sample size is calculated
- describe the sampling method
- discuss how to optimize the data quality
- discuss the ethical issues applicable to this type of study

---

KEY TERMS

Bias	Data quality	Sample size
Case selection	Imputation	Sampling
Chart review	Inter-observer agreement	Simple random sampling
Cohen's kappa	Missing values	

of emergency department patient records—that is, to carry out what is commonly called a **chart review**. However, the term "chart" is very specific and does not encompass all available sources of patient medical information, much of which is now recorded in aggregate form on electronic databases. For this reason, these studies are best described as medical record review (MRR) studies, a phrase that covers any study using pre-recorded, patient-focused data, such as physician and nursing notes, ambulance call reports, diagnostic tests, and so forth.[1,2] It should be noted that various study designs can use MRR for the purpose of data collection; these include certain observational methodologies such as case-series and case-control studies.

Advantages and limitations of medical record review studies

The obvious advantage to conducting an MRR is that the data have already been collected. This can save considerable time and resources. This method also makes it possible to address research questions that would be difficult to answer prospectively, such as the effects of harmful or beneficial exposures, the occurrence of rare events, and patterns of disease or behaviour over prolonged periods, to name a few examples.[2] However, despite the convenience, the use of pre-collected data can be a disadvantage, and researchers must understand the potential pitfalls before embarking on this kind of study. Typically, the data collected in medical records are not meant for research purposes and are not as valid or reliable as data whose collection is prospectively planned.[3] Clinical findings, such as whether a patient has a heart murmur or some other physical condition, are not consistently agreed upon or documented. Of course, some types of information found in medical records, such as demographic data and test results, are less open to interpretation and hence more reliable. The absence of some data is also a common problem and one that presents a major threat to the validity of MRR study results. The data sample in MRRs can also be biased by an absence of blinding and of randomization. These issues, along with potential solutions, are presented in the following sections.

Case selection

Because "cases" of interest in an MRR study have already occurred, the first challenge for the researcher is to identify those that are eligible for inclusion in the study. The method used to make this selection will depend on the research question. Presenting complaints and discharge diagnoses are not necessarily valid case-identification criteria unless they are integral to the research question, as in the following example: "Is pretest probability assessment of ED patients with a presenting complaint of leg swelling documented before D-dimer testing?" The study population in the resident's research question is emergency patients with suspected venous thromboembolism (VTE) who undergo D-dimer testing. Because "suspected VTE" is neither a presenting complaint nor a discharge diagnosis, the best way to accurately identify this population without reviewing the thousands of cases seen during the study period is to list all of the subjects who had D-dimer tests during their emergency department visit. The list will also contain, as we will see, many ineligible cases, but it should be possible to eliminate these cases using exclusion criteria established *a priori*.

Sample size calculation

The next question, then, is "How many cases are needed for the study?" That is, how many subjects are required to ensure that sufficiently precise estimates of the study measures of interest can be calculated?[4] As for any quantitative study, the method used to calculate sample size for MRR studies is determined by the statistical test to be used in the analysis of the primary outcome. For the resident's question, the sample size calculation is based on the desired reliability of the primary outcome (i.e., the proportion of charts with documentation of the pre-test probability). The resident decides that the reliability of her final results should have a confidence interval of 95%, which means that there is a 95% probability that the actual proportion of charts that include documentation of the PTP is within her predefined range of values.[5] Using an online calculator,[a] she is able to determine how many cases she needs to review to achieve this precision. Because of a variety of factors, such as the potential for error in ordering the test, not all of the patients who had D-dimer tests during their emergency department visit will be eligible. The resident understands the need to select a greater number of cases than was determined by her sample size calculation and estimates that about 5% will be ineligible. The reality is that she can't know with any degree of certainty what proportion of cases will be found ineligible, but at least she has anticipated the problem and compensated for the probable shortfall.

a See, for example, http://statpages.org/#Power

Sampling method

Now that the resident has a list of all potentially eligible cases, she needs to pick out the required number of cases from a list of hundreds. This is referred to as **sampling** (see also ch. 11). A common method of sampling is to select all of the consecutive cases within a given time frame. This is an acceptable approach if the period is long enough to account for seasonal variations or other temporal changes that are relevant to the research question. Bear in mind that sampling consecutive cases over a long period can result in the inclusion of more cases than are required.[6] For example, imagine that your sample size calculation has shown that your study requires 100 cases, and you see more than 100 potentially eligible cases each month. You would need to collect data only for a period long enough to meet the sample size requirement. However, if the clinical event in question is subject to seasonal variation, such as trauma or pneumonia, you would need to collect cases for a longer period of time (e.g., an entire year) to avoid time-period selection bias. This could mean collecting 12 times the number of cases needed for your final sample size. An alternative to consecutive case sampling, and the best non-consecutive sampling method for our case vignette, is **simple random sampling**. Simple random sampling provides an equal opportunity (probability) for each eligible case to be selected without **bias** and is best achieved by using a random number generator to identify the records for selection.[2] Random number generators are available online.[b] Other sampling methods, such as incidental selection (selection of the most easily accessible cases) and systematic selection (selection of every "nth" case), are more susceptible to bias and are best avoided.

Optimizing data quality

Generally speaking, each medical record is composed of different interpretations of different scenarios, often by different observers.[7-10] Moreover, the free-text format commonly used in patients' medical charts can be difficult to interpret. These shortcomings can create a larger-than-anticipated amount of erroneous and missing data. Therefore, the onus is on the researcher to demonstrate that the data have been extracted reliably and in an unbiased manner.[8] The first step the resident should take is to recruit others to extract the data, and thus avoid bias from her own opinions. She can further optimize the quality of her study data by applying several data extraction strategies. A description of the strategies used to avoid bias in data extraction is a requirement for publication in many peer-reviewed journals.[8] Some of the key strategies described in the literature are as follows:

- Train the data extractors.[11-13]
- Keep the data extractors blind to the study hypothesis or, in this case, the study objective.[8]
- Establish, *a priori*, unambiguous definitions for the study variables (e.g., PTP) and clear inclusion and exclusion criteria.[5,11]
- Create a study-specific computer data form (e.g., using Microsoft Access, Microsoft Corp., Redmond, WA).[14]
- Advise the data extractors at the beginning that their work will be checked for accuracy.[12]
- Check the reliability of the abstracted data in random samples.[15]
- Establish unambiguous rules regarding the management of missing or conflicting data.[16]

Missing information can lead to non-response bias in the results if the cases are simply deleted from the analysis. The impact of this will depend on the proportion of cases involved. One method of managing missing data and/or missing cases is **imputation**. This method substitutes some value for a missing value. For example, one could choose to substitute an average value of the variable in question for the missing value. Multiple imputation, which is typically reserved for large databases, is the multiple substitution of **missing values**.[17] Once all missing values have been imputed, the dataset can be analysed using standard statistical tests. There are no restrictions on the quantity of data that can be substituted, but the greater the proportion of imputed values, the less valid the results. Another method of managing missing values is by sensitivity analysis, in which the missing values are replaced with "best-case" and "worst-case" outcomes or values. An advantage of sensitivity analysis is that it can demonstrate the robustness of the results under different circumstances.

When two or more data extractors arrive at different versions of the same event, the researcher is faced with conflicting data. These discrepancies are often best resolved through consensus and, like the number of cases for which data are missing, should be reported in the results along with the

Designing

---

b See, for example, www.random.org/integers/

outcome(s) of their resolution. However, the readers of the study will also need to know to what extent the data extractors agreed in general. **Cohen's kappa** ($\square$) is the most commonly reported measure of **inter-observer agreement** for MRR studies. It is interpreted as the extent of agreement achieved compared with the total amount of agreement possible beyond chance agreement and is reported as a value from −1 (perfect disagreement) to 1 (perfect agreement).[18] As with many formulas, Cohen's $\square$ has its limitations; in some cases, other tests might be more appropriate.

Ethical issues

The patient health information that the resident intends to view, abstract and analyze is confidential. As such, she is required to abide by all of her hospital regulations regarding the privacy of patient information. She will most likely need to apply to her local Research Ethics Board for approval to conduct her study, and as a rule medical journals will not consider for publication any study that did not receive prior ethical approval (see also ch. 18). In some cases, however, institutional review boards provide blanket approval for quality improvement research deemed to present little risk to the patients whose data are used, and some medical journals will accept this practice, depending on the nature of the study. Regardless of the requirement for ethical approval, every effort should be made to ensure that patients are not identifiable in the presentation of their data.

Conclusion

Although MRR studies are not easy to conduct, they can often be completed in less time and at less expense than most prospective studies. MRR studies are recognized as a valid and valuable research design method in the medical literature, and recommendations for conducting and reporting them have been published. Residents who have taken the time to understand the limitations and methodological challenges of MRRs have published their studies in high-impact journals. ■

CASE POSTSCRIPT

The resident submits a study protocol to her institution's Research Ethics Board and obtains approval to proceed. With support from her supervisor and other content experts in the field, she develops a data collection form and trains two medical students to review the relevant patient records. Working with a final sample of 100 charts, as determined by her sample size calculation, she finds that adequate documentation of PTP was provided for only 10% of all patients with suspected DVT. Her findings are presented at a research meeting and prompt the creation of a standardized form for inclusion in selected charts that encourages clinicians to record the elements of a clinical probability assessment for DVT.

REFERENCES

1. Worster A, Haines T. Medical record review studies: an overview. *Israeli J Trauma, Intensive Care Emerg Med.* 2002;2(2):21–6.

2. Worster A, Haines T. Advanced statistics: medical record review (MRR) studies. *Acad Emerg Med.* 2004;11:187–92.

3. Burnum JF. The misinformation era: the fall of the medical record. *Ann Intern Med.* 1989;110(6):482–84.

4. Smith C, Mensah A, Mal S, Worster A. Is pretest probability assessment on emergency department patients with suspected venous thromboembolism documented before SimpliRED D-dimer testing? *CJEM.* 2008;10(6):519–23.

5. Last JM. *A dictionary of epidemiology.* 3rd ed. New York (NY): Oxford University Press; 1995.

6. Cummings SR, Newman TB, Hulley SB. Designing a cohort study. In: Hulley SB, Cummings SR, Browner WS, Grady D, Hearst N, Newman TB. *Designing clinical research: an epidemiologic approach.* 3rd ed. Philadelphia (PA): Wolters Kluwer/Lippincott, Williams & Wilkins; 2001. p. 101.

7. Worster A, Bledsoe RD, Cleve P, Fernandes CM, Upadhye S, Eva K. Reassessing the methods of medical record review studies in emergency medicine research. *Ann Emerg Med.* 2005;45(4):448–51.

Designing

8. Gilbert EH, Lowenstein SR, Kozoil-McLain J, Barta DC, Steiner J. Chart reviews in emergency medicine research: Where are the methods? *Ann Emerg Med*. 1996;27(3):305–8.

9. Lerner EB, Zachariah BS, White LJ. Conducting retrospective emergency medical services research. *Prehosp Emerg Care*. 2002;6(2 Suppl):S48–51.

10. Rangel SJ, Kelsey J, Colby CE, Anderson J, Moss RL. Development of a quality assessment scale for retrospective clinical studies in pediatric surgery. *J Pediatr Surg*. 2003;38(3):390–6.

11. Horowitz RI, Yu EC. Assessing the reliability of epidemiologic data obtained from medical records. *J Chron Dis*. 1984;37(11):825–31.

12. Reid JB. Reliability assessment of observation data: a possible methodological problem. *Child Dev*. 1970;41(4):1143–50.

13. Allison JJ, Wall TC, Spettell CM, Calhoun J, Fargason CA Jr, Kobylinski RW, et al. The art and science of chart review. *Jt Comm J Qual Improv*. 2000;26(3):115–36.

14. Banks NJ. Designing medical record abstraction forms. *Int J Qual Health Care*. 1998;10(2):163–7.

15. Beard CM, Yunginger JW, Reed CE, O'Connell EJ, Silverstein MD. Interobserver variability in medical record review: an epidemiological study of asthma. *J Clin Epidemiol*. 1992;45(9):1013–20.

16. Wu L, Ashton CM. Chart review. A need for reappraisal. *Eval Health Prof*. 1997;20(2):146–63.

17. Schafer JL. *Analysis of incomplete multivariate data*. Monographs on Statistics and Applied Probability 72. Boca Raton (FL): Chapman & Hall/CRC; 1997.

18. Cohen JA. A coefficient of agreement for normal scales. *Educ Psychol Measure*. 1960;20(1):37–46.

Designing

SUMMARY CHECKLIST

- ❑ Carefully consider the limitations and advantages of an MRR study before you start. Specifically, anticipate the data gaps you may encounter and their implications for the validity of your results.
- ❑ Devise a reliable method for identifying potentially eligible cases for screening.
- ❑ Frame your inclusion and exclusion criteria carefully to remove any ambiguity about case selection.
- ❑ Remember that unbiased sampling methods and appropriate sample size calculations are as important in MRR studies as they are in other forms of research.
- ❑ Take the necessary steps to optimize the quality of data collection: this will likely involve properly training those who will be reviewing the patient records, verifying data quality and reproducibility, and preventing bias by blinding the data abstractors to the study hypothesis.
- ❑ Set out the groundwork for successful chart review by establishing clear definitions for what needs to be collected and designing easy-to-use paper or electronic data collection forms.
- ❑ Remember that medical records contain privileged patient information and that research based on such records requires the approval of a Research Ethics Board both to safeguard the integrity of the work and to ensure that it will be eligible for consideration by a peer-reviewed journal.

Designing

13
Administrative database research

Carl van Walraven, MD, MSc, FRCPC

ILLUSTRATIVE CASE

A second-year Community Medicine resident wonders if there is an association between circulation of influenza virus and rates of hospital admissions for pneumonia, chronic lung disease and congestive heart failure. As a first step, he approaches faculty members with experience and expertise in accessing and analyzing the relevant provincial health databases.

Designing

■ **Administrative data are created in** multiple settings within the health system (e.g., in primary care practices, ambulatory clinics, hospital departments, nursing homes, and health authorities at the regional, provincial, federal and international level). Consider a patient who presents to the emergency department of a university teaching hospital with shortness of breath. Her demographic information and time of arrival are recorded in the patient registration system, her chest radiograph report is recorded in the hospital's diagnostic imaging system, and the dose and time of all medications she receives are recorded in the hospital's pharmacy system. Finally, the identity of the physician who assessed the patient and made the final diagnosis is recorded in the National Ambulatory Care Reporting System.[a] Thus, particular aspects of each patient's encounter are recorded in different datasets.

In administrative **database** research (ADR), these **health datasets** are linked by researchers to create a summary of each patient's encounter with various aspects of the health care system. This allows researchers to systematically study the interactions that groups of individuals have with

any portion of the system. These groups may be of any size, ranging from the patients of a walk-in clinic to a country's entire population. Administrative databases can also be used to define patient cohorts and determine whether patients encountered particular exposures and had specific outcomes. These capabilities give ADR the potential to answer important questions regarding associations and outcomes in health care.

However, it is difficult to define ADR purely in terms of the types of data it uses. Typically, ADR uses data collected to support the administration of health care by capturing

---

a   See http://secure.cihi.ca/cihiweb/dispPage.jsp?cw_page=services_nacrs_e

CHAPTER OBJECTIVES

After reading this chapter, you should be able to:
- describe what administrative database research is and is not
- identify research questions suitable for administrative database research
- describe the basic steps necessary to design and conduct an administrative database research project
- discuss the strengths and limitations of administrative database research

---

KEY TERMS

Administrative data	Data-sharing agreement	Electronic medical record (EMR)
Database	Electronic health record (EHR)	Health datasets

Designing

demographic information and calculating rates of service use, volume of procedures, diagnostic rates, and so forth. There is some uncertainty as to whether research that uses data in **electronic medical records** (EMRs) and **electronic health records** (EHRs) constitutes administrative health research in that sense. On the other hand, some data components of EMRs and EHRs, such as diagnostic or procedural codes, are identical to those typically found in administrative databases. Other components, such as laboratory test results or radiology reports, would be considered "gold standard" data; some investigators using such data (as in a medical record review) would not consider themselves to be doing ADR. For these reasons, a standard definition of ADR does not exist.

The type of data used in ADR demands that several particular steps be taken to plan a research project. First, you must determine whether the administrative data that you have in mind can actually answer your question. This requires discussion with someone who has an in-depth knowledge of those data. Factors to be considered in this step include data quality, database completeness and database duration (i.e., does the database go back far enough in time to answer your question?). Second, you must ensure that you, or another member of your research team, will be able to access the required data. If you cannot access the data, your project will be impossible. Last, you will need someone on your research team with sophisticated programming skills and an intimate knowledge of the database. Manipulating large datasets into an accurate analytical dataset requires extensive programming skills and an appreciation of the intricacies of each dataset used in the analysis. Without such a person, the project will be impossible.

Advantages of administrative database research

The several advantages that make ADR an attractive approach to many research questions can be described as follows.

ADR is relatively inexpensive. The bulk of most research budgets is spent on data collection, which requires dedicated staff and a great deal of time. Because administrative databases already exist, data collection and its associated costs can be avoided (assuming that no supplementary data collection is required). With the proviso that database and specialized biostatistical expertise are often required—

which could involve the investigator obtaining additional training, enlisting suitable collaborators or hiring expert consultants—ADR is relatively inexpensive.

ADR is relatively quick. In addition to being expensive, data collection can be very time-consuming. Since the data required for ADR already exist, delays related to data collection are avoided. Although time is required to examine and clean the data used in an ADR, this takes much less time than actually collecting the data.

ADR is often population-based. A frequent limitation of many research projects is the limited or unknown generalizability—the external validity—of the results. This limitation arises from the fact that most research is conducted on a sample, which can be a very small or non-random extract of the population that is purportedly being studied. ADR can avoid the limitation of poor generalizability if the databases that are used actually capture an entire, identifiable study population. For example, the Ontario Drug Benefits database can be used to conduct population-based research regarding out-of-hospital medication use among Ontarians aged 65 years and over. This is because covered medications dispensed to all of Ontario's seniors are captured in this database. Being able to conduct population-based research makes administrative databases especially relevant to researchers in population health and to policy-makers. Of course, if the databases being employed are relatively "focused"—such as a database covering a hospital's emergency department—the generalizability would be limited to those individuals who received care there.

ADR makes you independent. It is not uncommon for a research project to fail because a member of the team does not live up to his or her commitments. ADR can liberate you from this potential problem. With a few exceptions (see next section), there are very few barriers in ADR that stand between you and a completed project—assuming that you can formulate a good research question and critically review the relevant literature, as discussed in chapters 6 and 7, respectively. Minimizing the number of people upon whom you rely is essential to a successful research project and career (especially when you are just starting out).

ADR analyses can be repeated to monitor interventions. One of the most satisfying aspects of ADR is the fact that it draws upon databases that are continually updated. This is especially advantageous when one wants to monitor the effects of interventions that have been introduced to address problems identified through ADR. If the original analysis that identified the problem to be addressed by the new intervention has been recorded in a computer program, the effect of the intervention can be immediately—and repeatedly—determined by simply rerunning the analysis.

Potential disadvantages of administrative database research

The several notable potential weaknesses of ADR can be outlined as follows.

Data inaccessibility. Whether they cover a practice, department, institution or entire province, administrative databases contain personally sensitive information. Therefore, data custodians (i.e., the organization responsible for the data's security) will be appropriately risk-averse when it comes to providing researchers with access. Frequently, databases can be accessed only in a controlled manner, on-site at the organization responsible for them, and only after permission has been formally requested and approved. Accessing data within such organizations is usually feasible only if one is sponsored by or collaborates with a researcher within that organization. However, administrative data are generated at all hospitals and are usually much more available for one-time research projects. Such projects require approval from the local research ethics board and should involve a formal **data-sharing agreement** between the researcher and the hospital.

Poor or unknown data quality. Although data quality is a potential concern in all types of research, it is a particularly familiar theme in ADR. Administrative databases are usually created for a variety of reasons unrelated to the conduct of research (i.e., for administrative or clinical purposes). As a result, the priorities placed on information processing are very different from those required for ADR. Therefore, the accuracy of some administrative data required for a particular research question may be poor if those data are not important for the main purposes of the database and, as such, are not collected or maintained with the attention required for high-quality data.

Many administrative databases record diagnoses and procedures using codes. These codes are assigned by health records analysts after they have reviewed the applicable

health record in order to create classifications or groupings. Numerous steps occur between true diagnosis and the assignment of a code, and error is possible at any one of these steps. The published literature is replete with examples of codes being either insensitive or non-specific for a particular diagnosis or procedure that it supposedly represents. As a result, the inclusion of some proportion of inaccurate codes will yield results that differ greatly from those based on the actual entity represented by the code.

The problem of coding error is amplified by the large numbers of records that are screened for the presence or absence of the code of interest. The proportion of rows in an administrative dataset with a particular code can be very low. Trouble can arise when a disease with a very low prevalence (i.e., a low pretest probability) is combined with an imperfect test (such as a diagnostic code being used in the administrative database research study). The probability that someone who is assigned a given code truly has the disease it represents can be calculated by multiplying the pretest odds of the disease by the positive likelihood ratio of the code. When this calculation is made in cases where the condition is rare or the code is inaccurate, the probability that people with the code truly have the condition it is supposed to represent can be less than 50%.[1]

Because of the issue of coding inaccuracy, an ADR that requires a code to define the cohort, exposure or outcomes should be preceded by a study to determine the accuracy of the code as well as the frequency of the condition in question.[2] Both coding inaccuracy and the rarity of a condition will dramatically increase the risk of bias in ADR.

Poor data detail. When clinical researchers start using administrative databases for research, they are frequently struck by their lack of clinical detail. Even basic, commonly used clinical information (such as the patient's vital signs) are nowhere to be found in typical administrative databases. This lack of clinical detail can severely limit the type of research questions that can be answered with ADR. Two methods are commonly used to make up for this weakness: supplementing the information in the administrative database with data collected through some other means (e.g., a chart review); and linking pure administrative data with data from high-quality clinical data repositories, such as electronic medical records, which contain much more detailed clinical information.

The requirement for computer programming and statis-

tical expertise. Many steps will likely be required to modify administrative data into a suitable analytical dataset for your research project. A firm knowledge of a programming language that allows you to do this (e.g., SAS, SQL) is necessary to conduct ADR. Many people are scared off by the thought of learning how to program. If at all possible, these feelings should be repressed. Learning how to program does more than make independent ADR possible. It is a skill that will assist you in all research fields, since the vast majority of all research projects will have an analytical dataset. Being able to examine and analyze that dataset (which you will be able to do after learning how to program) is key to knowing your data and truly understanding your project. Many books and courses are available to teach you how to program common languages. (Two examples are given in Additional Resources.)

A high level of statistical knowledge and expertise is often required. ADR may involve repeated data measures that are often collinear and, as such, require special analytic techniques. It is often not feasible for individual researchers to learn these, which means that you will either need to seek out a biostatistician to join the research team as a collabora-

tor or to acquire sufficient project funding to hire a consultant with the necessary biostatistical expertise.

A final "limitation" of ADR arises from the fact that administrative datasets enable large sample sizes and, for that reason, the results of most inferential analyses will be statistically significant. As a result, it is essential that researchers pay more attention to the clinical importance and practical significance of the differences seen between populations as opposed to the statistical significance of such differences.

Conclusion

Administrative database research holds many important advantages, especially for junior researchers, provided that appropriate support is available from one or more suitable senior researchers. However, it is important to keep the notable limitations of ADR in mind when you consider using this methodology to answer your research question. ■

CASE POSTSCRIPT

To examine the association between circulation of influenza virus and rates of hospital admissions for pneumonia, chronic lung disease and congestive heart failure, the resident identified, approached and collaborated with several established health services researchers who enabled his access to the provincial influenza surveillance and hospital discharge databases. With this assistance, particularly that of a biostatistician with expertise with time-series analyses, the study was successfully completed and published[3] in a widely respected peer-reviewed journal.

REFERENCES

1. van Walraven C, Bennett C, Forster AJ. Administrative database research infrequently used validated diagnostic or procedural codes. *J Clin Epidemiol.* 2011;64(10):1054–59.

2. Schneeweiss S, Avorn J. A review of uses of health care utilization databases for epidemiologic research on therapeutics. J Clin Epidemiol. 2005;58(4):323–37.

3. Upshur RE, Knight K, Goel V. Time-series analysis of the relation between influenza virus and hospital admissions of the elderly in Ontario, Canada, for pneumonia, chronic lung disease, and congestive heart failure. Am J Epidemiol. 1999;149(1):85–92.

ADDITIONAL RESOURCES

Cody R. *Learning SAS by example: a programmer's guide.* Cary (NC): SAS Press; 2007.

Delwiche LD, Slaughter SJ. *The little SAS book: a primer.* 4th ed. Cary (NC): SAS Press; 2008.

- Both of these references provide an excellent introduction to the SAS programming language and application.

EXERCISE

List some research questions that may be suitable for administrative database research. List some that would not be.

SUMMARY CHECKLIST

❑   Select a question that you might use administrative data to address.
❑   List the advantages and disadvantages of this approach for your specific question.

Designing

Designing

14
Health professions education research

Jason R. Frank, MD, MA(Ed), FRCPC

ILLUSTRATIVE CASE

A 2nd-year Emergency Medicine resident knows that she will soon need to start a research project as a requirement for her program. Although most of her colleagues are doing medical record reviews of clinical problems, she is not particularly interested in following suit. What is really on her mind is her concern about the radiology curriculum in her residency program. She feels more at ease reading musculoskeletal and chest films than brain CT scans, for example, and wonders whether other residents share her concern that the program has gaps that need to be addressed. However, she has no idea how she would explore this question or even if it is an acceptable topic for scholarly research.

■ **The daily lives of front line health** care professionals provide ample evidence of the successes and challenges of health professions education (HPE). In every clinical encounter, we witness the abilities of other health care professionals; sometimes, we contemplate the limits of our own competence. HPE is a both a field of scholarship and an enterprise focused on the preparation of health care professionals to meet the needs of the patients and communities they serve. **The spectrum of health professions education** spans undergraduate training (e.g., MD, DDSc and BScN programs), postgraduate (e.g., residency) education leading to certification and practice, further advanced training (e.g. fellowships), lifelong continuing professional development, and faculty development in academic health science centres (see Fig. 14.1). As a scholarly field and an enterprise, HPE explores the most effective curricula and systems to ensure that patients and societies are best served by competent and caring health professionals. Everything from admissions decisions to teaching methods, curriculum topics, assessment tools, program evaluations and more are part of this subject area. The discipline is in fact multi-dimensional, and its aspects are pervasive in the work of all those involved with the various aspects of health care.

CHAPTER OBJECTIVES

After reading this chapter, you should be able to:
- define health professions education (HPE)
- define HPE research
- describe four broad categories of HPE research
- describe the typical areas of interest of those involved in HPE research
- describe typical methods used in HPE research

KEY TERMS

Assessment	Kirkpatrick's four-level framework
Cohen's d	Needs assessment
Competencies	Program evaluation
Instructional methods	Spectrum of health professions education

---

Figure 14.1
The spectrum of health professions education

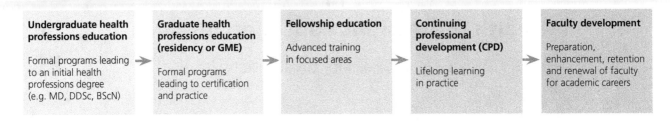

Undergraduate health professions education	Graduate health professions education (residency or GME)	Fellowship education	Continuing professional development (CPD)	Faculty development
Formal programs leading to an initial health professions degree (e.g. MD, DDSc, BScN)	Formal programs leading to certification and practice	Advanced training in focused areas	Lifelong learning in practice	Preparation, enhancement, retention and renewal of faculty for academic careers

Designing

Health professions education research is a legitimate domain of scholarship, to which numerous journals,[a] texts (see Additional Reading) and careers are devoted. If HPE plays a critical role in preparing health care professionals to serve society, then HPE research provides insights and evidence to guide that education. This chapter provides an introduction to the field and an overview of the kinds of HPE research studies you might be interested in contributing to. All of the principles and essential steps involved in any research study, and all of the major methodologies described in this guide, are relevant to HPE research studies. However, the subject areas of HPE and the contexts in which they are explored make HPE research unique.[1–3]

Categorizing health professions education research studies

What kinds of studies are addressed by health professions education research? Both quantitative and qualitative methods belong here, as does research focused on either an underlying theory or a practical everyday problem.[4] Although there are many ways of conceptualizing research in this field,[5,6] one simple way is to categorize HPE research into four areas according to the broad questions being asked (see Table 14.1). These four areas of questioning are outlined in the following sections.

What to teach, learn or assess?

The studies in this category answer questions about what belongs in the curriculum of a health care professional. What should be taught? What should be learned? What should be assessed? These questions can be thought of as dealing with "content issues" or "inputs." Contemporary research in this area is concerned with, among other things:

- the identification and characterization of **competencies** needed by a group of health care professionals in a given setting or context
- group consensus processes to create statements on priority curriculum elements
- the identification of gaps between identified priority abilities of professionals and their current abilities in a population (**needs assessment**)
- the characterization of existing or innovative curricula or **assessment** systems.

These studies are essential to ensure that health professions education is focused on the priorities that are most relevant to the needs of the patients and populations served by graduates. Without this body of work, curriculum content is often left up to each individual teacher or program director in an ad hoc manner. Neufeld and colleagues call this kind of research focusing on "demand-side medical education."[7]

How should we teach, learn or assess?

This category deals with **instructional methods** or techniques used to assess a health professional's competence. Akin to case reports in the clinical literature, studies in this area are often descriptions of curricula, tools or systems, including:

- descriptions of existing or innovative curricula
- descriptions of teaching or learning methods
- descriptions of assessment tools and processes
- historical studies on health professions education

These kinds of studies may be declining in the HPE research literature, giving way to increasing emphasis on the next category, namely studies that evaluate objective and subjective outcomes related to curricular approaches.[6,8]

---

a   E.g., *Academic Medicine, Medical Education, Medical Teacher, Advances in Health Sciences Education, Gerontology & Geriatrics Education, Journal of Dental Education, International Journal of Nursing Education Scholarship,* and *Journal of Nursing Education.*

■   **Table 14.1: Categories of health professions education (HPE) research studies**

Category	Areas of interest	Methods
What to teach, learn, or assess? These studies seek to describe or identify what should be taught, learned or assessed by a given group of health professionals in a given context.	• Needs assessments (perceived, observed, societal, epidemiologic, institutional) • Group consensus statements • Descriptions of curricula • Descriptions of assessment strategies	• Surveys • Delphi and other consensus methods
How to teach, learn, or assess? These studies seek to describe, clarify, and identify instructional or assessment methods for the health professions.	• Descriptions of curricula • Teaching/learning techniques • Teaching/learning innovations • Assessment techniques / tools • Assessment innovations • History of some aspect of HPE	• Educational case studies • Historical studies
What works? These studies explore the outcomes of curricula, programs and systems in HPE.	• Program evaluations • Validation of assessment tools • Effectiveness of teaching approaches • Descriptions of outcomes or effects • History of some aspect of HPE	• Controlled educational trials • Goal-based evaluations • Responsive evaluations • Expert reviews • Focus groups and other qualitative methods • Cohort studies • Case-control studies • Historical studies
Why does it work? These studies clarify why a given element of HPE does or does not contribute to a certain impact or outcomes. They contribute to our understanding of underlying theories or concepts related to HPE.	• Theory/concept building • Theory/concept testing • History of some aspect of HPE	• Controlled educational trials • Cohort studies • Case-control studies • Focus groups and other qualitative methods • Historical studies

Designing

What works?

Increasingly, scholars in health professions education have been focusing their attention on characterizing the effectiveness of elements of the HPE enterprise. This is considered to be part of the commitment to be accountable to the populations served by the health care professions.[3] These studies often try to solve pragmatic problems in the field and represents perhaps the majority of contemporary published papers. This is the domain of **program evaluations** of all kinds, using qualitative or quantitative methods, or both. In this category one can find studies on:

- the effectiveness or impact of existing or innovative curricula
- the effectiveness of teaching or learning methods
- the effectiveness of assessment tools and processes
- historical perspectives on health professions education

Program evaluations use an enormous variety of methodologies. For any study, the selection of the most appropriate method should be determined by the nature of the question being asked. For example, "goal-based" or program-oriented evaluations compare the actual outcomes of a program design with its intended outcomes. "Responsive" or participant-oriented evaluations focus on the intended or unintended effects of a program as perceived by stakeholders. So-called "connoisseur" evaluations rely on reviews by experts in a field.[9] Epidemiological approaches are also relevant here, including controlled trials, systematic reviews, cohort studies and case-control studies. These approaches to health professions education research are sometimes considered the most robust, given their focus on outcomes and their use of methods that are similar to those applied in the clinical research literature. Regardless, HPE research is certainly a broad and varied domain of activity that is essential to informing the advancement of health professions education as a field and the structure and function of HPE as an enterprise.

Why does it work?

The final category includes studies that often use methods similar to those used to address the question "What works?" but focus instead on what Cook and colleagues call "clarification."[5] These studies are useful in informing the development of conceptual frameworks within health professions education, making predictions from theories applied to HPE, and testing hypotheses in HPE.[5,10] A wide variety of studies and methods can be found here. Nevertheless, this category is often neglected by HPE scholars, a fact that is decried by some authors.[5,11–13]

Conducting a health professions education research project

Doing research in health professions education involves the same fundamental steps and principles described elsewhere in this guide. However, context is especially critical to HPE research: more than is the case, for example, with research on physiological phenomena, the validity, reliability and generalizability of HPE studies are affected by the settings and the population studied. By way of emphasis, the following list outlines some important elements to consider in conducting research related to HPE.[14,15]

1. **Question the curricula around you.** Does the teaching, learning and assessment in your professional environment work well? What elements could be better? Are the most appropriate topics being taught? How do you know whether the graduates of a given program are competent? Viewing your own environment through these lenses can help identify important problems to explore in a scholarly fashion.

2. **Review the relevant health professions education research literature.** There are thousands of published studies going back more than a century related to health professions education. These include papers published in major general medicine journals[b] and in HPE journals.[c] There is also an extensive grey litera-

ture of HPE reports. It is essential to conduct a thorough literature review to ensure that you are aware of what has already been done and what theories, concepts or hypotheses have already been explored. Major search databases are the same as those discussed in chapter 7, with the addition of ERIC.[d] Consultation with a research mentor who is familiar with this literature and enlisting the help of a librarian can save you months of searching.

3. **Carefully frame an appropriate health professions education research question.** To be effective, your research question should be tightly focused and clearly state the relevant population, variables and context of the study (see also ch. 6).

4. **The research question usually dictates the most appropriate methods.** The methods you selected for your study should be practical, and may need to involve both quantitative and qualitative approaches. Because it is difficult to control variables in educational research, randomized controlled trials are relatively infrequent in this field.

5. **Consider carefully the population of interest.** Bias can easily be introduced at this step in any study. Which population of health care professionals is most appropriate for your question? Which aspect of the spectrum of health professions education is relevant? Is your sample size adequate to enable you to make generalizable conclusions about the population?

6. **Select outcomes carefully.** These should not only match the goals of the study (e.g., a written test for a study of change in knowledge) but, wherever possible, should try to connect an intervention to "higher order" outcomes such as change in behaviour. **Kirkpatrick's four-level framework** is often cited as a guide to selecting outcomes. Of these levels, Kirkpatrick suggests that level 1—participant reaction or satisfaction—is the most basic and most commonly measured. Beyond this are three more types of outcomes: change in knowledge, change in behaviour, and im-

---

b E.g., *JAMA*, *Journal of General Internal Medicine*, the *New England Journal of Medicine* and *The Lancet*.

c E.g., *Academic Medicine*, *Advances in Health Science Education*,

Evaluation in the Health Professions, *Medical Education*, *Medical Teacher* and *Teaching and Learning in Medicine*.

d ERIC—the Education Resources Information Center—is an online digital library of education research and information; see www.eric.ed.gov

pact. For health professions education research, the latter can be thought of as patient- or population-level outcomes (e.g., improved diabetes control).[16]

7. **Consider validating your instruments.** Although many instruments already exist to measure health professions education research outcomes of relevance, few are validated. This limitation greatly weakens some studies. Can you use a pre-existing tool for your population and context? If you have to create a new one, how can you reassure a peer reviewer of its validity and reliability?

8. **Carefully consider effect size.** Data analysis in health professions education research studies is not always focused on *P* values. Statistical significance is often less important than educational importance and impact. Your study protocol should define a priori what constitutes a meaningful difference. Where the literature does not provide a benchmark, start with careful reasoning and, if possible, expert consensus. **Cohen's d** is a statistical measure that is sometimes used for the analysis of educational impact.[17]

9. **Be mindful of differing perspectives on the ethics of health professions education research.** Some Research Ethics Boards (REB) do not consider HPE program evaluations to need a certificate of ethical review. Others are very strict in considering any HPE research study that involves human subjects to be in need of full review. Regardless of the local REB's perspective, you must follow standard procedures to protect your subjects from any potential harm arising from their participation in the study. You should also bear in mind that many HPE journals will require evidence of ethics approval.

10. **Be cautious in interpreting your data.** No study is perfect, and so be circumspect in considering what your data really show. What are the limitations of your methods? What do you think is generalizable beyond your setting, context or population? How can your study reinforce or refute accepted beliefs, or generate new hypotheses and concepts? What does your study contribute to the field?

Conclusion

Research in health professions education is a dynamic, rapidly growing field of scholarly endeavour that informs and explores all aspects of preparing health professionals for practice. It is a legitimate area of inquiry, even for novice researchers, and its results can inform improvements to myriad aspects of the education and training of health care professionals. ∎

CASE POSTSCRIPT

Fortunately for the resident, her next shift is with a clinician-educator faculty member. After discussing the resident's research interest with her, the faculty member agrees to serve as her supervisor on a project that will be designed to explore radiology teaching in the EM program. After further discussion with her supervisor, and after reading relevant chapters of this guide, the resident settles on conducting a national needs assessment survey of program directors and residents in Emergency Medicine. Her conclusions are presented during her department's research day and form the basis for recommendations that are adopted by the residency training committee the next year.

REFERENCES

1. Norman G. Research in medical education: three decades of progress. *BMJ.* 2002;324(7353):1560–2.

2. Harden RM, Grant J, Buckley G, Hart IR. BEME Guide no.1: Best Evidence Medical Education. *Med Teach.* 1999;21(6):553–62.

3. Dauphinee WD, Wood-Dauphinee S. The need for evidence in medical education. *Acad Med.* 2004;79(10):925–30.

4. Albert M. Understanding the debate on medical education research: a sociological perspective. *Acad Med.* 2004;79(10):948–54.

5. Cook DA, Bordage G, Schmidt HG. Description, justification and clarification: a framework for classifying the purposes of research in medical education. *Med Educ.* 2008;42(2):128–33.

Designing

6. Regehr G. Trends in medical education research. *Acad Med*. 2004;79(10):939–47.

7. Neufeld VR, Maudsley RF, Picring RJ, Walters BC, Tunbull JM, Spasoff RA, et al. 1993. Demand side medical education: educating future physicians for Ontario. *CMAJ*. 1993;148(9):1471–7.

8. Chen FM, Bauchner H, Burstin H. A call for outcomes research in medical education. *Acad Med*. 2004;79(10):955–60.

9. Fitzpatrick JL, Sanders JR, Worthen BR. *Program evaluation: alternative approaches and practical guidelines*. 4th ed. Boston: Pearson / Allyn and Bacon; 2011.

10. Bordage G. Conceptual frameworks to illuminate and magnify. *Med Educ*. 2009;43:312–9.

11. Regehr G. It's NOT rocket science: rethinking our metaphors for research in health professions education. *Med Educ*. 2010;44(1):31–9.

12. Bunniss S, Kelly DR. 2010. Research paradigms in medical education research. *Med Educ*. 2010:44(4):358–66.

13. Gibbs T. Durning S, Van Der Vleuten C. Theories in medical education: towards creating a union between educational practice and research teaching. *Med Teach*. 2011;33:183–7.

14. Shea JA, Arnold L, Mann KV. A RIME perspective on the quality and relevance of current and future medical education research. *Acad Med*. 2004;79(10):931–8.

15. Cook DA, Bowen JL, Gerrity MS, Kalet AL, Kogan JR, Spickard A, et al. Proposed standards for medical education submissions to the *Journal of General Internal Medicine*. *J Gen Intern Med*. 2008;23(7):908–13.

16. Kirkpatrick DL, Kirkpatrick JD. *Evaluating training programs: the four levels*. San Francisco: Berrett-Koehler; 2006.

17. Kenny DA. *Statistics for the social and behavioral sciences*. Boston: Little Brown; 1987.

EXERCISES

1. Brainstorm some questions or problems you perceive from your experiences in health professions education. Are any of them worthy of an HPE research study?

2. Select one of the problems you identified in the exercise above. Do any published studies examine this problem? If so, what populations and contexts do they involve?

3. Select any study from one of the major health professions education journals mentioned in this chapter. Critique its methods. Do you agree with its conclusions?

SUMMARY CHECKLIST

- ❏ Discuss your interest in health professions education research with a qualified education research mentor.
- ❏ Identify some important problems to explore in an HPE research study.
- ❏ Select the category of HPE research study.
- ❏ Review the HPE research literature.
- ❏ Carefully frame an appropriate HPE research question.
- ❏ Select methods that are feasible in your context.
- ❏ Define the population of interest.
- ❏ Carefully select outcomes.
- ❏ Define and describe the Kirkpatrick levels involved.
- ❏ Consider validating any instruments.
- ❏ Carefully consider effect size.
- ❏ Carefully design your analysis.
- ❏ Submit your proposal for REB review, as appropriate.
- ❏ Interpret your results in the context of the HPE research literature.

15
Systematic reviews

Thomas A. Lang, MA

ILLUSTRATIVE CASE

For her master's thesis, a nursing student is considering a research project that will explore the effects of nurse staffing levels on patient outcomes in acute-care hospital settings. Her advisor suggests that she conduct a systematic review on the topic. Because she is unfamiliar with how to carry out a systematic review, her supervisor suggests several resources (including this guide) for her to review before their next meeting.

■ **A systematic review is a planned,** comprehensive, and reproducible summary of research results on a specified topic.[1] Systematic reviews are conducted according to a written protocol, developed in advance, that carefully defines the research question to be addressed, the desired characteristics of the research needed to answer the question, and the details of the search strategies that will be used to find articles reporting this research. The protocol also specifies criteria for selecting the articles to be reviewed from among those identified in the search, the specific variables for which data will be abstracted from each article, and the methods used to reduce the risk that these selection processes will bias the study. Finally, the results are compiled into evidence tables so that they can be interpreted in the context of all similar studies. In some circumstances, the numerical results can be pooled statistically in what is called a **meta-analysis**. The planned and systematic nature of these reviews helps to reduce bias, and because their results are intended to be reproducible, the internal validity of these reviews can be verified.

In contrast, **narrative reviews** are usually prepared by experts in the field who draw only on their personal reading, experience and judgment to summarize the topic. Thus, a narrative review is neither systematic nor reproducible; different experts may cite different evidence for different reasons, have different experiences, and reach different conclusions. Narrative reviews also rarely allow the results of individual studies to be pooled or synthesized statistically in any valid fashion.

CHAPTER OBJECTIVES

After reading this chapter, you should be able to:
- list at least three ways in which systematic reviews differ from narrative reviews
- list three uses of systematic reviews
- describe the steps in conducting a systematic review
- identify at least three sources of information about systematic reviews

---

KEY TERMS

Ancestry searches	Grey literature	MOOSE Statement	Realist reviews
Clinical trial registries	Hand searches	Narrative reviews	Risk of bias table
Cochrane Collaboration	Heterogeneity	Pearl-growing	Scoping reviews
Data abstraction	Inter-rater agreement	PRISMA Statement	Selection bias
Evidence tables	Intra-rater agreement	Publication bias	Sensitivity analyses
Forest plot	Meta-analysis	Rapid reviews	Summary of findings table

Some variations on systematic reviews are becoming more common. **Rapid reviews** are abbreviated systematic reviews designed to be completed in a few weeks to a few months, as opposed to the 6 to 12 months generally required to conduct a typical full systematic review. Time is saved by limiting the scope of the literature search, having a single investigator select studies and abstract data, not evaluating sources for bias, and so on. These reviews can be useful for answering certain types of clinical and policy questions, but they do not replace full systematic reviews.[2]

Scoping reviews assess the general characteristics of a problem. They are a form of "reconnaissance" or planning done in advance of a full study to help inform its design. Scoping reviews may or may not be systematic. They often include a wider range of study designs or sources than a comparable systematic review and are less concerned with the methodological quality of the included studies or with combining them into a single result. Instead, they are concerned with what these studies can contribute to future research efforts, such as information about ranges or trends.[3]

Realist reviews are essentially systematic reviews of qualitative data from a variety of sources, including interviews, observations and published research. Their purpose is to identify, test or refine possible explanations about what interventions or programs work, in what respects, for whom, how, and in which circumstances. Traditional systematic reviews might focus on, say, a program's effectiveness, whereas realist reviews focus on why the program is or is not effective. The goal is to provide a detailed, realistic and practical understanding of complex activities that can be applied in planning and implementing programs.[4]

Systematic reviews demand the same scientific rigour required of all health research. Because they are the product of a specific research methodology, they follow many of the same principles of inquiry, and involve design and execution issues that are similar to those of other research methods. In addition, because they do not necessarily require a well-funded research infrastructure and extensive research experience, they can often be undertaken by clinicians early in their careers,[5] although the amount of time, expertise and work that a good systematic review entails should not be underestimated.

The value of systematic reviews

Systematic reviews have several purposes.[1] For example, they can be conducted to:

- summarize a large and complex body of literature on a topic;
- clarify the strengths and weaknesses of studies on a topic;
- assess the consistency of results across studies;
- identify and attempt to explain the reasons for conflicting reports in the literature;
- document the need for further study; and
- collect the data needed to plan large clinical trials, such as the expected variance of the outcome of interest, typical patient accrual rates, sources of bias, and so on.

Meta-analyses based on systematic reviews can also be useful to:

- provide a quantitative estimate of a treatment effect;
- improve the precision of an estimated treatment effect;
- detect smaller treatment effects than have been reported in individual studies; and
- investigate variations in treatment effects through subgroup (stratified) analyses.

The Cochrane Collaboration

Perhaps the single most important resource for health-related systematic reviews is the **Cochrane Collaboration**.[a] Founded in 1993 and named after the British epidemiologist Archie Cochrane, the Cochrane Collaboration is an international not-for-profit organization that supports evidence-based practice by producing, disseminating and updating systematic reviews and meta-analyses of health care interventions. Through its website and regional centres, the Collaboration offers training and resources for conducting and reporting systematic reviews[6] and provides information for researchers, clinicians, policy-makers and patients. It also maintains the Cochrane Database of Systematic Reviews, which archives systematic reviews, meta-analyses and their associated protocols. Similar databases are maintained by the University of Adelaide's Joanna Briggs Institute,[b] which archives systematic reviews and meta-analyses on health care practices and outcomes, and by the Campbell Collaboration Library of Systematic Reviews,[c] which archives systematic reviews and meta-analyses in the fields of education, crime, justice and social welfare.

---

a   See www.cochrane.org
b   See www.joannabriggs.edu.au/about/home.php
c   See www.campbellcollaboration.org/

Conducting a systematic review

Systematic reviews, by definition, are secondary, retrospective studies of original research. They should, like all studies, be rigorously designed and conducted. As are other research designs, they are subject to error, confounding and bias,[7] all of which need to be minimized through careful planning and attention to detail. The steps in conducting a systematic review are described briefly below. More detailed information on all aspects of conducting systematic reviews is available from the *Cochrane Handbook*.[6]

The research question

Systematic reviews, like other research methods, require a testable hypothesis or a focused research question. The hypothesis or research question usually has several parts—the PICOT components described in other chapters of this guide (see especially ch. 6): a **P**atient (or population) with a problem or diagnosis; the **I**ntervention, exposure, or diagnostic test to be evaluated; a **C**omparator (e.g., no treatment, placebo, standard treatment); an **O**utcome; and a **T**ime period of interest. Sometimes there is also a setting of interest (e.g., intensive care units, Japan, submarines). For example: "In varsity high-school football players (the setting and population), is athletic taping or strapping (the intervention) more effective at preventing injury or re-injury of the ankle (the outcome) than not taping (the comparator), given advances in taping technology in the past 5 years (the time frame)?"

The scope and even the feasibility of conducting a systematic review on a hypothesis can often be assessed by determining how many and what types of studies are available for review. If the literature on the question is vast, the question can be narrowed to make the review more manageable. If the literature is sparse—usually an important finding in itself—the question can be changed or the project abandoned before more resources are spent.

The research protocol

Once the hypothesis has been determined, a protocol for conducting the review must be written. The protocol should identify in detail the search strategies to be used to find articles, the eligibility criteria for selecting which articles to review, the categories of data to be abstracted from them, and the process by which differences between reviewers in article selection and data abstraction will be addressed. Increasingly, especially on journal websites and in registries, such as those managed by the Cochrane and Campbell collaborations, protocols are being published with the systematic reviews or are otherwise made available to researchers who want to further evaluate or replicate the review.

Sample selection: the search strategy

The "sample" for a systematic review—which, ideally, will be a "census" of all eligible articles of interest—usually consists of published articles from the indexed scientific literature. Other types of data can and often should be included. Sometimes referred to as **grey literature**, these sources include unpublished dissertations, technical reports and conference proceedings that may or may not have been peer reviewed. The protocol for sample selection specifies how the articles are to be identified and the criteria they must meet to be included in final sample for review.

A health sciences librarian should create, or at least assist with, the search strategy (by identifying the index terms and Boolean operators that determine how the terms will be combined) and identify the databases to be used in the literature search (see ch. 7). Although MEDLINE is the largest database of published articles in the health sciences, a thorough review will include several others, such as such as Excerpta Medica's biomedical and pharmacological database, Embase; the Cumulative Index to Nursing and Allied Health Literature (CINAHL); and the Web of Knowledge, an academic citation indexing and search service that includes thousands of scientific journals, patents and conference proceedings. Other strategies include **hand searches** (i.e., looking page by page through key print or online journals to find relevant articles), **ancestry searches** (i.e., examining the reference lists in selected articles to find other relevant studies), and **pearl-growing**, in which the key words or index terms (the "pearls") of a source article are used to locate similar articles ("growing the pearl").

The search strategy needs to be rigorous to minimize **selection bias**, or bias caused by a discrepancy between the set of all eligible studies and those that are actually identified as eligible. Studies can be missed if the search strategy is flawed, if not all relevant databases are searched, if studies published in some languages are not included, or if eligible studies are not identified because they are indexed incorrectly or inconsistently. To minimize the potential for **publication bias**—bias created by the fact that positive studies are more likely to be published than negative ones—the search strategy also often needs to include the grey literature. For example, 45% to 65% of meeting abstracts are not followed by the full reports of the studies they

Designing

represent.[8] Many of these studies may not have been published because their results were not statistically significant, and so failing to include them in a review can bias the results. For the same reason, **clinical trial registries** should be searched to determine whether the results of registered trials have been published as anticipated.

In addition to addressing the hypothesis, included studies are usually restricted to certain study designs (e.g., only randomized controlled trials), study characteristics (e.g., only studies with at least 1 year of follow-up), date of publication (e.g., within the past 5 years), populations enrolled (e.g., patients with dementia), interventions used (e.g., antidepressants), specific endpoints or outcomes (e.g., pain relief, survival), or logistical realities (e.g., the time, cost and accuracy of translating articles published in other languages).

Studies included in reviews need to be assessed for quality. This assessment used to be based on any of several more-or-less objective scales or checklists, but these are no longer recommended. The current thinking from the Cochrane Collaboration is that a subjective assessment of the risk of bias is more realistic and useful. This assessment is recorded in a **risk of bias table**, which documents the results and allows others to verify the results.[6]

To create a risk of bias table, investigators evaluate six "domains" of a study:

1. How the randomization sequence was generated (the source of random numbers)
2. How the allocation sequence (the order in which patients are to be assigned to treatment groups) was kept secret from investigators ("allocation concealment")
3. How blinding was accomplished

4. Possible bias caused by the incomplete reporting of outcome data
5. Possible bias caused by the selective reporting of outcomes
6. Other issues that pose a threat to the validity of the study

An example is how the "blinding" domain might be assessed (Table 15.1). Investigators describe specifically how each study addressed each domain (Table 15.2); develop specific criteria for judging whether the likelihood of bias is high, low, or uncertain (Table 15.3); and then assign a judgment.

These assessments can then be used to conduct **sensitivity analyses,** in which individual aspects of the review are assessed to determine how much each affects the results. If the results change markedly when studies with, say, a higher risk of bias are included in the review, the results are said to be "sensitive" to study quality, and the conclusions of the review can be interpreted, presented and even stratified accordingly.

The included studies comprise the sample and are listed in the published review, if space permits, or published online. A list of excluded articles and the reasons for their exclusion is often published as well (sometimes as an online-only appendix) or are otherwise made available to any researcher who might want to replicate or validate the review. To determine whether identified articles meet the study's inclusion criteria, each article is often assessed independently by two reviewers. Differences in choices are usually resolved by consensus or with the aid of a third party.

■ **Table 15.1: A sample description of the blinding domain in an assessment of the risk of bias**

Domain	Description	Question to be answered
Blinding of participants	Describe measures used to blind study participants and personnel from knowing the group assignment of each participant. Describe any efforts to determine whether blinding was effective.	Was knowledge of group assignment adequately prevented during the study?

■ **Table 15.2: A sample summary descriptions and comments for assessing the risk of bias in blinding**

Domain	Description
Blinding of participants	"The placebo lozenge was identical to the active treatment, save that the active ingredient had been removed."
	Comment: Blinding was clearly attempted
Blinding of participants	"Patients were blinded to group assignment."
	Comment: Side effects were pronounced enough to eliminate any effectiveness of blinding

■ **Table 15.3: Sample criteria for determining the degree of possible bias in the blinding domain**

Risk of bias	Criteria for assessing the risk of bias
High	Blinding is possible and desirable but not reported
Low	Blinding is described in detail and its effectiveness is confirmed at the end of the study
Unclear	Blinding is claimed but details are not provided; other research by these authors has used blinding successfully.

Data collection

When the articles to be included in the review have been identified, the specified data are abstracted from each of them, usually by two or more trained abstractors working independently with a standardized and pre-tested data form. A third rater is often necessary to resolve any differences in the values abstracted by the primary raters. As a result, **inter-rater** and **intra-rater agreement** is usually assessed to identify any possible bias created by differences in judgment.

Data abstraction is not necessary straightforward. For example, although the size of the treatment and control groups may be readily apparent, the proportion of males and females or the number of patients actually completing certain phases of the trial might have to be computed from other numbers. Also, key data are often missing and cannot be obtained from the study authors.

Data analysis and interpretation

Once abstracted, the data are organized into one or more **evidence tables**. Typically, evidence tables in systematic reviews may show more qualitative data (Table. 15.4), whereas tables in meta-analyses may show more quantitative data (Table. 15.5). Once organized into evidence tables, the data can be interpreted in the context of data from similar studies, providing a more evidence-based form of interpretation than is possible in traditional narrative reviews. Under some circumstances, the numerical results of the individual studies can be pooled statistically in a meta-analysis to help further interpret the results. If so, the results are often presented in a characteristic **forest plot** that shows the estimates and confidence intervals for the individual studies as well as the pooled estimate and its confidence interval (Fig 15.1).

In addition, the variation among studies is often assessed statistically with measures such as Cochran's Q (or Cochran's chi-square) test or I^2, to determine whether it is within the range expected by chance or whether it indicates **heterogeneity** among the study results; that is, whether the observed variation among study results is greater than expected by chance.[9] For example, I^2 ranges between 0% and 100%, with lower values indicating less heterogeneity. Results found to be significantly heterogeneous usually warrant further examination, often through planned subgroup analyses, in an effort to identify potential explanations. When heterogeneity is high among studies, their results are usually not combined. In any event, systematic reviews and meta-analyses require competent statistical support, which, as in all research, should be sought before the research is planned in detail.

Designing

■ **Table 15.4: An evidence table showing qualitative data from a systematic review of the effects of nurse staffing on institutional financial outcomes**

Study (year)	Internal validity Design Duration (mo) Potential bias*	External validity Age of data Hospitals (n) Nurse units (n) Patients (n)	Effects on institutional financial outcomes	Clinical grade† Statistical grade‡
Collins 1981	Prospective 10 High	1989 1 1 –	**Changing from team nursing to all RN staffing, mean h/d of nursing sick leave dropped from 1.24 to 0.48 h/d** (*P* = 0.02). p. 35	1 1
			Changing from a team model of nursing to all RN staffing, mean h/d of overtime dropped from 0.79 to 0.39 h/d (*P* not reported). p. 35	1 ?
Brett 1993	Prospective 9 Moderate	1981 1 3 –	**A 17% reduction in RN minutes/patient/shift (16 min, from 96 to 80 min), after moving to team nursing, lowered average acuity-adjusted costs per patient day by $8, $13 and $88 on the 3 nursing units** (*P* < 0.04). p. 39	1 1
Harrison 1983	Prospective 10 Low	1985 1 3 –	**Nursing model (skill mix) had no significant effect on total cost/patient day.** The mean cost was $22.12 on the Primary Nursing unit (100% RN), $21.59 on the Modular Nursing unit (50% RN/ 50% LPN), and $20.19 on the Team Nursing unit (50% RN/ 25% LPN/ 25% aides) (*P* not reported). p. 180	0 0

* Potential bias was graded as moderate unless the presence or absence of a design or analytic feature seemed to make the study more or less subject to bias.

† Three investigators independently graded the clinical importance of each finding. Differences were resolved in discussion. 0 = the finding was not considered to be clinically important; ? = the finding may or may not be clinically important; 1 = the finding was considered to be clinically important.

‡ Statistical grades: 0 = The *P* value was > 0.05, was not reported, or the results were described as not being statistically significant.

1 = The *P* value was < 0.05, or the results were described as being statistically significant.

RN = registered nurse; LPN = licensed practical nurse

■ **Table 15.5: An evidence table showing qualitative data from a systematic review of the effects of nurse staffing on institutional financial outcomes**

Study (year) Notes	Control group			Treatment group			Difference between rates, %
	n	Drop-outs	Event rate, % (n/n)	n	Drop-outs	Event rate, % (n/n)	
Early cancer							
Aaron (1989) Isolated disease	74	14	8 (5/61)	78	8	17 (11/63)	−9
Carty (1990) Isolated disease	23	3	10 (2/20)	27	2	12 (3/25)	−2
Edwards (1990) Comorbid disease	82	6	7 (5/76)	79	4	8 (6/75)	−1
Advanced cancer							
Fellow (1991) Comorbid disease	31	9	9 (2/22)	31	6	4 (1/25)	5
Halleron (1992) Isolated disease	55	7	2 (1/48)	51	4	4 (2/47)	−2

Designing

Figure 15.1: A fictitious example of a **forest plot** showing the point estimates (the closed squares) and the 95% confidence intervals (the horizontal lines) for individual studies in a meta-analysis. Smaller studies have wider confidence intervals (indicating less precise estimates), and larger ones have narrower intervals (indicating more precise estimates). The pooled estimate (the open diamond) reflects the pooled sample sizes and thus has the narrowest confidence interval. The area of each square is proportional to the number of events in the study. A risk ratio of 1 means that the risk of the treatment group is the same as that of the control group. Values less than 1 indicate a reduced risk in the treatment group, and values greater than 1 indicate an increased risk. When the outcome is expressed as a risk ratio, confidence intervals that cross 1 indicate that that result was not statistically significant at the 0.05 level. The confidence interval for the pooled estimate shown does not cross 1, indicating a statistically significant overall result.

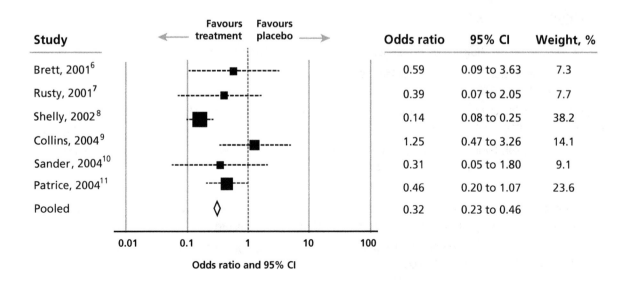

Study		Odds ratio	95% CI	Weight, %
Brett, 2001[6]		0.59	0.09 to 3.63	7.3
Rusty, 2001[7]		0.39	0.07 to 2.05	7.7
Shelly, 2002[8]		0.14	0.08 to 0.25	38.2
Collins, 2004[9]		1.25	0.47 to 3.26	14.1
Sander, 2004[10]		0.31	0.05 to 1.80	9.1
Patrice, 2004[11]		0.46	0.20 to 1.07	23.6
Pooled		0.32	0.23 to 0.46	

Odds ratio and 95% CI

The review can also include a **summary of findings table**, which presents the main findings of a review as well as indications of the quality of evidence, the magnitude of the treatment effect and the sum of available data on the main outcomes.[6] In addition, the Grades of Recommendation, Assessment, Development, and Evaluation (GRADE) ranking system can be used to indicate the general quality of the findings in a systematic review or meta-analysis.[6]

Publication of the results

The final stage of any research is publication. The **PRISMA Statement**[10] presents guidelines for reporting systematic reviews and meta-analyses of randomized controlled trials, and the **MOOSE Statement**[11] presents guidelines for reporting systematic reviews and meta-analyses of observational studies. Many journals require that these guidelines be followed as a condition of publication.

Conclusion

For clinicians focused on patient care, conducting systematic reviews can provide an in-depth understanding of a topic that will support clinical decision-making. For researchers, conducting systematic reviews can provide an in-depth understanding of the current knowledge about a topic and can be an important first step in planning original research studies. Systematic reviews will make both of these groups of health professionals familiar with the literature on the topic: who is publishing in this area; what endpoints are commonly assessed; what sources of error, confounding and bias need to be considered; and what results tend to be common. Finally, systematic reviews can be relatively inexpensive to conduct and can provide even new investigators the opportunity to make important contributions to the literature. ■

CASE POSTSCRIPT

Working with a medical librarian, the student designs a strategy for searching the literature. The search identifies 2897 titles. After screening the abstracts of these articles, the student decides to retrieve 490, 43 of which meet the inclusion criteria she and her supervisor have identified. She then abstracts data on the same variables from these articles, organizes the data into a series of evidence tables, and compares the results of all 43 studies. Examining the evidence tables, she notes that all studies had adjusted for patient case mix and nursing skill mix. She finds some evidence that richer nurse staffing is associated with lower failure-to-rescue rates, lower inpatient mortality rates, and shorter hospital stays. Further, total nursing hours and skill mix do appear to affect some important patient outcomes.

REFERENCES

1. Lang TA, Secic M, editors. *How to report statistics in medicine.* 2nd ed. Philadelphia (PA): American College of Physicians; 2006.
2. Watt A, Cameron A, Sturm L, Lathlean T, Babidge W, Blamey S, et al. Rapid versus full systematic reviews: validity in clinical practice? *ANZ J Surg.* 2008;78(11):1037–40.
3. Rumrill PD, Fitzgerald SM, Merchant WR. Using scoping literature reviews as a means of understanding and interpreting existing literature. *Work.* 2010;35(3):399–404.
4. Pawson R, Greenhalgh T, Harvey G, Walshe K. Realist review–a new method of systematic review designed for complex policy interventions. *J Health Serv Res Policy.* 2005;10 Suppl 1:21–34.
5. Lang T. Systematic reviews as research assignments for training physicians. *Acad Med.* 2004;79:1067–72.
6. Higgins JPT, Green S, editors. *Cochrane Handbook for Systematic Reviews of Interventions* Version 5.1.0 [updated March 2011]. The Cochrane Collaboration. 2011. Available from: www.cochrane-handbook.org
7. Olsen O, Middleton P, Ezzo J, Gøtzsche PC, Hadhazy V, Herxheimer A, et al. Quality of Cochrane reviews: assessment of sample from 1998. *BMJ.* 2001;323(7317):829–32.

8. Scherer RW, Langenberg P, von Elm E. Full publication of results initially presented in abstracts. Cochrane Database Syst Rev. 2007 Apr 18;(2):MR000005.

9. Higgins JP, Thompson SG, Deeks JJ, Altman DG. Measuring inconsistency in meta-analyses. *BMJ*. 2003;327(7414):557–60.

10. Moher D, Liberati A, Tetzlaff J, Altman DG; PRISMA Group. Preferred reporting items for systematic reviews and meta-analyses: the PRISMA Statement. *PLoS Med*. 2009;6(7):e1000097.

11. Stroup DF, Berlin JA, Morton SC, Olkin I, Williamson GD, Rennie D, et al.; Meta-analysis of Observational Studies in Epidemiology (MOOSE) Group. Meta-analysis of observational studies in epidemiology: a proposal for reporting. *JAMA*. 2000;283(15):2008–12.

ADDITIONAL RESOURCES

Barza M, Trikalinos TA, Lau J. Statistical considerations in meta-analysis. *Infect Dis Clin North Am*. 2009;23(2):195–210.

Callcut RA, Branson RD. How to read a review paper. *Respir Care*. 2009;54(10):1379–85.

- A good overview regarding completing and critiquing "review papers."

Centre for Reviews and Dissemination. *Systematic reviews: CRD's guidance for undertaking reviews in health care*. York (UK): University of York; 2009. Available from: www.york.ac.uk/inst/crd/pdf/Systematic_Reviews.pdf

Crumley ET, Wiebe N, Cramer K, Klassen TP, Hartling L. Which resources should be used to identify RCT/CCTs for systematic reviews: a systematic review. *BMC Med Res Methodol*. 2005 Aug 10;5:24.

Egger M, Davey Smith G, Altman D, editors. *Systematic reviews in health care: meta-analysis in context*. London: BMJ Books, 1995.

- A dated but excellent source of information on systematic reviews.

Equator Network: Enhancing the QUAlity and Transparency Of health Research. Available from: www.equator-network.org/.

- This site has links to guidelines for reporting studies using any of several research designs.

Higgins J, Thompson S, Deeks J, Altman D. Statistical heterogeneity in systematic reviews of clinical trials: a critical appraisal of guidelines and practice. *J Health Serv Res Policy*. 2002;7(1):51–61.

Hunt M. *How science takes stock: the story of meta-analysis*. New York: Russell Sage Foundation; 1997.

- A good history of systematic reviews and their application in several areas.

Ioannidis JPA, Lau J. The impact of high-risk patients on the population risk and on the population treatment effect. *J Clin Epidemiol*. 1997;50:1089–98.

Ioannidis JP, Lau J. Pooling research results: benefits and limitations of meta-analysis. *Jt Comm J Qual Improv*. 1999;25(9):462–9.

Ioannidis JP, Lau J. State of the evidence: current status and prospects of meta-analysis in infectious diseases. *Clin Infect Dis*. 1999;29(5):1178–85.

Jüni P, Altman DG, Egger M. Systematic reviews in health care: assessing the quality of controlled clinical trials. *BMJ*. 2001;323(7303):42–6.

Jüni P, Witschi A, Bloch R, Egger M. The hazards of scoring the quality of clinical trials for meta-analysis. *JAMA*. 1999;282(11):1054–60.

Khan KS, Kunz R, Kleijnen J, Antes G. Five steps to conducting a systematic review. *J R Soc Med*. 2003;96(3):118–21.

Manchikanti L, Datta S, Smith HS, Hirsch JA. Evidence-based medicine, systematic reviews, and guidelines in interventional pain management: part 6. Systematic reviews and meta-analyses of observational studies. *Pain Physician*. 2009;12(5):819–50.

Margaliot Z, Chung KC. Systematic reviews: a primer for plastic surgery research. *Plast Reconstr Surg*. 2007;120(7):1834–41.

Sagoo GS, Little J, Higgins JPT. Systematic reviews of genetic association studies. *PLoS Med*. 2009;6(3):e1000028.

Simon SD. *Statistical evidence in medical trials: What do the data really tell us?* Oxford: Oxford University Press; 2006.

- See especially chapter 5, on systematic overviews and meta-analysis.

Designing

Sweet M, Moynihan R. *Improving population health: the uses of systematic reviews*. New York: Milbank Memorial Fund and Centers for Disease Control and Prevention; 2007.

Treadwell JR, Tregear SJ, Reston JT, Turkelson CM. A system for rating the stability and strength of medical evidence. *BMC Med Res Methodol*. 2006 Oct 19;6:52.

Wallace BC, Schmid CH, Lau J, Trikalinos TA. Meta-Analyst: software for meta-analysis of binary, continuous and diagnostic data. *BMC Med Res Methodol*. 2009 Dec 4;9:80.

Yuan Y, Hunt RH. Systematic reviews: the good, the bad, and the ugly. *Am J Gastroenterol*. 2009;104(5):1086–92.

Zwahlen M, Renehan A, Egger M. Meta-analysis in medical research: potentials and limitations. *Urol Oncol*. 2008;26(3):320–9.

Designing

EXERCISE: ASSESSMENT QUESTIONS

1. What is the difference between a narrative review and a systematic review?

2. What is the difference between a systematic review and a meta-analysis?

3. What are the PRISMA and MOOSE statements?

4. How is quality assessment of studies used in a systematic review?

5. What is the Cochrane Collaboration?

SUMMARY CHECKLIST

❑ Thinking about your research topic, list the ways in which a systematic review would be useful.
❑ Do the same for a narrative review.
❑ Using the PICOT framework, select a specific question to explore in a systematic review.
❑ What kind of question will you choose? Why?
❑ Write a detailed systematic review research protocol, including your search strategy and sources. Refine it with the help of a librarian or methodologist.
❑ Pilot your search. Refine again.
❑ Conduct your search.
❑ Carefully label the records you find, using a system to track each one.
❑ Screen your initial results for relevance, following your a priori criteria for further in-depth review. Flag results that are relevant background material for your later write-up of the project.
❑ Screen your included results in more detail and keep those that meet all your criteria.
❑ Analyze your data according to your plan.
❑ Report your findings, keeping in mind published guidelines for the reporting of systematic reviews.

16
An introduction to qualitative research

June C. Carroll, MD, CCFP

Fiona Alice Miller, MA, PhD

ILLUSTRATIVE CASE

A resident notices that the staff physicians in her clinic take differing approaches to the management of diabetes, and that not all follow the most recent guidelines of the Canadian Diabetes Association. She would like to understand how physicians feel about clinical practice guidelines and how they decide whether or not to use them. It seems to her that the best way to approach these questions would be through a qualitative study, but she has no experience with this kind of research. She would like to know more about qualitative methodology and how it can be applied.

The first and most important step in undertaking a research project is to formulate a research question. Whatever that question may be, it should inspire your curiosity and intellectual passion, for you will be expending a great deal of time and energy in the effort to answer it. It is also important to determine what methodology offers the best approach to your question. This chapter will help you determine whether a qualitative approach is suited to your research project.

What is qualitative research?

Qualitative research helps us understand social phenomena, including beliefs, behaviours, practices and interactions.[1] Whereas quantitative research attempts to measure phenomena, to identify quantity and size, or to investigate the cause-and-effect relationships between measured phenomena, qualitative research examines the "What?" "Why?" and "How?" of the social world: the meanings people make of their experiences, and the nature and social significance of their actions.[2] It is a naturalistic approach that studies people and social processes as they are, rather than under experimental conditions. Qualitative research gathers data from and about people using interviews, focus groups, observation (participant and non-participant), document analysis and related techniques.[3] Qualitative research is defined by the use of an inductive approach to analysis (although deductive strategies can also be used), drawing on multiple or rich accounts to describe a phenomenon or to generate theories or hypotheses about it.

CHAPTER OBJECTIVES

After reading this chapter, you should be able to:
- list the types of research questions most appropriate for qualitative research;
- identify ways to conduct a qualitative study, either as an independent project or in tandem with a quantitative study;
- describe qualitative methodologies and methods, together with their advantages and disadvantages;
- identify approaches to qualitative data analysis; and
- list techniques to ensure credibility in qualitative research.

KEY TERMS

Case studies	Grounded theory	Redundancy
Document analysis	Immersion/crystallization	Reflexivity
Ethnography	In-depth interviews	Sampling
Field observation	Participant observation	Writing as a method of inquiry
Focus groups	Qualitative description	

When should you use a qualitative approach?

In deciding whether a qualitative methodology offers the best approach to your research question, consider the following:

- Qualitative research can be used to explore phenomena and generate theories about them, or to describe or evaluate initiatives such as policies, programs or organizational developments.
- Qualitative research can be used to supplement quantitative work, to bring detail to or illuminate findings, or to help explain unexpected or confusing results (e.g., studies with negative results, low response rates or high drop-out rates).
- Qualitative approaches are often the best choice for the study of "social or psychological phenomena such as behaviours, motivations, perceptions and expectations."[1] They are used when social context is seen as important.
- Qualitative research is sometimes undertaken in advance of a quantitative study to explore the meaning of phenomena, determine how the issues under study are perceived, identify useful outcome measures, generate hypotheses, suggest the existence of confounding factors, or develop relevant and answerable survey questions.

Philosophical orientation

The rise of qualitative research methodologies has been accompanied by a great deal of discussion and debate about the nature of the knowledge they generate. Quantitative researchers have sometimes been skeptical of the value of qualitative research, while some qualitative researchers have argued that their research adopts a perspective toward knowledge that is incommensurate with quantitative methods, rendering mixed-method approaches impossible.[4] The polarization of these views has diminished over time, and health services and clinical researchers are increasingly attuned to the contributions that qualitative approaches can make. Nevertheless, debates continue about the extent to which qualitative research requires a specific philosophical orientation and a commitment to a specific theoretical framework.[3]

All researchers can benefit from exploring the philosophy of science and the particular role of their own work in constructing knowledge. However, for the purposes of this chapter we take the pragmatic view that qualitative methods can generate useful and transferable knowledge about the social world, both alone and in combination with quantitative approaches, and that this can be done without sustained philosophical attention to the nature of knowledge and reality.[5] However, for those interested in a fuller discussion of the theoretical underpinnings of qualitative research, the work by Greene,[4] Cohen and Crabtree,[6] Mays and Pope,[7] Glanz and colleagues[8] and Teddlie and Tashakkori[9] provides a good starting-point.

Qualitative research methodologies

Once you have decided that qualitative research is the best way to answer your research question, it is important to choose which specific approach to use. Different methodological frameworks are useful for answering different sorts of questions[3] and will guide the particular methods you use in data collection and analysis. Consider how different types of questions are addressed by different qualitative approaches:

1. **What is the culture of this group?** This type of question is often addressed through the research methodology called **ethnography**, which involves "studies of the values, beliefs and practices of groups."[1] The method typically used is **participant observation**, by which the researcher is present in the phenomenon being studied and records his or her observations in detailed field notes. As an example, this methodology might be used to understand the way of life of first-year residents in a particular specialty. The goal would be to understand the behaviours and beliefs that characterize the culture of the group. The analysis moves beyond description to "reveal or explain social patterns or observed conduct."[1] This method is quite time-intensive, as it typically involves "lengthy participation or immersion in the everyday life of a chosen setting."[10]

2. **What is going on here?** Questions of this type are sometimes examined through **case studies**, which examine complex phenomena in context. A "case" might be an individual, a program, an organization, a community or region, or an event. By providing a holistic and detailed look at single or multiple cases, these studies help to explain how contextual factors shape the phenomena being studied. Case studies typically use multiple data sources, including inter-

Designing

views, observation and documents, and are often presented as a narrative description. They can also incorporate quantitative data.[11,12] Case studies are commonly used in evaluative or policy analysis research; examples would be a study of the introduction of a new funding model for primary care (e.g., capitation) that explores staff expectations and experiences, change processes, and influences on implementation and outcomes.[5,13]

3. **What does this experience mean?** Various qualitative approaches (e.g., grounded theory, phenomenology, ethnomethodology) seek to explore how people experience the world and the meaning they make of it. An example of this type of study might be an analysis of prenatal screening that aims to explore how women understand screening, what it means to them and how it affects the experience and social process of pregnancy or motherhood. Interviews or focus groups are typical techniques used within this approach.

Qualitative methods: Which is appropriate?

The specific methods you use for data collection and analysis in a qualitative study should be appropriate to the research question and your particular methodologic framework. Data may derive from observation, in-depth interviews, focus groups, documents, or a combination thereof.

- **Field observation** is used to "record social phenomena directly and prospectively."[14] The observer can be a participant in the phenomenon under study (participant-observer) or a non-participant. In either case, the researcher spends time in the environment under study and records observations and interactions in field notes.
- **In-depth interviews** may be chosen when the research question requires detailed probing of feelings or behaviours, or when the researcher is exploring particularly sensitive experiences that informants may be more willing to discuss privately than in a more open setting. For example, individual interviews might be used to understand why physicians don't follow certain practice guidelines. Individual interviews can also be used for practical reasons: for example, key informants can be interviewed in their own offices at a time convenient to them.

- **Focus groups** are often used as a means of data collection if the research question is likely to evoke a range of views and the researcher wants to elicit interaction, debate and rich discussion among participants about the research question. Because of their more public nature, focus groups provide insight into shared meanings and beliefs but can make it difficult to delve into individual or contrary experiences. Focus groups require a facilitator skilled in managing group dynamics.
- **Document analysis** can include the examination of records of organizations (e.g., meeting minutes, annual reports), individuals (diaries, blogs), or groups (newsletters, newspapers, websites). These can be used to help explain the context for a case or the culture of a group, or to elicit feedback from an individual about her or his experiences (e.g., using an educational brochure to elicit reactions from women to their experience of prenatal screening). Researchers must think through their reasons for selecting certain documents and not others, and how they should read and interpret their content in light of what is known of their origin or history.

Qualitative methods: Collecting data
Field observation

The researcher engaged in field observation spends time in a "natural" setting—that is, a setting in which the phenomena under study actually take place. By doing so, the researcher can experience, explore and seek to represent the social life and social processes of that setting. Further, the duration and frequency of the researcher's on-site presence can foster the development of a respectful relationship and rapport with people in that setting. Data are collected through extensive field notes written on a regular basis to capture phenomena as they occur or shortly thereafter. In ethnographic studies, researchers interview people in their setting; although these interviews share features with qualitative interviewing more generally, the ongoing contact and emerging rapport characteristic of the ethnographic approach give the researcher an opportunity to conduct repeated interviews that enable a rich "exchange of views."[15]

Interviews and focus groups

In-depth interviews are usually conducted only once per individual and last from 30 minutes to several hours.[16] They typi-

Designing

cally involve one respondent, although pairs or small groups might be interviewed in cases where this is more comfortable for the respondents (e.g., a married couple, a key informant with a helper). It is important for the interviewer to rapidly develop a rapport with the interviewee. Researchers who choose this approach would benefit from reading about techniques to achieve the various stages of rapport.[16–20]

Focus groups ideally comprise 6 to 8 people; groups with fewer than 5 participants tend not to generate enough interaction, and groups of more than 10 will usually not give each participant enough time to speak. Answering a research question will usually require 4 to 6 focus groups, and a minimum of 4 is usually needed to reach redundancy or saturation (see definition in section on sampling). Focus groups usually last from 1 to 2 hours.

Conducting an interview/focus group. Interview and focus group discussions are typically "semi-structured," meaning that they are loosely organized around a series of questions that define an area to be explored. Questions should be open-ended to encourage discussion; questions that can be answered with a "yes" or "no" are to be avoided. Questions should also be sensitive and clear, and should not inadvertently suggest an expected answer. It is important that the interviewer/facilitator enable participants to go below the surface in their commentary and explore the phenomenon in detail. The interviewer/facilitator should probe the participants' meaning, rather than taking it at face value. Questions such as "Tell me more about …" or "Can you tell me what you mean by …" can be helpful to richly explore the topic. The interviewer/facilitator should try not to talk very much, focusing instead on facilitating the conversation of others. It is important to ensure that everyone has a chance to speak on a topic, to be accepting of divergent opinions, and to not assume agreement.

Researchers should develop a guide listing relevant questions and probes to help organize the interview or focus group. In some situations, these guides can be circulated before the session, for example to enable key informants to gather relevant materials that can better inform the discussion. Open discussion during an interview or focus group session is conducive to eliciting answers to questions about behaviour or experiences, opinions, beliefs, and feelings, but it is less suited to obtaining answers to questions about factual matters or demographics. Such questions are often included in a short questionnaire administered to participants either before or after the interview or focus group session.

Interviews and focus groups are typically recorded on audiotape, so that discussions can be transcribed in full. A good recording system is therefore essential, and a back-up system is advised: technical failure has resulted in the loss of many a researcher's data. In addition, researchers should make notes on important points, thoughts, and the mood or tone of responses, as well as on non-verbal behaviour, as these field notes can complement the analysis.

In interviews or focus group sessions, it is important to consider participants' needs and convenience; attention should be given to practical considerations such as parking, child care, an accessible location, refreshments, and reimbursement for time, expenses, etc.

Sampling

Although participants for qualitative research can be obtained through random sampling, it is more common to use "purposive sampling"—that is, to recruit participants from groups whose views or experiences the researcher anticipates will be relevant to the phenomenon under study.[1,21,22] Purposive sampling often involves "maximum variation sampling," which aims to maximize the range of types of informants by relevant criteria (e.g., age, gender, race, socioeconomic status, urban or rural location, organizational affiliation, occupation, social role, etc). It might also be important to sample for "extreme" cases, "typical" or "ideal" cases, or "negative" cases that are the "exception to the rule."[22] Sampling strategies depend on the research question and will sometimes need revision as the research progresses. Theoretical sampling involves efforts to purposefully recruit respondents who can address issues the researcher identifies in the data collected to that point, to explore them in more detail, or to confirm or deny their relevance.

An alternative to purposive sampling is convenience sampling, in which the pool of potential participants is so small or so difficult to access that the researcher recruits those who are available. This is often the case for "key informants"—that is, individuals who play a significant role or have special knowledge about the phenomenon under study, such as key policy-makers, program directors and others.[16] In these cases, a "snowball" sampling strategy may be used, wherein future potential respondents are identified by existing participants. Whatever sampling technique you choose, it is critical to justify your choice and to provide a full description of your sampling strategy in the methods section of your research report.

In contrast to quantitative methodology, there is often no predetermined sample size in qualitative research. Data collection and analysis usually occur iteratively, such that the analysis of the initial interviews, focus groups or field notes informs subsequent data collection efforts. Researchers read and analyze data as they are generated, consider the findings, and highlight topics that need clarification or questioning in further depth.[23] This ongoing analysis informs subsequent data collection—that is, both the sampling and the questions being asked.[16] Interview or focus group guides are often modified as a result of this process. In addition, sampling strategies often become more theoretical. Sampling stops when there is **redundancy** on core issues—that is, no new trends or themes are being uncovered and a thorough understanding of the phenomenon under study has been reached. This is called "saturation." As a rule of thumb, Guest and colleagues[24] suggest that 6 to 12 interviews will be needed when the sample comprises a relatively homogeneous group.

Analyzing qualitative data

Data, data preparation and data organization

Data for a qualitative study typically consist of audio- or videotapes of interviews or focus groups, transcripts of those tapes, field notes made by the researcher, documents collected by the research team, and notes taken during the ongoing analysis meetings.

To aid analysis, interviews and focus group sessions should be transcribed word for word, with wide margins for coding, one line space between each speaker, individual speakers identified by code such as letters or numbers, lines and pages numbered, and the date and place of the interview or focus group clearly noted.

Some researchers use computer software programs such as Ethnograph (Qualis Research, Colorado Springs, Colo.) or NVivo (QSR International, Cambridge, Mass.) to assist with data management. These programs do not perform the analysis but help with data organization and basic coding and retrieval of data. Sections of text can be grouped under coded categories or themes for ease of review or cross-referencing.

Data analysis

Broadly speaking, qualitative data analysis involves efforts to synthesize and make sense of a volume of qualitative material to reveal "core consistencies and meanings."[5]

Qualitative data analysis generally involves inductive reasoning to identify patterns, themes and categories in the data. With an inductive approach, findings emerge from the interaction between the researcher and the data, rather than being deduced using an existing framework. Although inductive strategies are typical, qualitative researchers may also use deductive approaches to test theories or hypotheses, or a mix of inductive and deductive strategies, in which sensitizing concepts or theories are used alongside more open explorations of the data to search for new patterns or thematic interpretations.

The key analytic strategy is classification to identify patterns, categories or themes and code the data accordingly. The process is iterative: initial classification schemes are refined through ongoing review and analysis of the data.

Common features of qualitative analysis

In line with the work of Miles and Huberman,[25] the basic tasks of qualitative analysis can be categorized as follows:

- assigning codes to field notes or transcripts;
- writing any remarks in margins;
- identifying similar phrases, themes, patterns and differences;
- taking these commonalities and differences and themes back into the field for further data collection;
- gradually constructing themes or generalizations that describe the patterns in the data; and
- comparing these generalizations against constructs or theories.

The various approaches used in qualitative data analysis reflect different theoretical assumptions. They vary by the degree to which the researcher seeks to make inferences about the data: for example, low-inference interpretations stay close to the data, while high-inference interpretations seek to generate wider conclusions, typically through the development of conceptual frameworks or theories. Analytic approaches also differ by the extent to which the researcher draws on a pre-existing set of ideas, concepts or hypotheses in the data analysis: purely inductive approaches seek to limit their reliance on pre-structured analytics, while mixed inductive/deductive approaches use pre-structured themes or theories as sensitizing concepts or hypotheses to facilitate the analytic process. A further difference is the degree to which the analysis is formalized through an

Designing

analytic method or technique; some approaches recommend specific sets of analytic procedures, while others offer less formal guidance and rely more explicitly on the researcher's expertise and insight.

An example of a low-inference analytic strategy is **qualitative description**. This approach aims to provide "a comprehensive summary of events in the everyday terms of those events."[26] Interpretation stays close to the data, rather than generating more abstract or theoretical interpretations. Among high-inference analytic strategies, **grounded theory** encourages the use of a strictly inductive approach to build theory, rather than describing events or testing theory; further, grounded theory involves a systematic set of analytic steps through a process of constant comparison, including various types of classification or "coding" to identify, group and select themes and then build typologies and theories.[27–29] Other high-inference approaches offer less technical guidance about the analytic process. Proponents of **writing as a method of inquiry** recommend close engagement with the data through the process of constructing a written text. Similarly, **immersion/crystallization**[16,30] requires that "the analyst repeatedly immerses him or herself into the text in reflective cycles until interpretations intuitively crystallize."[16]

The readings suggested at the end of the chapter provide more detailed information on qualitative methods of analysis.

Ensuring quality in qualitative research

There is much debate about how to evaluate the quality of qualitative research. Many researchers (especially in Europe) endorse the concepts of reliability and validity, while others (especially in North America) suggest that a comprehensive assessment of trustworthiness is more appropriate. Whatever terms are used, we would emphasize the importance of rigour in the design and conduct of the research to ensure quality, rather than solely the use of evaluative criteria that assess the relevance or transferability of the findings once the research is complete.[31] Thus, the quality of qualitative research depends on the careful use of an appropriate study design, including data sources, sampling strategies, data collection methods and analytic approaches. It relies also on the expertise and integrity of the researcher, and the researcher's understanding and appreciation of the nature and limits of qualitative inquiry.

Researchers should strive to produce a plausible and coherent analysis of the phenomenon being studied. In addition, it is important to describe the study design in sufficient detail in any publication or presentation, so that another trained researcher could be confident that the steps in the data collection and analysis process were rigorous and fair, and that the findings were sound and supportable.

Because the quality of qualitative research depends on the ability of the researcher, it is essential for researchers to exercise what is called **reflexivity**, the "recognition of the influence a researcher brings to the research process."[22] Researchers must be aware of their use of theory or sensitizing concepts, and of any biases or preconceived ideas about the results of the research that they bring to the process. In fact, to make these biases transparent, qualitative researchers may wish to include (and journal editors may require) an explicit description of the researchers' background and preconceived ideas regarding the topic under study and how these perspectives may have potentially influenced the conduct, analysis and reporting of the study. In addition, the researcher needs to give thought to power relationships between himself/herself and the study participants and to differences in gender, ethnicity and socioeconomic status that might influence the research question, methodology or analysis.[16,22] For example, women living in shelters who have experienced intimate partner violence might find it difficult to share their experiences of medical care with physician-researchers, whom they may perceive as having idyllic relationships and as being from a different social class.

Several techniques are used in qualitative research to help safeguard the quality of the research findings.[6] Journal reviewers will look for the following techniques, which should be built into your methods and analysis where appropriate.

- **Audit trail.** Clearly document all stages in your research process, including decision points and insights that you gain along the way.
- **Methods.** Clearly explain and justify the methods you used to generate data; you may need to explain why, for example, you preferred a focus group to an interview strategy.
- **Sampling strategy and size.** Present a clear argument to justify your sampling strategy. This will include discussion of the type of sampling (purposive, convenience), the rationale for your selection or exclusion of certain types of individuals, organizations

or documents, as well as a justification of the size of your study sample. You will likely need to explain how you arrived at the redundancy or saturation of data.

- **Quality of analysis**
  - To minimize researcher bias and enrich the analysis, have several members of the research team code the data independently and meet to discuss emerging themes.
  - If anything seems unclear in the analysis, collect more data to try to understand the phenomenon; this will mean going back to the transcripts or to the participants themselves for clarification.
  - During the data collection and analysis phases of your research, actively look for "negative" cases or "outliers" that run counter to emerging themes, which might require you to modify or revisit your analysis. This is sometimes called "confirming-disconfirming sampling."[22]
  - Support key findings with quotations from transcripts or field notes in your research report.
- **Triangulation.** The use of multiple approaches can strengthen a study. Triangulation can involve the use of multiple sources for data relevant to the research question (i.e., documents, charts, interviews, literature) and looking for convergence or support for emerging theories.[6] It can also involve the use of multiple methods, investigators or theoretical perspectives.[5]
  - In health research, it is common to pursue triangulation through multidisciplinarity, by including members from a range of disciplines on your research team to bring a range of vantage points to the interpretation of data and enhance your analysis.
- **Member checking**
  - Where appropriate, present your findings to the study participants (or a sample) to determine whether your findings and interpretations ring true to them.[1]

Ethical considerations

As with all research involving human subjects, ethical approval from a Research Ethics Board is required for a qualitative study. Qualitative data often consist of personal reports of experiences or key informants' distinct professional experiences. There may therefore be a particular need

for attention to privacy and confidentiality issues, as careless reporting could mean that research participants are identifiable by an informed observer even though they are not named.

Writing a qualitative paper

Qualitative papers can be written in accordance with the conventional IMRAD structure of scientific publications: Introduction, Methods, Results, Analysis and Discussion, although the Results section is often termed Findings in qualitative research. When written for non-medical and non-scientific journals, qualitative papers often dispense with the IMRAD sequence in favour of a more thematic or narrative approach; for example, it is not uncommon to see findings reviewed alongside a discussion of their meaning and significance. In addition, such papers are often longer; for example, they may include extensive quotations from the primary data, and may incorporate a more detailed discussion of the relevant theoretical literature. Some recent examples of qualitative research papers are outlined in Table 16.1. These papers highlight different aspects of qualitative research methods or analysis and provide examples of how to conduct qualitative research projects and write up the results.

Evaluating the quality of your report

Various authors offer tips on ensuring that your research report is as rigorous as possible and will stand up to the scrutiny of journal editors.[1,6,7,22] As you assess the quality of your work, consider the following questions:

- **Introduction**
  - Is the research question stated clearly?
  - Have you explained why your research question is important and what new information your study will provide?
- **Methods**
  - Have you justified your decision to use a qualitative approach?
  - Have you justified your sample selection and described your sampling technique?
    - Do you explain clearly how the study participants were selected?
    - Do you explain why the range of cases or settings was appropriate?
  - Was the methodologic approach described in sufficient detail that the reader would be able

Designing

Designing

■ **Table 16.1: Examples of qualitative research papers**

Citation	Method	Comment
Lau et al.[32] Patients' adherence to osteoporosis therapy: exploring the perceptions of postmenopausal women	Focus groups	Good example of iterative process of methodology and analysis. Provides a good description of steps taken to ensure rigour (minimization of researcher bias, and triangulation); good demonstration of analytical method (development of code book; use of qualitative data retrieval computer program); and good presentation of findings (factors influencing adherence and adherence strategies are mapped onto medication-taking process).
Lee et al.[33] Exploring family physician stress: helpful strategies	Interviews	Provides a good description of technique used for purposive and maximum-variation sampling; good analysis and discussion using systems theory; good use of figures to illustrate findings.
Pottie et al.[34] Integrating pharmacists into family practice teams: physicians' perspectives on collaborative care	Exploratory focus groups	Good example of iterative process: issues related to collaborative practice with pharmacists that emerged from the focus group analysis were used to inform the development of a semi-structured interview guide for individual interviews
Schaufel et al.[35] "So you think I'll survive?": a qualitative study about doctor-patient dialogues preceding high-risk cardiac surgery or intervention	Observational study based on dialogue between patients with serious heart disease and their physicians	Good example of analysis based on audiotaped transcripts of dialogue
Vikis et al.[36] Teaching and learning in the operating room is a two-way street: resident perceptions.	In-depth interviews	Provides a good example of an interview guide. The interplay among thematic categories is well illustrated in a figure.
Wilkes et al.[37] Patient experience of infertility management in primary care: an in-depth interview study	In-depth interviews	A good example of qualitative data analysis. Data are categorized into emerging themes using constant comparison including • open coding (labelling) • axial coding (categorization) • selective coding (core categories/themes) Includes the development of concept diagram describing findings.

to determine whether it was appropriate for the research question?
— Were the study methods described in enough detail that a trained researcher could be confident that the steps in the data collection and analysis process were true to the methodology and that the findings were sound and supportable?
— Do you explain any iterative processes used in collecting and analyzing data?
— Do you explain how you addressed researcher bias and used techniques of reflexivity?
— Have you included a statement giving details of Ethics Review Board approval for your study?

- **Findings**
  — Have you justified the themes and interpretations presented in your analysis and supported them with data (i.e., appropriate quotations)?
  — Have you explained how your findings relate to your hypothesis, to existing theoretical frameworks or to theory development?

- **Discussion**
  — Are the limitations of your study discussed?
  — Is your research described in sufficient detail that the reader can judge how your findings might be applied to other settings?

Conclusion

Qualitative research is a valuable approach that can help us come to a better understanding of experiences, behaviours, cultures, phenomena and events. It is important to conduct qualitative research with the same attention to methodological quality as is expected in quantitative research. Well-executed qualitative studies can reward both researchers and readers with rich detail and fresh insights to guide their understanding, inform practice and policy development, and support and guide further rigorous qualitative and quantitative research. ∎

Designing

REFERENCES

1. Wright JG, McKeever P. Qualitative research: its role in clinical research. *Ann R Coll Physicians Surg Can*. 2000;33:275–80.

2. Pope C, Mays N. Qualitative methods in health research, editors. In: Pope C, Mays N, editors. *Qualitative research in health care*. Oxford (UK): Blackwell Publishing; 2006. p.1–11.

3. Kuper A, Reeves S, Levinson W. An introduction to reading and appraising qualitative research. *BMJ*. 2008;337:a288.

4. Greene JC. Is mixed methods social inquiry a distinctive methodology? *J Mix Methods Res*. 2008;2(1):7–22.

5. Patton MQ. *Qualitative research & evaluation methods*. 3rd ed. Thousand Oaks (CA): Sage Publications; 2002.

6. Cohen DJ, Crabtree BF. Evaluative criteria for qualitative research in health care: controversies and recommendations. *Ann Fam Med*. 2008;6(4):331–9.

7. Mays N, Pope C. Qualitative research in health care: assessing quality in qualitative research. *BMJ*. 2000;320(7226):50–2.

8. Glanz K, Rimer BK, Viswanath K, editors. *Health behavior and health education: theory, research, and practice*. 4th ed. San Francisco (CA): Jossey-Bass; 2008.

9. Teddlie C, Tashakkori A. Major issues and controversies in the use of mixed methods in the social and behavioural sciences. In: Teddlie C, Tashakkori A, editors. *Handbook of mixed methods in social and behavioral research*. Thousand Oaks (CA): Sage Publications; 2003. p. 3–50.

10. Pope C. Conducting ethnography in medical settings. *Med Educ*. 2005;39(12):1180–7.

11. Byrne D, Ragin CC, editors. The SAGE handbook of case-based methods. Thousand Oaks (CA): Sage Publications; 2009.

12. Yin RK. *Case study research: design and methods*. 4th ed. Thousand Oaks (CA): Sage Publications; 2009.

13. Stake RE. *The art of case study research*. Thousand Oaks (CA): Sage Publications; 1995.

14. Giacomini MK, Cook DJ. Users' guides to the medical literature: XXIII. Qualitative research in health care A. Are the results of the study valid? Evidence-Based Medicine Working Group. *JAMA*. 2000;284(3):357–62.

15. Heyl BS. Ethnographic interviewing. In: Atkinson P, Coffet A, Delamont S, Lofland J, Lofland L, editors. *Handbook of ethnography*. London: Sage Publications; 2001. p. 367–83.

16. Dicicco-Bloom B, Crabtree BF. The qualitative research interview. *Med Educ.* 2006;40(4):314–21.

17. Briggs CL. Learning how to ask: A sociolinguisitic appraisal of the role of the interview in social science research. Cambridge (UK): Cambridge University Press; 1986.

18. Miller WL, Crabtree BF. Depth interviewing. In: Crabtree BF, Miller WL, editors. *Doing qualitative research*. 2nd ed. Thousand Oaks (CA): Sage Publications; 1999. p. 89–107.

19. Rubin HJ, Rubin IS. Listening, hearing and sharing social experiences. In: *Qualitative interviewing: the art of hearing data*. Thousand Oaks (CA): Sage Publications; 2005. p.1–18.

20. Spradley J. *The ethnographic interview*. New York: Holt, Rinehart & Winston; 1979.

21. Barbour RS. Making sense of focus groups. *Med Educ.* 2005;39(7):742–50.

22. Kuper A, Lingard L, Levinson W. Critically appraising qualitative research. *BMJ.* 2008;337:a1035.

23. Pope C, Ziebland S, Mays N. Qualitative research in health care. Analysing qualitative data. *BMJ.* 2000;320(7227):114–6.

24. Guest G, Bunce A, Johnson L. How many interviews are enough? An experiment with data saturation and variability. *Field Methods.* 2006;18(1):59–82.

25. Miles MB, Huberman AM. *Qualitative data analysis: an expanded sourcebook*. Thousand Oaks (CA): Sage Publications; 1994.

26. Sandelowski M. Whatever happened to qualitative description? *Res Nurs Health.* 2000;23(4):334–40.

27. Glaser BG, Strauss AL. The discovery of grounded theory: strategies for qualitative research. Chicago: Aldine Publishing; 1967.

28. Lingard L, Albert M, Levinson W. Grounded theory, mixed methods, and action research. *BMJ.* 2008;337:a567.

29. Creswell JW. *Qualitative inquiry and research design: choosing among five approaches*. 2nd ed. Thousand Oaks (CA): Sage Publications; 2007.

30. Richardson L, St. Pierre EA. Writing: A method of inquiry. In: Denzin NK, YS Lincoln YS, editors. *The SAGE handbook of qualitative research*. 3rd ed. Thousand Oaks (CA): Sage Publications; 2005. p. 959–75.

31. Morse JM, Barrett M, Mayan M, Olson K, Spiers J. 2002. Verification strategies for establishing reliability and validity in qualitative research. *Int J Qual Methods.* 2002;1(2):1–19.

32. Lau E, Papaioannou A, Dolovich L,Adachi J, Sawka AM, Nair N, et al. Patients' adherence to osteoporosis therapy: exploring the perceptions of postmenopausal women. *Can Fam Physician.* 2008;54(3):394–402.

33. Lee FJ, Brown JB, Stewart M. Exploring family physician stress: helpful strategies. *Can Fam Physician.* 2009;55(3):288–9.e1–6.

34. Pottie K, Farrell B, Haydt S, Dolovich L, Sellors C, Kennie N, et al. Integrating pharmacists into family practice teams: physicians' perspectives on collaborative care. *Can Fam Physician.* 2008;54(12):1714–17.e5.

35. Schaufel MA, Nordrehaug JE, Malterud K. "So you think I'll survive?": a qualitative study about doctor-patient dialogues preceding high-risk cardiac surgery or intervention. *Heart.* 2009;95(15):1245–9.

36. Vikis EA, Mihalynuk TV, Pratt DD, Sidhu RS. Teaching and learning in the operating room is a two-way street: resident perceptions. *Am J Surg.* 2008;195(5):594–8.

37. Wilkes S, Hall N, Crosland A, Murdoch A, Rubin G. Patient experience of infertility management in primary care: an in-depth interview study. *Fam Pract.* 2009;26(4):309–16.

ADDITIONAL RESOURCES

Atkinson P, Coffey A, Delamont S, Lofland J, Lofland L, editors. *Handbook of ethnography*. London: Sage Publications; 2001.

- This is a comprehensive reference work for ethnographic research across the social sciences, including both introductory overviews and detailed critical essays.

Braun V, Clarke V. Using thematic analysis in psychology. *Qual Res Psychol.* 2006;3(2):77–101.

- This article provides clear guidelines for those wanting to start a thematic analysis or to conduct one in a more deliberate and rigorous way.

Designing

Crabtree BF, Miller WL. *Doing qualitative research*. 2nd ed. Thousand Oaks (CA): Sage Publications; 1999.

- This introductory textbook offers an excellent overview of qualitative research methods along with chapters on strategies for data collection and analysis.

Denzin NK, Lincoln YS, editors. *The SAGE handbook of qualitative research*. 3rd ed. Thousand Oaks (CA): Sage Publications; 2005.

- This text is considered an essential reference—perhaps the definitive reference—for qualitative research.

Giacomini MK, Cook DJ. Users' guides to the medical literature: XXIII. Qualitative research in health care A. Are the results of the study valid? Evidence-Based Medicine Working Group. *JAMA*. 2000;284(3):357–62.

- This paper describes how to assess the validity of qualitative research reports, including assessment of sampling, methods and comprehensiveness of data collection, analysis and findings.

Glesne C. *Becoming qualitative researchers: an introduction*. 4th ed. Englewood Cliffs (NJ): Prentice Hall; 2010.

- This text is a very informative and readable guide to the design and conduct of qualitative research.

Kuper A, Reeves S, Levinson W. An introduction to reading and appraising qualitative research. *BMJ*. 2008;337:a288.

- This excellent introduction to qualitative research includes a list of definitions of key terms used in qualitative research and a brief outline of theoretical approaches to qualitative research.

Liamputtong P, Ezzy D. 2005. *Qualitative research methods*. 2nd ed. Oxford (UK): Oxford University Press; 2005.

- This text is a very readable guide to the design and conduct of qualitative research, with a particular focus on health.

Mays N, Pope C. Qualitative research in health care. Assessing quality in qualitative research. *BMJ*. 2000;320(7226):50–2.

- This article gives a detailed description of ways to improve validity in qualitative research and includes a list of questions to pose in evaluating a qualitative study.

Miles MB, Huberman AM. *Qualitative data analysis: an expanded sourcebook*. Thousand Oaks (CA): Sage Publications; 1994.

- This practical sourcebook on qualitative research provides detailed information on qualitative data analysis.

Schwandt TA. *The Sage dictionary of qualitative inquiry*. 3rd ed. Thousand Oaks (CA): Sage Publications; 2007.

- As its title suggests, a dictionary/reference of qualitative research.

Wright JG, McKeever P. Qualitative research: its role in clinical research. *Ann R Coll Physicians Surg Can.* 2000;33:275–80.

- This is a good general article on the role of qualitative research, differences from quantitative research, and a brief overview of qualitative methods.

Designing

EXERCISES

1. Describe the difference between qualitative and quantitative methodology.

2. Review a qualitative research paper and see if you can list the steps taken to ensure quality of the data and the analysis.

Designing

SUMMARY CHECKLIST

- ❑ Considering your research question, list ways in which a qualitative approach would be useful—or not so useful.
- ❑ Select a qualitative method relevant to your research question.
- ❑ Write a draft protocol defining all elements, including the target population, sampling, data collection, data organization and analysis.
- ❑ Consider any ethical issues arising from your protocol.
- ❑ Review your draft protocol with a qualitative methodologist. Revise.
- ❑ Write up your results, being mindful of published guidelines for qualitative analyses.

17
Writing a research protocol

Vicky Tagalakis, MD, MSc

ILLUSTRATIVE CASE

During the two years you have spent as an Internal Medicine resident at an ambulatory clinic, you have observed the results of different approaches to blood pressure monitoring. You form a hypothesis that patients whose blood pressure is managed with the use of a 24-hour ambulatory blood pressure monitor are more likely to achieve target blood pressure than patients whose blood pressure is managed by office-based manual sphygmomanometry alone. An extensive search of the literature reveals that very little research has been done on this topic. Your supervisor, an active researcher in hypertension and cardiovascular disease, is enthusiastic about your idea and proposes that you conduct a study to investigate it. Having formulated your research question, reviewed the medical literature, discussed your research question and proposed a study plan with your supervisor, you are now preparing to write a research protocol so that you can apply for a grant to fund your study.

Proposing

■ **A research protocol is a detailed** plan that will help you to formalize and operationalize your research ideas, map out how the study will be carried out, act as a reference to ensure all members of the research team adhere to the methods outlined, and provide reference points for monitoring the study's progress and evaluating its outcomes. Proficiency in protocol writing is an acquired skill. Although some people are naturally better at it than others, anyone can benefit from the simple tips described in this chapter.

Start writing early. You should begin to write your protocol at least four months before the grant submission deadline. This will give you time to search the medical literature, seek advice, and revise your research question and study plan. Leaving the writing process to the last few weeks before the deadline won't leave you enough time to obtain and act upon input from collaborators and experts in the field, or to address the issues that will inevitably come to light during the writing process as you focus on the details of your protocol.

Organize a team of collaborators and advisors early. The input, feedback and advice that your team can provide during the preparation and review of your written protocol are invaluable. They can help you refine your study question and objectives, advise you on methods, and provide you with tools and resources. Once the protocol is written, they can provide feedback on the content, giving particular

CHAPTER OBJECTIVES

After reading this chapter, you should be able to:
- describe the major components of a research protocol
- apply useful tips for writing a good research protocol
- develop good research protocol writing practices

KEY TERMS

Ascertainment bias	Intervention bias	Referral bias
Co-intervention bias	Measurement bias	Selection bias
Contamination bias	Non-respondent bias	SMART
Information bias	Outcome variables	Withdrawal bias
Instrument bias	Recall bias	

attention to clarity and coherence. Their input should address four key questions:

- Is the research question sufficiently clear and refined to serve as an anchor for the research endeavour?
- Are the proposed study design and methodology adequate to answer the research question(s) and achieve the study objective(s)?
- Are the design and methodology feasible (e.g., is the sample size adequate)?
- Is there sufficient detail and instruction to ensure that the study is replicable?

If the answer is yes to all four questions, then you have succeeded in developing a well-thought-out and well-written protocol that the reviewers will appreciate.

Get the writing style right. When you apply to a granting agency for funding, remember that your research protocol is one of many that reviewers will have to read and rank. So, make it enjoyable to read! Aim for writing that is clear, concise, interesting, easy to read, and free of spelling and grammatical errors. Make sure your reasoning is logical and precise. You want to engage the reviewers with your ideas, not to distract them with errors and convoluted thinking. Get advice from your supervisor about writing style, and ask him or her for examples of well-written protocols that have been successful at grant competitions. These should give you an idea of effective structure, writing style and flow, and the level of language to use. Also consult guidebooks and resources on grant and protocol writing (see Additional Resources) for the principles of good expository writing, such as starting each paragraph with a strong topic sentence and using, where possible, the active rather than passive voice (see also ch. 29).

Know the requirements and instructions of the granting agency. Early in the writing process, become familiar with the granting agency's requirements and instructions for submitting an application, which can take far more time to complete than you might expect. Moreover, non-adherence to the rules can lead to your application being disqualified. There are usually instructions pertaining to length, formatting and the components to include (e.g., investigator CVs, an abstract, a budget) as well as other requirements (e.g., the application deadline, required signatures, number of copies). These instructions vary according to the granting agency and are available for reference on their respective websites.

Once you have formulated your research question, searched the literature, sought input and feedback from your collaborators and supervisor, devised a plan for your research study, looked at examples of other protocols, and referred to the granting agency's website for guidelines and instructions, you are ready to start writing the protocol.

The components of a research protocol

Although requirements vary from one granting agency to another, research protocols are most commonly structured as follows:

- project title
- project summary (up to one page)
- statement of the problem (up to one page)
- research proposal (about 75% of the allotted pages)
  — background
  — research objectives
  — study design and method
  — statistical analyses
  — sample size calculation
- ethical considerations
- the role and expertise of team members (about 200–250 words)
- study timeline (about 50–100 words)
- strengths and limitations (about 250–300 words)
- anticipated results and implications (about 300 words)
- references

Each of these components is discussed in the following sections.

Project title

The title should be concise and clearly convey the central research objective, including the population to be studied. In the case of a randomized clinical trial, the intervention to be studied or tested should also be described. Avoid using acronyms and other abbreviations in your title. For our case example, the project title might be:

Comparison of ambulatory blood pressure monitoring vs conventional clinic-based manual sphygmomanometry for attainment of target blood pressure in patients with newly diagnosed hypertension.

Proposing

Project summary

As the first section (after the title) that the reviewers will read, the project summary occupies a key position in your protocol. In your summary, you should aim to (1) arouse interest in your project; (2) convince the reviewers of its importance; and (3) provide a brief but concise overview of your research plan, including its objective(s) and proposed study design and methods. A well-written summary can go a long way toward establishing your project as credible and worthy of funding. If you have completed pilot research in the area of your proposed study, include a statement summarizing this work, the progress achieved, and how it naturally leads to or supports your current proposal (see ch. 21).

Statement of the problem

The purpose of this section is to provide, in a succinct form, a justification for your proposed research and explain why it is important and merits funding. Typically, it begins by describing the current situation and then outlines gaps in, or the inconclusiveness of, existing evidence. It may also question existing knowledge in light of recent evidence from other studies—perhaps even from your own preliminary work.

To use our example, your statement of the problem might explain that preliminary data from your clinic show that only 60% of patients have achieved their target blood pressure by 6 months after the initiation of antihypertensive drug therapy, and that this success rate is consistent with rates reported in published studies. You emphasize the importance of attaining target blood pressure with regard to primary and secondary prevention of cardiovascular endpoints such as stroke and heart disease. Typically, when patients are first started on antihypertensive therapy, their blood pressure is checked every 6–8 weeks during the first 6 months. At these follow-up visits, patients have their blood pressure measured with a manual sphygmomanometer (3 measurements 5 minutes apart). Alternatively, they can have an ambulatory monitor placed for 24 hours; this is returned by the patient the next day so that the measurements can be retrieved. Your exhaustive literature search shows that 24-hour ambulatory blood pressure monitoring is as reliable as monitoring with a manual sphygmomanometer. You then hypothesize that, in patients with newly diagnosed hypertension, management by 24-hour ambulatory blood pressure monitoring will lead to higher rates of target blood pressure attainment at 6 months compared with management by manual sphygmomanometer monitoring.

Research proposal

Background. The background section extends the statement of the problem with an in-depth review of the current state of knowledge on the topic—including your pilot work and preliminary results—and the rationale for your study. For example, you should indicate why your research question is compelling, why your approach to it is ideal, and why you and your team are well positioned to do this research. There are three important parts to the background section:

1. **A restatement of the main study question and/or hypothesis** and how it relates to health priorities locally and/or universally (e.g., attaining target blood pressure can have an impact on the prevalence of cardiovascular diseases, such as stroke and heart disease, which impose a significant burden on society). In this example, one might propose the following:

   In patients with hypertension who are followed in an outpatient clinic, does routine monitoring with sphygmomanometry as compared with scheduled 24-hour ambulatory monitoring result in a higher proportion of patients achieving predetermined blood pressure targets?

2. **An extensive literature review** that describes the current evidence and/or knowledge of the research problem or question, identifies gaps in that knowledge, and states what questions or controversies remain unresolved. It is important to enlist a health librarian to help with your literature search (see ch. 7): a systematic and thorough search at the start of the research process is invaluable and can save time later if you want to refine your research question or objectives and thus need to re-consult the literature.

3. **A convincing argument to justify your study** and thus persuade the reviewers that it should be funded. You must be able to outline clearly why your study should be done; what knowledge will be obtained and how it will contribute to the existing evidence to address knowledge gaps and/or controversies; the potential benefits of your study to the scientific and health services community and to patients; and how feasible it is for your study, given its proposed methodology and design, to answer the research question and/or hypothesis.

Proposing

Research objectives. Your research objectives arise from your study question(s) and/or hypothesis. These objectives should be stated clearly and concisely, specifying what is to be described, measured, determined, identified and (in the case of a study hypothesis) confirmed or disproven. Both general and specific objectives should be identified. Beware of formulating too many objectives, or objectives that cannot feasibly be achieved within the scope of your project. Research grants are often ranked poorly if the research objectives are not attainable on the basis of the study plan. They should be **SMART**: **S**pecific, **M**easurable, **A**chievable, **R**elevant and **T**imely.[1]

General objective. Your statement of the study's general objective should encapsulate what will be studied and the knowledge you expect to gain. For example:

Our goal is to determine whether 24-hour ambulatory blood pressure monitoring results in better blood pressure control than blood pressure monitoring by clinic-based manual sphygmomanometer in patients with newly diagnosed hypertension.

Specific objectives. Your description of specific objectives should make the general objective more precise with respect to measurable endpoints and should preview elements of the study design. For example:

1. *To determine and compare the proportion of patients with newly diagnosed hypertension who attained target blood pressure at 6 months with 24-hour ambulatory blood pressure monitoring vs office-based manual sphygmomanometry.*
2. *To determine the percentage change in mean arterial pressure at 6 months after initiation of therapy compared with at the start of therapy in patients whose hypertension was managed with 24-hour ambulatory blood pressure monitoring vs patients whose hypertension was managed with office-based manual sphygmomanometry.*

Study design and methods. The methods section describes in a concrete and objective manner the procedures that will be used to achieve your study objectives. It is the manual of operations and hence a very important part of the protocol. It should contain sufficient detail and instruction so that if another investigator were to repeat your study he or she would obtain comparable results. It is universally accepted by the scientific community that the methods section should include a detailed description of the following:

- the study design
- the study population
- the method of recruitment
- operational definitions of variables, including outcomes to be studied
- the proposed intervention (if applicable)
- data collection methods and management
- sample-size calculations
- proposed statistical analyses

Some of these items are described further below.

Study design. This subsection should identify the study design chosen (e.g., case-control, experimental/interventional study). If a less robust design has been chosen (e.g., case-control as opposed to a prospective cohort study), then an explanation as to why this design was chosen in preference to other possibilities should be provided (e.g., because of resource limitations or ethical considerations).

We will carry out a randomized clinical trial whereby consecutive patients referred to an Internal Medicine clinic for hypertension management will be randomly assigned to periodic monitoring of blood pressure with a 24-hour ambulatory blood pressure monitor vs manual sphygmomanometer during a 6-month treatment period.

Study population. Be as clear as possible in your description of the population in which your study will be carried out. Also describe the source population from which the study population is derived, as well as the sampling methods used to obtain the study population (e.g., a random sample from a larger population, or a series of consecutive patients attending a clinic). Provide details on the following, as appropriate for your study design:

- the study group definitions, e.g., cases vs controls in a case-control study); unexposed vs exposed individuals (in a cohort study); control vs experimental group (in an interventional study);
- inclusion and exclusion criteria, recruitment and enrolment procedures and, if applicable, matching factors for cases and controls;
- methods of randomization and allocation.

Reviewers will always pay close attention to the study population to assess the potential generalizability and relevance of results and to detect **selection** or **ascertainment**

bias, which occurs when some members of the source population are less likely to be included in the study than others and, as a result, the study fails to represent equally all groups of individuals from the source population.

Operational definitions of all variables. It is important to provide operational definitions of all variables to be studied, especially outcomes. Give a clear description of what type of variables will be studied, what is understood by each variable, and how data on variables will be collected, recorded and analyzed. You should also explain the validity and reliability of the proposed definitions and measurements.

In our example, blood pressure–related measurements are the primary **outcome variables**, but you would also need to specifically state whether the mean, systolic or diastolic pressure will be measured. Moreover, you would need to provide a clear description of the procedure and process for recording blood pressure by both manual sphygmomanometer and 24-hour ambulatory blood pressure monitoring (e.g., Who will record the blood pressure by manual sphygmomanometer? Will it be measured in both trial arms? How frequently will blood pressure measurements be done by either method? Which brand model will be used for 24-hour ambulatory blood pressure measurements? Has this model been validated? Is it reliable across different study populations?) Definitions that are standardized and/or well described in the literature should be described briefly, with supporting references.

Protocols whose operational definitions are imprecise—e.g., "Demographic variables will be considered" or "Blood pressure will be measured according to standard clinic procedures"—do not receive favourable rankings from reviewers, since the relevance of the variables to the study objectives cannot be assessed. Moreover, vague or incomplete descriptions of variables do not allow for the uniform execution of a study protocol across different sites.

Data collection. It is essential to describe in detail how data will be collected and recorded. Describe your data collection methods (e.g., patient interview, chart review, self-administered questionnaire), who will be collecting the data (e.g., research nurse, each participant), and the data collection instruments you will use (e.g., questionnaires, interview guide, medical record extraction form). If these procedures have been standardized and described in the literature, provide and describe the pertinent references. If these procedures and instruments have previously been tested by you or your research team, include details on your findings with regard to the accuracy and reproducibility of their measurements or results.

You should also describe in the data collection section the methods you propose to use to safeguard your data against biases that may threaten the validity of your research and render your results inaccurate. Common sources of bias to consider are described in Textbox 17.1.

Data management. This section should describe your procedures for data entry (e.g., who will enter the data, whether data entry will be blinded, and what software will be used) along with the measures you will take to ensure the completeness and accuracy of the information being entered (e.g., duplicate entry of data, cross-validation).[a] You should also describe where the data will be stored and what security measures will be undertaken to protect patient confidentiality, such as storing information securely in a locked filing cabinet in a locked office or using password protection on a secure computer network.

Statistical analyses. This section, which describes your proposed data analyses, is best written in conjunction with a statistician. It should include details on the variables to be used to compare the groups, a description of your summary measures (e.g., odds ratio, risk ratio, hazard ratio), your methods of analyses (e.g., *t* test, logistic regression analysis, survival analysis), a justification of adjustments for predefined confounders, and a description of how you will deal with missing data. This section should also specify the alpha level to be used (the cut-off probability value for statistical significance) and whether two-tailed statistical tests will be used. The statistical software that you intend to use should also be referenced.

Sample size calculation. Early in the planning stages of your study and before you begin to write your research protocol, enlist the help of a statistician to assist with issues such as determining an appropriate sample size to ensure that your

Proposing

---

a   "Duplicate data entry" refers to the process whereby data from case report forms obtained in a study are independently entered by two individuals and compared to ensure the accuracy of entry. "Cross-validation" describes a process where either the source material for data entry into spreadsheets or the content of the spreadsheets themselves are reviewed by study personnel (usually an investigator or coordinator) to ensure accuracy.

TEXTBOX 17.1: SOURCES OF BIAS[2]

SELECTION BIAS

This bias results from a systematic error in the procedures or factors used in the selection of subjects, such that the study sample is unrepresentative of the population of interest. This means that the observed association between, for example, an exposure and disease, is different for those who actually participated in the study and those who should theoretically have been eligible for inclusion but did not participate. **Referral bias**, which occurs because people who are referred to a study are often different from non-referred individuals, and **non-respondent bias**, which occurs because subjects who choose to respond to a call to participate in research studies are generally different from those who do not respond, are among the various types of selection bias.

MEASUREMENT (OR INFORMATION) BIAS

This bias results from a systematic error in the collection of information or data. Its consequences will vary, depending on how the inaccurate data relate to the study exposure and/or outcome(s) of interest. Examples of measurement bias are **recall bias** (e.g., cases—individuals identified as having the disease under study—tend to recall past exposures more completely and accurately than controls) and **instrument bias** (which occurs when a study instrument such as a faulty sphygmomanometer leads to inaccurate measurements being recorded; because it affects all study groups equally, the resulting measurement error will tend to bias the study result toward the null, underestimating any real difference).

INTERVENTION BIAS

This type of bias arises from a systematic error in how an intervention (as in a randomized controlled trial) is carried out, or in the manner in which the study groups were exposed to the intervention. Examples of intervention bias include **contamination bias**, which occurs when members in the control group inadvertently (or not so inadvertently) receive the intervention or treatment, thus minimizing the difference in outcome between the intervention and control groups, **co-intervention bias**, which occurs when interventions other than the study treatments are applied differently to the study and control groups (this is a serious problem when double-blinding is absent), and **withdrawal bias**, which occurs when outcomes for subjects who leave the study (drop-outs) are substantially different from the outcomes of those who remain in the study.

TEXTBOX 17.2: PITFALLS IN PROTOCOL WRITING*

- Starting too late.
- Failing to provide a clear research question.
- Setting too many objectives, or objectives that are beyond the scope of the project.
- Failing to provide the context or "big picture" of your research.
- Failing to present a clear and precise rationale for your approach.
- Failing to cite key studies or present a thorough review of the knowledge in your topic area.
- Giving too much detail on minor issues and not enough on major ones.
- Writing in a rambling style.
- Making mistakes in grammar and spelling.
- Failing to provide a sample size calculation and power calculation.

*See also the "Ten common research pitfalls" listed at the end of chapter 1.

Proposing

study will have sufficient statistical power. The statistician can help with the writing of this and the other analytical parts of the methods, which should describe your sample size calculation and include details on how you arrived at the estimates of difference to be detected (e.g., the minimum difference in percentage change in mean arterial blood pressure expected between the two study groups) and the statistical assumptions made regarding the distribution of variables and your chosen levels of significance, as well as references for your methods of calculation.

Ethical considerations

Ethical considerations apply to all types of health research, ranging from experimental intervention trials to database studies. As a result, you should specify whether approval has been received, is pending, or will be sought from an appropriate ethics review committee. If such approval is not necessary (as in a meta-analysis of published data), then you must state that this is the case and explain why. Moreover, you should also describe any ethical issues related to your study: these might pertain to recruitment strategies, inclusion and exclusion criteria (e.g., the participation of vulnerable subjects such as children, or exclusions based on race or sex), potential risks and benefits to study participants (especially in intervention studies), the de-linking of identifying information when working with administrative databases, and any issues concerning the rights of subjects. You should also include, in an appendix, the consent forms you intend to use and any approval letters from ethics committees, if these are available at the time of your grant submission.

Team members

In this section, you should identify the members of the research team and describe in specific terms their role on the team and the expertise they bring to the project. You want to be able to convince the reviewers that your team is well positioned and equipped to see the study to a successful and timely completion. Three main roles in a typical research team are as follows:

Principal investigator. The principal investigator is primarily responsible for the intellectual direction of the research project and oversight of the execution of the protocol. The principal investigator also assumes administrative responsibility (e.g., fund allocation, hiring of study personnel, research ethics submission) for the project. Some studies may have two or more "co-principal investigators."

Co-investigator. Co-investigators work closely with the principal investigator and make a significant contribution to the intellectual direction and conduct of the research. Some co-investigators may bring very specific expertise to the team (e.g., methodological or statistical).

Collaborator. The main role of collaborators in a research project is to provide a specific service (e.g., access to equipment, provision of specific reagents, training in a specialized technique, statistical analysis, or access to a patient population).

Study timeline

It is important to specify the estimated time, usually in weeks to months, required for completion of the various stages of your study (e.g., time for patient recruitment, time for data collection and entry, time for analysis, etc.). This will help the reviewers to gauge the feasibility of your study and assess the duration of the funding support that will be needed. For example:

This study will require 3 years (36 months) for completion: 2 months for hiring and training of study nurses and the development of a computerized data entry form; 24 months for recruitment of patients and follow-up, 4 months for data entry and cleaning, and 6 months for completion of data analysis and manuscript preparation.

Strengths and limitations

It is good practice to highlight the strengths of your proposal and to indicate its limitations and how these will affect your study. As the reviewers read your protocol, they will identify limitations and will inevitably have something to say (since it is much easier to criticize someone else's protocol than to write one). It is therefore to your advantage to anticipate and pre-empt criticism by identifying those limitations yourself, assessing their potential impact, and suggesting alternative strategies along with their advantages and disadvantages. The reviewers will appreciate that you are being proactive and can anticipate and address pitfalls and obstacles.

Anticipated results and implications

This paragraph is the last section of the protocol and is meant to summarize and emphasize the significance of your research in terms of its anticipated results and implications. When writing this section, try to answer the following question: "How will results of your study be useful to clinicians and patients, to policy makers, the medical community at large, and to future research efforts?" Some researchers consider the questions, "So what?" and "Who cares?" as they write this section. Although this is a small paragraph, it is the last thing the reviewers read, and you want to leave them with the impression that your area of research is important and should be funded! For example:

Hypertension is a major public health problem affecting 1 in 3 adult Canadians. The results of this study will improve the management of blood pressure in outpatient clinics by ...

References

Refer to and follow the granting agency's specifications and instructions with regard to the formatting of references. Enter your references into a citation management software package such as Endnote or Reference Manager right from the start of the writing process; this will save you time in the long run. Most university or hospital libraries offer workshops on using referencing or citation software.

Conclusion

Clearly, writing a good research protocol requires starting early, being organized, focusing on timelines, reading and thinking critically, recruiting help from others (e.g., librarians for literature searches, statisticians for analysis, methodologists for study design and conduct), seeking guidance from supervisors, mentors and collaborators—and, most importantly, committing time and attention to the writing process. These elements will help you avoid the pitfalls listed in Textbox 17.2. Often the most difficult part is simply to get started! ■

Proposing

REFERENCES

1. Singh S, Suganthi P, Ahmed J, Chadha VK. Formulation of health research protocol—a step by step description. *NTI Bulletin* 2005;41(1–2):5–10. Available from: http://medind.nic.in/nac/t05/i1/nact05i1p5.pdf

2. Hulley SB, Cummings SR, Browner WS, Grady DG, Newman TB. *Designing clinical research: an epidemiologic approach.* 3rd ed. Philadelphia: Lippincott Williams & Wilkins; 2007.

ADDITIONAL RESOURCES

Fathalla MF, Fathalla MMF. *A practical guide for health researchers.* Cairo: World Health Organization Regional Office for the Mediterranean; 2004. Chapter 5: Writing the research protocol; p. 65–71. Available from: www.emro.who.int/dsaf/dsa237.pdf

- An extensive and practical guide on the entire research process, including how to plan the research, write the protocol, apply for funding, implement the study, analyze and interpret the data, report the results, and write and publish a scientific paper.

McInnes R, Andrews B, Rachubinski. *Guidebook for new principal investigators: advice on applying for a grant, writing papers, setting up a research team and managing your time.* Ottawa: Canadian Institutes of Health Research. Institute of Genetics. Available from: www.cihr-irsc.gc.ca/e/27491.html

- An excellent overview of how to write research protocols for grant applications.

Pan American Health Organization. *Guide for writing a research protocol.* Washington (DC): The Organization; n.d. Available from: www.paho.org/English/HDP/JDR/RPG/Research-Protocol-Guides.htm

- A very good overview of the main steps in developing a research protocol.

University College London Hospitals: NHS Foundation Trust. *Guidelines for completing a research protocol for observational studies.* London: Medical Statistics Unit, University College London Hospitals R&D Directorate; 2006. Available from: www.sld.cu/galerias/pdf/sitios/revsalud/guidelines_for_observational_studies.pdf

- An overview of writing research protocols for observational (non-intervention) studies (e.g., case-control or cohort) and the biases that should be addressed.

SUMMARY CHECKLIST

- ❑   Gather all the information you will need to write your protocol, including any specific formats for target audiences.
- ❑   Give your project a clear, explicit title.
- ❑   List the members of your research team and their role (investigator, co-investigator, collaborator).
- ❑   Write a brief project summary.
- ❑   Write a succinct problem statement.
- ❑   Write up your background statement, using the results of your literature review to justify your study.
- ❑   Clearly articulate SMART research goals.
- ❑   Describe your study design, including appropriate details about your population, settings, relevant variables, recruitment, any interventions, etc.
- ❑   Describe how you will collect and manage your data.
- ❑   Describe your data analysis methods and any relevant calculations.
- ❑   Describe how ethical issues will be managed.
- ❑   Construct a realistic study timeline.
- ❑   Describe anticipated results and their significance.
- ❑   Describe the strengths and weakness of your approach.
- ❑   If applicable, create a budget for your project.
- ❑   List your references in an appropriate format.
- ❑   Show your protocol to your team and mentors. Revise.

Proposing

Proposing

18

Getting to "approved": Concepts, guidelines and processes in ethics applications

Julia Spence, MD, MSc, FRCPC

ILLUSTRATIVE CASE

A third-year surgical resident is asked by his supervisor, who has expertise in medical education, to work on a research project with her. The proposed project will randomly assign junior surgical residents to one of two educational programs to teach chest tube placement in the trauma care setting. One group will be trained using a high-fidelity trauma simulator (educational intervention group); the other will be trained using a simple model of a chest wall (control group). All junior surgical trainees at two hospitals will be asked to participate. After the training phase of the study, participants will perform a simulated trauma resuscitation in which they will be required to place a chest tube. A trained observer masked to the group assignment will assess performance using a validated checklist. Residents will be given feedback on their performance. Funding for the project is available, and so no formal grant application is needed. However, the supervisor asks the resident to start work on a submission for Research Ethics Board review and institutional approval. The resident is not sure what this involves.

■ **Although applying for ethics** approval for your research proposal can be a daunting prospect, it affords an opportunity for you to consider your project from an indispensable perspective: that of the participant. Clinical science cannot progress without the participation of willing patients and healthy volunteers; however, because this participation almost invariably involves some degree of **risk**, the ethical oversight of health sciences research is crucial. This chapter will explain why ethical review is needed, outline national and international standards that guide ethics review, discuss the basic ethical principles of research involving human participants and describe the process of obtaining Research Ethics Board and institutional approval for a research project.

Why is ethics review required?

The development of generalizable knowledge in clinical health science requires research involving real people,

whether they are patients or healthy volunteers. The ethical conduct of this research demands that both researchers and those who oversee research find a balance between, on the one hand, protecting research participants to the point where research becomes impossible and, on the other hand, exposing participants to needless or unacceptable risks. It is also important to understand that research does not

Proposing

CHAPTER OBJECTIVES

After reading this chapter, you should be able to:

- discuss the research ethics application and review process
- list important components of ethics review
- describe issues that should be discussed with research participants during the consent process
- list applicable national and international guidelines for the conduct of research
- describe the role of research administration in the ethics approval process

---

KEY TERMS

Assent	Conflict of interest	Privacy	Tri-Council Policy Statement
Autonomy	Confidentiality	Research administration	Vulnerable populations
Benefit	Informed consent	Research Ethics Board (REB)	
Beneficence	Justice	Respect for persons	
Concern for welfare	Minimal risk	Risk	

necessarily benefit the individual participant: rather, *it aims to benefit society as a whole*. Research participation is, therefore, fundamentally altruistic. This is in contradistinction to the commonly held belief that individuals will directly benefit from participation in research (i.e, "the therapeutic misconception."[1])

In addition to having no guarantee of **benefit**, those who participate in research are at risk of being exploited. Formal ethics review seeks to minimize this possibility by ensuring the independent assessment of all proposed studies. The review process aims to ensure that the potential risks of research are acceptable in light of the potential benefits and that those risks and benefits are distributed fairly among all eligible groups. It is imperative that potentially **vulnerable populations** not be unjustly burdened by participation in research that might not be of benefit to them.

A key function of ethics review is to ensure that there is an adequate process to obtain **informed consent**. Participants must be given sufficient information regarding the purpose, methods, risks and benefits of the research project, and about their rights and obligations, so that they can make an informed decision about whether to participate. The principles of informed consent will be discussed in more detail later in the chapter.

Standards for the ethical conduct of health sciences research

Many regulatory frameworks for research oversight arose in response to infamous examples of abuse of vulnerable research participants.[1-4] Foundational documents include the *Declaration of Helsinki*,[5] the *Belmont Report*,[6] those portions of the United States *Code of Federal Regulations* concerning the "protection of human subjects,"[7,8] and the Council for Biomedical Research Involving Human Subjects (CIOMS) *International Ethical Guidelines for Biomedical Research Involving Human Subjects*.[9]

In Canada, the field of research policy and research ethics review is relatively new; most guidelines have been in place only since the late 1990s. Central among these is the *Tri-Council Policy Statement: Ethical Conduct for Research Involving Humans* (*TCPS*).[10,11] Canadian researchers are obligated to comply with applicable regulations (related to both federal and provincial/territorial legislation) as well as to the *TCPS*. Because regulations and guidelines are updated regularly, it is important to be aware of the fact that ethics policies can evolve, even over the course of a project.

As a researcher, you are responsible for understanding and applying not only the ethics guidelines and regulations for the jurisdiction in which you are carrying out your project, but also those associated with the conditions of your funding. This applies to grants accepted from government sources from other countries. For example, research funded by the US government, or conducted at institutions receiving US government funding, must comply with applicable US federal regulations in addition to the *TCPS*.

The Tri-Council Policy Statement

In 1998, the Canadian Institutes of Health Research (formerly known as the Medical Research Council), the Natural Sciences and Engineering Research Council of Canada, and the Social Sciences and Humanities Research Council of Canada adopted the *TCPS*; amendments followed in 2000, 2002 and 2005,[10] and a second edition was released in 2010.[11] The *TCPS* sets out a standard for the conduct of research involving human subjects in Canada. As a condition of funding from any of the three councils, it is required that, at a minimum, researchers and their institutions apply the ethical principles and the articles of this policy for all research conducted under its auspices.

The *TCPS* supports and encourages research; however, the need for generalizable knowledge must be balanced by respect for human dignity. The second edition describes three principles: respect for persons, concern for welfare, and justice (international guidelines and earlier versions of the *TCPS* have also framed the first two of these concepts in the language of **autonomy** and **beneficence**).[10]

- In the context of research, the principle of **respect for persons** incorporates the obligation to respect the autonomy of individuals in order to ensure that they are able to make decisions without interference or undue influence. This principle recognizes that participation in research can be direct, or through the use of data or biologic materials, indirect. Furthermore, researchers are obligated to protect those who, by virtue of impaired decision-making capacity, have diminished autonomy.
- The principle of **concern for welfare** implies that individuals and groups who participate in, or are affected by, research must be protected from exploitation and unacceptable risk. The best possible balance between risks to participants and potential societal benefits of a proposed study must be sought.

Proposing

- The principle of **justice** relates to the obligation to treat potential participants fairly and equitably and to ensure that groups are neither unduly burdened with the risks of research nor denied the benefits and knowledge gained by research.

The application of these principles maximizes the benefits and minimizes the harms of research; this in turn helps to engender public trust in the scientific process, which in itself is beneficial to society.

The *TCPS* provides guidance for researchers and REBs in the following areas:

- research ethics framework and review
- informed consent and departures from general principles of informed consent
- fairness and equity in research participation
- privacy and confidentiality
- conflicts of interest
- multi-jurisdictional research
- research involving Aboriginal peoples
- qualitative research
- use of human biological materials
- human genetic research
- clinical trials

Tip

Many REBs require that an ethics tutorial, such as the one offered by the Tri-Council or the US National Institutes of Health, be completed before a project can be approved and funding released.

A summary and tutorial for the *TCPS* document can be found at www.pre.ethics.gc.ca/eng/education/tutorial-didacticiel/

A similar course is available from the NIH at http://phrp.nihtraining.com/users/login.php

The Royal College of Physicians and Surgeons of Canada also provides an excellent resource at http://rcpsc.medical.org/bioethics/extended-primers/research-ethics-full_e.php

Guidelines for clinical trials

Clinical trials are research studies that assign human participants or groups to health-related interventions. Because of the time and resources necessary to complete clinical trials, they are not usually carried out by trainees. In some cases, trainees might be involved with clinical trials being carried out to seek regulatory marketing approval for investigational drugs or devices, or for novel, unapproved uses of drugs and devices; such studies must be conducted in compliance with Canadian federal regulations.[12] If applicable, researchers should also be knowledgeable about the International Conference on Harmonisation – Good Clinical Practice (ICH–GCP)[a] guidelines, which have been adopted by Health Canada.[13] Good Clinical Practice (GCP) is an international ethical and scientific quality standard for designing, conducting, recording and reporting trials that involve the participation of human subjects. Canadian researchers should also be compliant with the *Declaration of Helsinki*[5] and the *CIOMS International Ethical Guidelines for Biomedical Research Involving Human Subjects*.[9]

Tip

Many REBs and institutions require certification of study investigators and staff in Good Clinical Practice (GCP) guidelines before they undertake a clinical trial. Many one-day accredited courses are available.

Research Ethics Board Review

What is a Research Ethics Board?

Research ethics review is essentially a peer review process. The members of a **Research Ethics Board** (REB) meet regularly and discuss proposed research projects from the viewpoint of the potential participants. Institutions appoint the REB to review the ethical acceptability, scientific validity and feasibility of all research involving humans conducted within their jurisdiction or under their auspices.[11] REBs are independent and accountable for their decisions. Although the number of members and their areas of expertise will depend on the range and volume of research within their institution, in Canada the minimal require-

Proposing

---

a The full name of the ICH is the International Conference on Harmonisation of Technical Requirements for Registration of Pharmaceuticals for Human Use. See www.ich.org/home.html

ment for an REB is five members, who must include (1) at least two members with research expertise, (2) one who is knowledgeable in ethics, (3) one who is knowledgeable in the law, and (4) one who has no affiliation with the institution (community member). Ad hoc advisors may be appointed to provide scientific expertise required for specific proposals.

Tip

Many REBs will allow researchers to observe a meeting; many request or require principal investigators to present and discuss their protocols, especially in the case of ethically challenging research. However, researchers are not allowed to observe deliberations or voting directly related to the review of a project with which they are associated.

What types of studies must be reviewed by an REB?

According to the *TCPS* (Article 2.1), all research that involves human subjects requires review and approval by an REB before it can be initiated. Research involving human remains, cadavers, tissues, biological fluids, embryos or fetuses must also be reviewed by an REB. However, research about living individuals that is based on legally accessible and publicly accessible information (e.g., a systematic review, documents, records, etc.) does not always require ethics review (Article 2.2).[11] Performance reviews or testing within normal educational requirements should not be subject to REB review. Quality assurance/improvement (QA/QI) projects might not require review, and many institutions provide specific guidance to determine whether a project is considered QA/QI or research.

Tip

If, given the nature and scope of your proposed project, you are in any doubt about the requirement for ethics review, seek guidance from your local REB.

What do REBs consider when they conduct a review?

The three principles of *respect for persons, concern for welfare* and *justice* provide the foundation for all research ethics review. On the basis of these principles, REBs consider the

specific issues related to each protocol. The review process allows REBs and investigators to identify issues that may affect participants, to balance differing perspectives, and to consider potential solutions. Many REBs are moving toward a model of greater collaboration with both researchers and potential research participants, through both formal and informal mechanisms.

Independent review allows the project to be examined from the participant's viewpoint. Regardless of how well intentioned they are, researchers have multiple, legitimate interests (including expeditious study completion, funding, career interests) that may be perceived to be in conflict with the interests of participants. Independent review helps to ensure that the best interests of participants are protected. It seeks to maximize the societal value of research while minimizing risks and ensuring that those who agree to participate will be treated with respect. In so doing, independent review also ensures a greater level of public accountability. At a minimum, the issues outlined in the following sections will be considered by an REB in the course of a review.

Tip

Seek guidance from your institutional REB as you develop your protocol. A non-scientific colleague may also provide valuable content and language guidance when developing a proposed consent form.

The research question. Research in the health sciences is of value to society when it leads to potential improvements in health or health care. Without this potential for societal value, research participants may be assuming risk to no purpose. The importance of the question addressed by a research project is thus an important ethical consideration.

Tip

Many REBs request a lay summary of the protocol that clearly defines the research question. Ensure that your summary is written in language suitable for a non-scientific audience. This ensures that all members of the REB, both scientific and non-scientific, will understand the significance of your project.

Proposing

Scientific validity. Although some investigators might feel that it is not the business of an REB to evaluate the scientific merits of a study, scientific validity is fundamental to the ethical conduct of research. REBs should ensure that members with expertise in research and methodology are present during the review process to ensure that scientific validity is competently considered. Unless a research project has a clear potential to generate reliable and valid results that are generalizable to the greater population, it does not warrant the exposure of participants to any potential risk.

Risks and benefits. It is clear that participation in virtually any research project entails risk, however minimal that risk may be. In Canada, **minimal risk** research is defined as research in which the probability of possible harms implied by participation is no greater than that encountered by the participant in those aspects of his or her everyday life that relate to the research.[11]

An integral component of the REB review process is the discussion of potential risks and benefits as well as proposed mechanisms to minimize potential risk and maximize potential benefit. The potential risks and benefits of research should be discussed in lay terms during the informed consent process. Risks are not limited to physical risks: they may include psychological, social, economic and privacy risks. Where available, risk estimation should be based on current data. Similarly, the potential benefits of research should be described to the participants. Commonly provided secondary benefits, such as remuneration, the provision of specialized care or increased surveillance, should not be considered part of the risk-benefit evaluation, since they do not justify risky research. The overall benefits to society are assumed and are generally not included in the REB discussion or consent process.

Participant selection and recruitment (see ch. 20). Participant selection and recruitment must ensure the fair selection of participants and the equitable distribution of research risks and benefits. Study participants should be drawn from the least vulnerable population that will enable valid conclusions to be reached. Some potential participants may have vulnerabilities related to cognitive ability, age, clinical status, social marginalization, economic disadvantage or incarceration. These participants should not be recruited *specifically* because of these conditions; however, potentially vulnerable participants *may* be recruited if the knowledge gained from their participation is likely to

directly benefit those in similar circumstances. In short, vulnerability is minimized and study integrity is maximized by ensuring that the target group for participation is appropriate for the study question, design, risks and benefits.

Partnerships. Researchers must consider, and work corroborative with, the communities they serve. This may entail involving patients or community members in the planning and conduct of a study. At the conclusion of the research, the community is also entitled to fair and, in some cases, tangible benefits of the research. Expectations in this regard should be discussed before the project is begun.[11]

Respect for participants. It is important that individuals are treated with respect throughout all the phases of a study, including during recruitment (regardless of whether participation is agreed to or declined), study participation and follow-up, and after the formal commitment has ended. Researchers must not limit their responsibility to the monitoring of individuals during the trial (e.g., for adverse reactions, adverse events, change in status), but also must consider halting the trial if aggregate outcomes from the current study or data obtained from other sources raise safety concerns or make the study unnecessary. Researchers must also respect the choice of any participant who decides, at any time, to withdraw from the study.

At the end of the study, participants and concerned communities should be informed about the outcome of the research. Having assumed the risks associated with research participation, they have a right to understand the results and their implications for health care and health care policies.

Consideration should also be given to the ongoing care of research participants at the time of trial completion. This may require referrals to primary care providers and, in more complex situations, ongoing arrangements for access to medication, interventions or treatments that should have shown to benefit the participants or research population.[5,13]

Having respect for participants also means following a fair and thorough process for obtaining informed consent, respecting privacy, and keeping personal information confidential. These important ethical requirements are discussed in the following sections.

Informed consent. The informed consent process is fundamental to the ethical conduct of research. It recognizes the autonomy of individuals with decision-making capacity. For the researcher and the research participant, the dis-

Proposing

cussion that occurs during the recruitment and consent process provides an opportunity to discuss the study design as well as the rights and obligations of the participant.

The imbalance of power between researcher and participant, and the potential for participants to be unduly influenced by that imbalance, should always be considered, especially when a treating physician is conducting a study that involves his or her own patient population. An established patient-physician relationship can make research participants particularly vulnerable during the informed consent process.

Consent documents must disclose information relevant to the research study in a complete and accurate fashion while striking a balance between exhaustive disclosure and readability. Standard components of a consent form are provided in Table 18.1. Most REBs are able to provide sample consent forms that demonstrate suggested wording and formats.

For the informed consent process to be valid, the potential participant must have the capacity to understand and appreciate the information presented. He or she must voluntarily agree to participate without being unduly influenced or coerced. In some contexts the approval of leaders (e.g., households, school principals, elders, etc.) might need to be obtained before individuals are contacted; however, each individual must provide independent consent for participation. For persons from whom consent cannot be obtained, whether for reasons of age, mental capacity or severe loss of function, strategies must be developed to obtain informed consent from legally authorized representatives and to give opportunities for potential participants to refuse participation or to **assent** to participation. That is, some individuals who do not have the capacity for genuinely informed consent might have sufficient capacity to determine that they do not want to participate, or, with the guidance of a surrogate decision-maker, may be able to assent to participate. Provision for assent is commonly included in ethics applications for studies that recruit minor and/or adolescent participants, in conjunction with the informed consent of the legally authorized representatives of potential participants. In certain circumstances, waiver of consent may be permitted (e.g., for chart reviews in which privacy protection has been maximized). In specific situations—such as those involving emergency care, when the prospective participant cannot provide consent, immediate intervention is required, and the research may provide a real possibility of benefit, REBs may permit

research to be conducted without free and informed consent or with delayed consent. Consent for ongoing participation must be obtained at the earliest opportunity after enrolment. Guidance should be obtained from the *TCPS*[11] and local applicable regulations.

Tip

Most REBs will provide sample consent forms. In general, consent forms should be written at a reading level appropriate for the proposed study population. Ensure that they are proofread carefully before submission.

Local REBs will provide guidance regarding waiver of consent, substitute decision-makers, and consent in emergency health care situations. Be sure to obtain the guidance you need early in the planning stages of your study.

Privacy and confidentiality. Issues of **privacy** and **confidentiality** arise with respect to research participants and the sponsors of research.

First, respect for the privacy of research participants and the confidentiality of their personal data is not only ethically imperative but, at many sites, is subject to federal, and/or provincial or territorial legislation. Researchers are responsible for the security of any personal information, including health information, that they collect throughout the life of the study and sometimes for many years beyond: that is, during the recruitment, enrolment, collection, analysis, storage and destruction of data.[12] This obligation applies to identifying or identifiable information, such as names, address, full postal codes, telephone and fax numbers, email and IP addresses, URLs, health card numbers, images, social insurance numbers, medical record numbers, dates of birth, and any health-related information. Investigators must be in compliance with the duties set out in locally applicable federal, provincial and territorial legislation, the *TCPS* and local applicable policies. An excellent resource for privacy-related issues is the document *Best Practices for Protecting Privacy in Health Research*[12] as well as the *TCPS*.[11]

Second, researchers must also consider the impact of any contractual obligations with sponsors with respect to the confidentiality of data and proprietary information.[14,15] Such agreements can set limits on the right of initial analysis

Proposing

■   **Table 18.1: Elements commonly included in letters of information and/or research participant consent forms**

Item	Explanation
Study title	Full title and working title
Principal investigator	Name, credentials and contact information
Co-investigators	Names, credentials and contact information
Study coordinator	Names, credentials and contact information
24-hour contact	Name of someone whom the participant can contact with urgent questions or concerns about the study at any time
Study sponsor	In general, as defined in ICH–GCP
Conflict of interest	Declaration as consistent with institutional policy
Study information	
Introduction	General information about the specific research as proposed
Background and purpose	Information about why the study is being conducted, and about the standard (non-experimental) treatment
Description of the methods	What will happen during the study, how may people will take part, the responsibilities of participants, and details about study visits and procedures
Potential harms	The potential harms of participation, both significant and common. Literature should be used, when possible, to provide estimated rates of occurrences. This section may include reproductive risks, or these may be listed separately.
Potential benefits	The potential benefits of individual participation
Alternatives to participation	Other choices available to the potential participant
Privacy and confidentiality	The impact of the study on the privacy and confidentiality rights of the participant
Communication with primary care or treating doctor	How the results and therapy with be communicated with the participant's doctor, if this is agreed to by the participant
Costs of participation/reimbursement	Any costs, reimbursement and remuneration associated with participation
In case of injury, illness or harm	Recourse available in the case of harm
Participation and withdrawal	An explanation that participation is voluntary, and that the participant has the right to withdraw without penalty
New findings or information	What the participant may expect with regard to being informed of new findings or information that has a bearing on the study
Study results	How (or whether) study results will be communicated to the participant
REB contact information	Information about the Research Ethics Board review and contact information in case the participant has any questions regarding his or her rights
Statement of consent and signatures	Frequently contains a summary of the rights and obligations of the participant. The signature of the participant and of a witness to the consent procedure or to the signature is frequently obtained. This section may also require that the person who obtained consent sign and dates the consent form.

Proposing

and interpretation of the clinical trial dataset. As part of ensuring the integrity of their research, it is important for researchers to seek assurances that their contractual rights and obligations are consistent with local standards, policies and the *TCPS*. As will be discussed later in the chapter, review by your institution's **research administration** office will ensure that institutional policies are met regarding confidentiality agreements and privacy-related issues arising from transfers of personal information and biological material, and from the publication of findings.

What should I do if I need to change my protocol or study procedures?

REBs make decisions regarding the acceptability of suggested departures from originally approved research.[11] In general, there are three categories to consider: (1) unanticipated or unexpected events; (2) changes from the approved protocol arising from ongoing feedback; and (3) unavoidable, single-incident deviations from the approved protocol. All protocol amendments must be reviewed and approved by the approving REB. *Issues of safety should be addressed immediately by the research team and reported promptly to the REB.*

Tip

Participant safety is paramount. Immediate changes to a protocol that are necessary to ensure patient safety should be implemented, and REBs should be notified as soon as possible.

What is involved in continuing ethics review?

The REB is responsible for making a final determination as to the nature and frequency of continuing ethics review. At a minimum, an annual status or end-of-study report is required. Annual renewal may require, but is not limited to, documentation regarding the conduct of the study, including the number of participants recruited, timelines, adverse events, unanticipated findings and an update regarding the current literature.

Conflict of interest

A **conflict of interest** can arise when activities or situations place persons or institutions in a real, potential or perceived conflict between their duties or responsibilities related to

research and their personal, institutional or other interests. *Conflicts of interest—also called "competing interests"—do not necessarily imply wrongdoing, and the recognition, disclosure and management of potential conflicts of interest mitigate the risk of scientific misconduct.* Conflicting roles, duties and responsibilities must be assessed to ensure that the interests of potential participants and the integrity of research are preserved. It is the responsibility of researchers, REB members and institutions to identify real, potential or perceived conflicts of interest associated with their roles and to establish mechanisms to declare and manage these issues as they arise.

Tip

It is your responsibility to be aware of your institution's guidelines and requirements for the declaration and management of conflicts of interest.

Clinical trial registration

Clinical trial registries permit web-based access to information regarding ongoing clinical trials so that information is available about trials and their results.[b] Trial registration is the accepted international standard. According to the TCPS, "All clinical trials shall be registered before recruitment of the first trial participant in a recognized and easily web-accessible public registry" (Article 11.3).[11] Trial registration helps ensure that all stakeholders—from patients, to clinicians, systematic reviewers, developers of clinical practice guidelines, and policy-makers—can make themselves aware both of ongoing trials and of the existence of trials whose results are never published. This awareness serves a number of purposes. Publication bias and selective reporting—that is, failure to publish negative studies or studies with less promising results—distort the body of available evidence.[16–18] Non-disclosure agreements with trial sponsors can contribute to the suppression of negative or inconclusive findings; trial registration, in tandem with the development of editorial policies that insist on registration and full access to data as a requirement for publication, seeks to combat this problem. As well as improving awareness of trial results, registration of ongoing trials helps researchers avoid unnecessary duplication and provides opportunities for collaborative work and the identification

---

b   Examples include www.clinicaltrials.gov and www.controlled-trials.com

Proposing

of potential research gaps. It is hoped that registration will also lead to improved quality of trials by identifying methodologic problems or bringing to light protocol changes made during the course of a trial. Finally, trial registration allows potential participants to identify trials that may be applicable to them.

In compliance with the requirements of the WHO and the International Committee of Medical Journal Editors, researchers should register their trial before they start to recruit participants, and provide their REB with the registration number.[16] According to the WHO, "a clinical trial is any research study that prospectively assigns human participants or groups of humans to one or more health-related interventions to evaluate the effects on health outcomes."[c]

One example of a clinical trial registration site is ClinicalTrials.gov. Open to over 170 countries, this site provides report summaries for registered clinical trials and observational studies. The site includes information on participant flow, baseline characteristics, outcome measures, statistics and adverse events as well as pertinent administrative information.[19] Although information may be submitted for any trial, according to the US Food and Drug Administration Amendments Act of 2007[d] the responsible party for a study must register and report results for trials, including, but not limited to, trials of drugs and biologics of controlled clinical investigations (excluding Phase I) or of a product subject to FDA regulations. In general, the most responsible party is required to submit "basic results not later than one year after the 'primary completion date' or the date that the final subject was examined or received intervention."

The role of institutional research administration

Institutions are responsible for *all* research conducted within their jurisdiction or under their auspices.[10,20] That is, they are responsible for the conduct of research conducted by their faculty, staff or students, regardless of where the research is conducted. Institutions are responsible for ensuring that research is conducted in compliance with applicable policies, guidance documents and regulations. This includes oversight related to funding, good clinical practice and privacy legislation. Institutions are also responsible for ensuring that research teams who apply for grants or agree to conduct research on behalf of a sponsor have appropriate access to resources and participants as well as the skills and knowledge necessary to conduct the research in an efficient and safe manner. In general, institutions receive and administer funds on behalf of research teams. It is essential, therefore, that institutional and ethics review be conducted.

To be eligible to receive and administer funds from the federally administered agencies (CIHR, NSERC and SSHRC), institutions must agree to comply with a number of agency policies set out as schedules to a Memorandum of Understanding between the agencies and institutions.[20] In a similar fashion, institutions that receive funding from US government sources must provide assurances that the use of the funding will be in compliance with the specified regulations.[20]

Clinical trial applications to Health Canada are required for studies intended for use in regulatory marketing approval in Canada. This includes Phase I, II and III clinical trials,[21] including trials that test the safety and effectiveness of marketed drugs outside the parameters of the approved indications.

Contracts and agreements

Your institution's research administration staff provide a variety of services on behalf of the institution and its researchers—including you. They have expertise in the preparation and review of agreements, including:

- clinical study agreements
- confidentiality/non-disclosure agreements
- material transfer agreements
- service provider/independent contractor's agreements
- peer-reviewed funding agreements
- basic science research agreements
- inter-institutional agreements
- intellectual property agreements (e.g., licence agreements)
- privacy/data sharing agreements

Review by institutional representatives ensures compliance with applicable policies, including those related to transfers of personal information and biological material, liability and publication.

Researchers must consider the impact of contractual obligations with sponsors, who may seek to limit the right of initial analysis and interpretation of the clinical trial

Proposing

---

c   WHO International Clinical Trials Registry Platform, www.who.int/ictrp/en/
d   See http://clinicaltrials.gov and http://prsinfo.clinicaltrials.gov/fdaaa.html

dataset. It is important that researchers ensure the integrity of their research. Assurances should be sought that contractual rights and obligations are consistent with local standards, policies and the TCPS. Review by institutional representatives ensures that institutional policies are met regarding agreements and privacy-related issues arising from transfers of personal information and biological material, and with regard to publication.

Insurance

Researchers who are contracted by third-party sponsors should ensure that appropriate insurance is in place that will cover any potential claims resulting from the project. Of note, in the case of peer-reviewed funding, the researcher's home institution is considered the sponsor and is therefore responsible for providing insurance.

Researchers should ensure that they have insurance coverage. They may be covered under institutional insurance, as employees. However, in the case of physicians, insurance may not be available in this fashion. It is your responsibility to contact your insurer, including the Canadian Medical Protective Association (CMPA), to inquire as to the type and nature of insurance coverage you have with respect to research, since not all types of projects may be covered.

Conclusion

Preparing a research ethics board and institutional application are essential steps in the conduct of research. Although it may be perceived as burdensome, it allows researchers to view a study protocol from the perspective of the participant, to minimize risks, and to maximize safety and the potential benefits of the research. Ethical principles should be considered when the protocol is being designed; ethics should not be an afterthought. The *Tri-Council Policy Statement: Ethical Conduct for Research Involving Humans*[11] provides important information for Canadian researchers. Those planning to conduct clinical trials should also seek specific training in the International Conference on Harmonization–Good Clinical Practice (ICH–GCP)[13] guidelines to ensure that regulatory requirements are met. Finally, researchers should be aware of both the implications and the obligations associated with funding sources. As applicable, all necessary contracts should be reviewed by your institution to ensure that any required agreements are in place. ■

Proposing

CASE POSTSCRIPT

Although the potential risks arising from participation in this research project appear to be minimal, various issues should be reviewed before the protocol is submitted to the REB. Although the staff supervisor may perceive the project as a quality improvement effort that does not require REB review, if the student intends to present or publish the results, and thus disseminate the information to a broader audience, it will likely be deemed research. If the trial is to be conducted at more than one site, investigators should make themselves aware of the protocol applications and policies for individual and multi-site reviews. (Of note, variability in REB review and requirements among sites may add to the logistical challenges, including the time necessary to obtain all required approvals.)

From a scientific perspective, the question appears to be important and scientifically valid.

How will residents be recruited for the study? The REB might consider residents to be a potentially vulnerable population insofar as they are in the process of completing mandatory training requirements. Might they feel pressured to participate in a study conducted by a colleague or staff supervisor? Would using a neutral third party (a research coordinator) to obtain consent help to minimize such influence? Is there a strong expectation on the part of the researcher that 100% recruitment will be achieved, or do the residents perceive such an expectation to exist?

The residents will likely have questions about the potential consequences of participating or not participating. They—like the REB—will want to know the risks and benefits. Will participation have an impact on their training? Will it affect their current or future evaluations? If it will (or is perceived to), how can this be managed? Will participants be permitted to withdraw from the study if they choose? If so, can they withdraw their data?

The protocol states that residents will be provided with feedback. Who will provide this feedback, and how? For example, is it appropriate for a resident colleague to have access to the performance ratings of his or her peers? Will the assessments become part of their permanent training record? Is this reasonable? What are alternative strategies?

What other privacy and confidentiality concerns need to be addressed? The researchers must give consideration to the number of residents available for the study, and to whether potentially identifying demographic data are being collected, grouped and reported in a manner that will maintain privacy. (In general, the minimum size for grouped data should be five, i.e., n = 5.)

How will consent be sought? Informed consent will be required if this is a research protocol. Consent guidelines for the respective REBs should be followed. The consent form should be checked for spelling, grammar and readability. In this case, the general reading skills of the participants will be felt to be high, and most REBs will allow for a more sophisticated description of the study, as well as of associated risks and benefits, privacy issues and the rights and obligations of the research participant.

Finally, in assessing the potential risks to participants and the ethical issues arising from the protocol, consideration should be given to holding a group discussion to enable adequate input from all parties before REB approval is sought.

Proposing

REFERENCES

1. Emanuel EJ, Wendler D, Grady C. An ethical framework for biomedical research. In: Emanuel EJ, editor. *The Oxford textbook of clinical research ethics.* 1st ed. New York: Oxford; 2008. p. 123–35.

2. Rothman DJ. Research ethics at Tuskegee and Willowbrook. *Am J Med.* 1984;77(6):A49.

3. Curtis H. Getting ethics into practice: Tuskegee was bad enough. *BMJ.* 2004;28;329(7464):513.

4. Goldby S. Experiments at the Willowbrook State School. *Lancet.* 1971;1(7702):749.

5. World Medical Association. *WMA Declaration of Helsinki—ethical principles of medical research involving human subjects.* October 2008. Available from: www.wma.net/en/30publications/10policies/b3/index.html

6. (US) National Commission for the Protection of Human Subjects of Biomedical and Behavioral Research. *The Belmont Report: ethical principles and guidelines for the protection of human subjects of research.* Washington: The Commission; 1979.

7. (US) Department of Health and Human Services. *Code of Federal Regulations.* 21 CFR 50, 1996 Oct 2. Report No. 61(192).

8. Department of Health and Human Services. *Code of Federal Regulations.* 45 CFR Part 46, Protection of Human Subjects. 15-1-2009. 20-1-2010.

9. Council for International Organizations of Medical Sciences (CIOMS). *International ethical guidelines for biomedical research involving human subjects.* Geneva: CIOMS; 2002. Available from: www.cioms.ch/publications/layout_guide2002.pdf

10. Canadian Institutes of Health Research, Natural Sciences and Engineering Research Council of Canada, Social Sciences and Humanities Research Council of Canada, *Tri-Council Policy Statement: Ethical Conduct for Research Involving Humans (TCPS),* 1998 (with 2000, 2002, 2005 amendments). Ottawa: Interagency Secretariat on Research Ethics; 2005. Available from: www.pre.ethics.gc.ca/eng/archives/tcps-eptc/Default/

11. Canadian Institutes of Health Research, Natural Sciences and Engineering Research Council of Canada, and Social Sciences and Humanities Research Council of Canada, Tri-Council Policy Statement: Ethical Conduct for Research Involving Humans, 2nd ed. Ottawa: Panel on Research Ethics; December 2010. Available from: www.pre.ethics.gc.ca/eng/policy-politique/initiatives/tcps2-eptc2/Default/

12. Canadian Institutes of Health Research. *CIHR Best Practices for Protecting Privacy in Health Research.* Ottawa (ON): The Institutes; 2005. Available from: www.cihr-irsc.gc.ca/e/documents/et_pbp_nov05_sept2005_e.pdf

13. International Conference on Harmonization of Technical Requirements for the Registation of Pharmaceuticals for Human Use. *Guidance for industry. Good clinical practice: consolidated guideline. ICH topic E6.* Ottawa: Health Canada; 1997. Available from: www.hc-sc.gc.ca/dhp-mps/alt_formats/hpfb-dgpsa/pdf/prodpharma/e6-eng.pdf

14. For case law examples and the Nancy Olivieri case see http://canadianhealthcarelaw.com/index.php?option=com_content&view=category&layout=blog&id=99&Itemid=83&lang=en

15. Naylor D. Early Toronto experience with new standards for industry-sponsored clinical research: a progress report. *CMAJ.* 2002;166(4):453–56.

16. DeAngelis C, Drazen JM, Frizelle FA, Haug C, Hoey J, Horton R, et al. Clinical trial registration: a statement from the International Committee of Medical Journal Editors. *CMAJ.* 2004;171(6):606–7.

17. Foote M. Clinical trial registries and clinical trial result posting: new paradigm for medical writers. *Biotechnol Annu Rev.* 2006;12:379–86.

18. Steinbrook R. Public registration of clinical trials. *N Engl J Med.* 2004;351(4):315–7.

19. ClinicalTrials.gov. About the ClinicalTrials.gov results database. Available from: www.clinicaltrials.gov/ct2/info/results

20. Memorandum of Understanding on the Roles and Responsibilities in the Management of Federal Grants and Awards. 2010.

21. Canada. Food and Drug Regulations (C.R.C., c. 870). Part C, Division 5: Drugs for clinical trials involving human subjects. Available from: http://laws-lois.justice.gc.ca/eng/regulations/C.R.C.,_c._870/page-397.html#h-251

Proposing

ADDITIONAL RESOURCES

The following websites and articles provide more information and case studies regarding research ethics.

Evolution of protections for research participants

University of Waterloo. Office of Research Ethics. *Evolution of protection of human participants in research* [updated 2009 March 26]. Available from: http://iris.uwaterloo.ca/ethics/human/resources/index.htm

The Jesse Gelsinger case (gene therapy/conflict of interest)

New York Times. See articles compiled at: http://topics.nytimes.com/topics/reference/timestopics/people/g/jesse_gelsinger/index.html

Johns Hopkins University lead paint study

Alliance for Human Research Protection. *Johns Hopkins University experiment on lead paint puts children in danger.* See articles compiled at: www.ahrp.org/children/HopkinsEndangers.php

The need for contract review and publication agreements

Naylor D. Early Toronto experience with new standards for industry-sponsored clinical research: a progress report. *CMAJ.* 2002;166(4):453–56.

Ownership of tissue, consent and contracts

Grady D. The lasting gift to medicine that wasn't really a gift. *New York Times.* 2010; Feb 1. Available from: www.nytimes.com/2010/02/02/health/02seco.html
- The case of Henrietta Lack's unknowing donation to science of the HeLa cell.

Skloot R. Taking the least of you. *New York Times.* 2006; Apr 16. Available from: www.nytimes.com/2006/04/16/magazine/16tissue.html?pagewanted=1
- For an important case concerning ownership of prostate tissue samples, see "The case that could change everything," p. 7.

Privacy

Canadian Institutes for Health Research. *CIHR best practices in protecting privacy in health research.* Ottawa: The Institutes; 2005. Available from: www.cihr-irsc.gc.ca/e/documents/et_pbp_nov05_sept2005_e.pdf
- An excellent resource for the management of privacy issues in the context of research.

The Tuskegee syphilis study

Tuskegee University. *Research Ethics: The Tuskegee syphilis study.* Available from www.tuskegee.edu/global/story.asp?s=1207598

White RM. Unraveling the Tuskegee study of untreated syphilis. *Arch Intern Med.* 2000;160(5):585–98.

Proposing

SUMMARY CHECKLIST

❑ Review the relevant institutional ethics statements for your jurisdiction (eg. TriCouncil, NIH). Complete any online tutorials that are available.

❑ Review your research protocol, and identify any ethical issues that it raises.

❑ Revise your protocol to incorporate the management of ethical issues, such as informed consent.

❑ Apply to all of the relevant REBs for your study, using the application forms they require.

❑ Note the number and details of your ethics certificates.

❑ Register your study, if applicable, in relevant databases.

❑ If you make any changes to your protocol, compose an amendment to inform your REB.

❑ Complete your regular review or end-of-study declaration for the REBs.

Proposing

19
Research funding and other resources

G. Mark Brown, MSc

Eddy S. Lang, MDCM, CCFP(EM), CSPQ

ILLUSTRATIVE CASE

A senior Pediatrics fellow is interested in investigating the prevalence of occult hypoglycemia among infants who present to the emergency department with vomiting and probable gastroenteritis. She soon realizes that gathering and analysing the data, and ultimately disseminating the results, will require significant resources. First, in order to achieve the requisite sample size, a method to screen and recruit a sufficient number of eligible families for inclusion in the study is needed. Second, some aspects of data entry and analysis will need to be contracted to someone with specialized expertise in this area. Third, if the project were to be accepted for presentation at the annual scientific meeting of the Canadian Paediatric Society, the costs of registration, travel and accommodation will need to be considered. Although some of the expenses of the project might be covered at no cost to the resident through her hospital or university, she will need to find a funding source to cover the rest.

■ Research requires funding. Even

simple projects need some degree of financial support along with human resources. If you are wondering "Where do I start?" or "Who can help me?" you are on the right track. However, the first step is to draw up a budget for your project. Indeed, this is a requirement of many Research Ethics Board applications. This chapter will provide a framework for planning resources, reducing costs and securing the necessary operating funds and human resources. Novice researchers often underestimate the resources needed to complete a study. Good will and the contributions of volunteer collaborators are helpful, but they are not sustainable. Nor do they cover material resources. Any experienced clinical researcher will confirm that, as with a home renovation, the successful completion of a project typically costs more than anticipated. Even the smallest of projects require some labour, by experts and others, along with access to technology, space and time. Although funding can be difficult to obtain, it is not impossible; in fact, in some cases novice researchers find it easier to access the resources they need than their senior colleagues do.

The costs of research

As the research road map presented in chapter 1 of this guide shows, questions of resources and funding present early and often in the course of research project. As a junior researcher, one of your first steps on the road is to identify and approach a potential supervisor—that is, a faculty

CHAPTER OBJECTIVES

After reading this chapter, you should be able to:

- describe the wide range of formal small-grant funding opportunities that are potentially available to support the research projects of health care trainees and residents
- discuss creative methods for enlisting human resources or accessing necessary infrastructure to advance a research project
- list other creative and potentially unconventional strategies for injecting funds or other financial and "in-kind" support into the conduct or dissemination of research

---

KEY TERMS

Budget	Human resources
Collaboration	Sources of funding
Financial requirements	Volunteers
Grants	

Proposing

Proposing

member who will guide and support you in the conduct of your research project (see ch. 3). Although finding an advisor with a strong publishing record is important, so too is evaluating his or her funding record. Does he or she have funding, or work with a research group or laboratory that routinely secures **grants**? If so, are these grants a potential source of funding for your project? For example, existing operating grants might provide funds for your proposed research in whole or in part. At a minimum, your supervisor should be able to provide suitable guidance for obtaining your own funding and help you to troubleshoot problems that arise. In the end, remember that funding is not the responsibility of the supervisor, although securing funding without the help of a supervisor is highly unusual.

Next, consider how your research question will be operationalized. As you assess your study design, as detailed in chapter 9, the key is to determine whether it is feasible. At the most practical level, this means having adequate money and personnel to do the job properly. Key to this is input from frontline research staff. Even if they are not directly involved in your project, experienced research staff can advise you about potential barriers to executing your study, and about possible solutions. If your study design is too ambitious, it is also likely to cost too much and to require too many people to be achievable.

Step 5 of the research road map—developing an outline for the project—is all about planning. Textbox 19.1 lists the human and other resources that might be needed for even a modest research project. Careful thought at this stage will not only prevent mistakes and spare you some headaches and cost overruns, but will also make your research experience more enjoyable and more rewarding.[1,2] A cornerstone of planning is the creation of a realistic budget: every grant application you write will require one.

Your methodology and research protocol will dictate most of your costs. Aside from the type of study you choose—a randomized controlled trial will be more expensive to conduct than a survey, for example—questions of cost arise from how the data collection and analysis will be done (and by whom), the sample size necessary to achieve adequate study power, who will handle the administration and paperwork, and whether outside consulting and specialized knowledge are needed. The greatest research costs are labour, labour, and labour. The amount that contracted work is worth is dictated by professional standards and local labour agreements. Again, it's always best to go to people with expertise in this area, such as your institution's

Human Resources department, to avoid any unpleasant surprises.

When the research is over and the results are analyzed, you aren't quite finished. Disseminating your study results will require time and energy, and can involve further expense. For example, is this work to be published? Where will it be presented, and in which formats? Is travel required?

Once you know what your costs are, you have done half the work of planning your project funding. Now you need to be aware of how you can cut costs and what funding is available. These issues are the focus of the remainder of this chapter.

TEXTBOX 19.1: POTENTIAL HUMAN AND FINANCIAL RESOURCE REQUIREMENTS OF RESEARCH

Human resources

Chart abstractors/reviewers
Data collection
Data entry
Enrolment and screening
Librarian: literature review
Statistician: study design and analysis
Study administrator

Financial requirements

Administrative and office supplies
Consultants: database, statistics
Enrolment and data collection
Printing and publication
Statistical software
Survey administration
Travel

Managing resources to cut costs

Human resources represent a potentially significant cost and an administrative challenge for any research project. However, there is a bright side, for this is also an area where, with the help of your supervisor and a little creativity, you can substantially cut costs.

Although this might be your first experience managing a research project, your supervisor should be familiar with the research process and the area of health your question probes. He or she should know whom to approach for help and what resources are available to facilitate your work.

Moreover, with a track record of successful funding, your supervisor should be able to guide you to the institutional, governmental and industry grants relevant to your study. You will also undoubtedly be surrounded by other residents or health care trainees with a wide range of backgrounds, some of whom may have significant research experience. Use their knowledge and experience to your advantage. A senior trainee might have won the grant you seek in a previous year and be able to provide you with valuable insights. Another might know how best to conduct a literature search; another, with a master's degree in epidemiology, might be willing to save you the cost of outsourcing statistical advice. Participate in journal clubs and other departmental activities where you are likely to develop your own expertise. And consider that, although your peers are busy people, they are also a potential source of volunteer labour.

Resource-sharing is the basis of **collaboration** and is often a means of reducing costs. Collaboration can bring needed expertise to a study, obviating the expense of outsourcing. It can also make use of existing capital and research infrastructure that might be impractical or impossible to duplicate on your budget. This is the same principal that allows many small, university-built satellites to get into space: they piggyback on the efforts of larger commercial outfits, who pay the bulk of the significant launch costs. In the field of health research, this could mean associating with a research network doing similar work (see ch. 4) and possibly aligning your research question with their interests. Of prime consideration in such relationships are questions of ownership of research, recognition and authorship (see ch. 3), expectations for which need to be discussed before the research begins.

Even more valuable than collaborators are **volunteers**, the majority of whom are interested students who can be invaluable to you: they generally have fairly flexible schedules and may be able to give you their time for a low rate— or even for free. Although they may have limited health care knowledge and often limited research acumen, students are always looking to gain relevant experience, particularly if they want to get into professional health care programs and/or graduate school.[3] Similarly, undergraduate medical students hoping to enter a particular specialty want to meet residents and staff to enhance their chances of being accepted. However, this is a two-way street. Health researchers have a vested interest in providing such research experience because it attracts students to their profession and field of study. It also develops a pool of research experience that

these same fields can tap later. Although volunteers can be sought from the generalist training programs, a more promising avenue is to seek out specialty-specific interest groups to focus your call for volunteers (e.g., an Emergency Medicine Interest Group). This is an attractive option when funding is very limited; an important caveat, however, is "You get what you pay for."

If you are lucky enough to have one in your department, Research Associate programs[4,5] are a unique resource for volunteer help. These programs are departmental or university-based organizations of volunteers, typically medical or nursing students, managed by experienced medical researchers. Volunteers receive training specific to their particular duties and fill many screening, study enrolment and data collection roles. They receive the same benefits as the student volunteers alluded to previously, but management by the program coordinator removes much of the administrative stress of coordinating what could be several students for your one study.

The budget

If you have been thinking about costs through the planning and development of your study design, most elements of the **budget** should already be determined. Now it is time to estimate the specific costs associated with each aspect of the project. Start with a list of everything you want and pare it down to what is absolutely necessary. Include a contingency budget for unforeseen expenses; with the proper planning and input from experienced personnel in this area, these should be minimal. Your budget should specify a minimum and maximum: your actual costs should fall somewhere in between. Discuss the budget with your supervisor and get his or her opinion on whether the total amount is feasible. Table 19.1 provides examples of budget items that might be involved in a resident research project, with cost estimates in 2010 Canadian dollars.

Formal funding mechanisms

Why seek formal funding? The simple answer is that a lot of this type of money is available. Another reassuring aspect is that the exercise of applying for formal funding forces you to go through a clearly laid-out process that, regardless of the outcome, will likely make any subsequent funding requests, formal or otherwise, easier to prepare. However, this type of financial support has other benefits as well. The

Proposing

Proposing

■   **Table 19.1: Sample budget items, with associated cost estimates**

Commercially available online survey program	$20–$50/month
Medical record search (first 100 free)	$3/chart
Use of prepared and validated data collection or survey tool	$250–$500
Survey methodologist A quantitative survey specialist will provide advice regarding survey methodology to ensure survey validity and maximize response rates.	$50–$80/hr
Statistical analyst To address study design and quantitative analysis; responsible for statistical programming and data analysis.	$50–$100/hr
Reference database To generate a database of studies retrieved through searches, select studies for inclusion in the study, and provide citations for a manuscript.	$150–$350
Duplication costs at $0.20/page. Distribution of information, assessment and data collection tools to study participants and reviewers. Distribution of studies to blinded investigators assessing items for inclusion.	$50–$500+
Administrative costs Acquiring contact information and correspondence (e.g., survey implementation); blinding investigators responsible for assessing studies for inclusion; organizing volunteer resources.	$25–$40/hr
Office costs Including occasional photocopies, printing, faxes, telephone contacts and teleconferencing.	$100
Database support An information technology specialist will generate and manage an electronic database of data retrieved from studies selected for inclusion.	$30–$40/hr
Travel and media preparation For presentation of the study findings at your specialty association's annual conference	$400–$1000
Poster for results dissemination	$250–$500

application process involves, peer review, giving you a valuable opportunity to obtain an expert opinion on your proposal. Weak proposals are often rightly turned back at this point. However disappointing this may be, it is better to discover the shortcomings of your project now, rather than after the money is spent with a poor result to show for it.

Formal applications also involve stepwise planning and deadlines that will help to get you on track, on time and off to a good start with your research. Finally, winning a grant often brings prestige and credibility. When seeking grants, look for resources designated for junior investigators, new researchers or residents and other health trainees.

Formal funding can have disadvantages, though. Application timelines are sometimes restrictive, forcing you to work according to someone else's schedule. Also, if you don't find out about the grant deadline with enough lead-time you might find yourself scrambling to pull everything together at the last minute—or being left out entirely. (Large portions of your project proposal can often be used to draft a grant application, saving valuable time when deadlines approach.) Also, no matter how worthy your proposal, you will likely be competing with numerous other applicants. Fewer than 50% of grant applications are successful. However, don't think of your work on an unsuccessful proposal as wasted; the documents you prepare for one application can often be tailored for another, and the time you invest in honing your ideas should enhance your next project's chances of success.

Examples of the many **sources of funding** are listed in the Additional Resources section at the end of this chapter. Important first-line sources are federal and provincial agencies that fund science, social science and medical research, often through an institute or foundation. These include the Social Sciences and Humanities Research Council (SSHRC), the Natural Sciences and Research Council of Canada (NSERC) and the Canadian Institutes of Health Research (CIHR). At the provincial level are organizations such as Alberta Innovates Health Solutions (a division of the Alberta Heritage Foundation for Medical Research), Ontario's Ministry of Research and Innovation, and Quebec's Fonds de la recherche en santé.

National societies and associations offer grants for research in specific fields. The Royal College of Physicians and Surgeons of Canada has a grant that targets resident research specifically, as do specialty societies such as the College of Family Physicians of Canada (CFPC) and the Canadian Association of Emergency Physicians (CAEP). Consider related specialties when your research project spans more than one field, as in our case scenario (the Pediatrics fellow could seek funding in both Pediatrics and Emergency Medicine). Check out the website of your national association for more information. In fact, spend some time on the website of your university, medical school or department. Universities usually have a research office dedicated to facilitating grant and funding efforts that can provide, as well as information on specific funding sources, grant mentoring programs and expertise to point you in the right direction.

Many private foundations exist to promote research and health care investment; these are usually affiliated with hospitals or disease-specific societies. Examples include the Canadian Cancer Society, the Heart and Stroke Foundation, the Kidney Foundation of Canada and the Alzheimer's Society of Canada. In Ontario, the Physicians' Services Incorporated Foundation is a unique physician-centred resource for grants. Certain specialties also have related foundations that offer research funding, such as the Canadian Foundation for Women's Health (the foundation of the Society of Obstetricians and Gynaecologists of Canada). However, specialties often have no direct relationship with related organizations, and an initial funding search might be broadened to find these funding opportunities (e.g., the Canadian Paediatric Society and the Sick Kids Foundation both provide awards and grants for Pediatrics research). Unless you have a specific organization in mind, use searchable databases of granting facilities—for there are literally thousands of foundations. Excellent resources include the Community of Science, Imagine Canada and GrantsNet. Moreover, many universities have a person designated as the grant advisor whose role it is to identify appropriate potential sources of funding for a given project.

Informal funding mechanisms

Not all sources of funding have to be organizations with formalized grants and grant application processes. Billing groups and "practice plans" are clinical practices in which physicians develop a pool of funds for a common use. Frequently this is to promote advancement of their field without the constraints of outside agencies. Consequently, research conducted through this mechanism must have relevance to clinicians. An example might be research that can help improve clinical efficiency, for example through novel triaging, the use of electronic databases or the development of clinical practice guidelines.

Industry is also a source of funding—one with deep pockets but a profit-making agenda. At issue with this mechanism are significant concerns related to ownership of the study results and potential conflicts of interest (see ch. 18). If you pursue industry sponsorship, you must ensure that your funding or grant is unrestricted. Local pharmaceutical companies and other biomedical manufacturers will often provide small (< $5000), unrestricted research grants to junior researchers who apply. An example might be a grant from an ultrasound manufacturer to assess how

Proposing

frequently ultrasound is used at the bedside in emergency departments. Review your university's requirements regarding the kind of legal agreements that must be in place before industry or other private funding may be accepted.

Finally, consider the graduate-student approach of begging and borrowing. The contacts you make in other labs, with other students and with other researchers open doors. Equipment is often not in use, space is sometimes unoccupied and people are frequently willing to do an hour or two of work simply for the experience.

Conclusion

Funding research takes time, effort and—most importantly—planning. However, the cost of research, whether financial or human, should not be seen as a major impediment. There are many sources of grants and a deep pool of expertise and labour to get the job done correctly, on time and on budget. ■

CASE POSTSCRIPT

Proper study design and the development of a solid research protocol would have averted most of the problems the Pediatrics fellow is now facing. However, if enough volunteers can be found to identify and recruit eligible participants for entry into the study, the project might still be feasible. Determining whether either the pediatric or emergency departments have Research Associate programs could solve the human resources and organizational challenges this represents. Data entry can be tackled in a similar manner, although analysis often requires specialized expertise. A collaborator may be able to provide this without additional cost, or the resident could spend some time learning the material herself. Finally, funding can be sought from appropriate organizations or the hospital's research foundation to cover the costs of study execution and the dissemination of results.

REFERENCES

1. Hebert RS, Levine RB, Smith CG, Wright SM. A systematic review of resident research curricula. *Acad Med.* 2003;78(1):61–8.

2. Barletta JF. Conducting a successful residency research project. *Am J Pharm Educ.* 2008;72(4):92.

3. Sparano DM, Shofer FS, Hollander JE. Participation in the academic associate program: effect on medical school admission rate. *Acad Emerg Med.* 2004;11(6):695–8.

4. Hollander JE, Valentine SM, Brogan GX Jr. Academic associate program: integrating clinical emergency medicine research with undergraduate education. *Acad Emerg Med.* 1997;4(3):225–30.

5. Hollander JE, Singer AJ. An innovative strategy for conducting clinical research: the academic associate program. *Acad Emerg Med.* 2002;9(2):134–7.

ADDITIONAL RESOURCES

National Organizations

Canadian Coalition for Global Health Research
www.ccghr.ca/default.cfm?control=funding&lang=e&subnav=roadmap

Canadian Health Services Research Foundation
www.chsrf.ca/funding_opportunities/index_e.php

Canadian Institutes of Health Research (CIHR)
www.cihr-irsc.gc.ca

- CIHR has a master list of funding opportunities that is updated on a regular basis.

Knowledge Translation (KT) Canada
http://ktclearinghouse.ca/ktcanada/education/funding

Natural Sciences and Research Council of Canada
www.nserc-crsng.gc.ca

- NSERC provides a list of new funding opportunities and general application information.

Royal College of Physicians and Surgeons of Canada
http://rcpsc.medical.org/awards/wightman_e.php

- K.J.R. Wightman Award for Scholarship in Ethics

Social Sciences and Humanities Research Council (SHHRC)
www.sshrc.ca/site/apply-demande/program_index-index_programmes-eng.aspx

- SSHRC provides a general page on programs available for researchers to apply to.

Provincial
Alberta Innovates Health Solutions
www.ahfmr.ab.ca/grants.php

Nova Scotia Health Research Foundation
www.nshrf.ca

Ontario Ministry of Research and Innovation
www.mri.gov.on.ca/english/programs/default.asp

Physicians' Services Incorporated Foundation
www.psifoundation.org/

Quebec Fonds de la Recherche en Santé
www.frsq.gouv.qc.ca/en/index.shtml

Medical schools and universities
The Research Institute of the McGill University Health Centre
http://muhc.ca/research/dashboard

University of Alberta: Research Services Office
www.rso.ualberta.ca

University of British Columbia: Office of Research Services
www.ors.ubc.ca/index.htm

University of Toronto: Research and Innovation Office
www.research.utoronto.ca/for-researchers-administrators/funding-sources

Disease and specialty-specific funding
Alzheimer Society of Canada
www.alzheimer.ca/english/research/resprog-awards09.htm

Proposing

Canadian Association of Emergency Physicians
www.caep.ca/template.asp?id=16A0191B258246CDB2FF9FD2FD4FEBCC

Canadian Heart and Stroke Foundation
www.heartandstroke.com/site/c.iklQLcMWJtE/b.3479073/k.99CA/Funded_Research.htm

College of Family Physicians of Canada
www.cfpc.ca/Family_Medicine_Resident_Awards/

Kidney Foundation of Canada
www.kidney.ca/Page.aspx?pid=362

Obstetrics and Gynaecology—Canadian Foundation for Women's Health
http://cfwh.org/index.php?page=research-funding&hl=en_CA

Pediatrics—Canadian Pediatric Society
www.cps.ca/english/Residents/Grants.htm

Sick Kids Foundation
www.sickkidsfoundation.com/grants/

Foundations

Chronicle of Philanthropy
http://philanthropy.com/grants

Community of Science
http://fundingopps.cos.com
- The Community of Science site provides a wealth of resources for the world's researchers including links to funding opportunities.

Council on Foundations
www.cof.org

Foundation Center
http://foundationcenter.org

GrantsNet
http://sciencecareers.sciencemag.org/funding
- This site allows you to search through thousands of funding opportunities in nearly all scientific and medical fields.

Imagine Canada
www.imaginecanada.ca
- A searchable database of thousands of Canadian foundations and grants; requires a subscription to access, which many universities hold.

Proposing

SUMMARY CHECKLIST

- ❑ List all of the resources needed for your research project. Review them with your supervisor and team and revise.
- ❑ Create a budget that describes the amounts and the flow of resources for the project.
- ❑ List all of the relevant sources of funding for the project. Prioritize them.
- ❑ Apply for funding.
- ❑ Ensure all funds are managed professionally and accounted for.
- ❑ Create a report summarizing all your resources used for the project.
- ❑ Return unused funds.

20
Sampling, recruiting and retaining study participants

Kaberi Dasgupta, MD, MSc, FRCPC

ILLUSTRATIVE CASE

A second-year resident in Internal Medicine is interested in learning more about factors that influence adherence to antibiotic therapy and their impact on the likelihood of recurrent infection and antibiotic resistance. He has framed a research question as follows: "Among patients from the inpatient clinical teaching unit discharged home on oral antibiotic therapy, does a follow-up visit with the treating resident increase the likelihood of adherence to antibiotic therapy?" He expects that the results of his study might alter the discharge planning approach at his institution and beyond.

■ **A clinical study that relies on** primary data collection always presents a challenge. There are many threats to both the internal and external validity of a study that can limit the scientific validity of the findings and thus the conclusions that may be drawn from them. The process of clinical research is time-consuming and can be frustrating. Nonetheless, a well-designed primary study involving the collection of clinical data can provide valuable information, as well as much satisfaction to the researcher. Moreover, clinical research in its many forms—including clinical trials, prospective cohort studies, case-control studies and cross-sectional studies—are the only means of addressing some kinds of research questions.

Defining the study population

Clinical research requires the participation of a sample of real people. Constructing that sample involves, in the first place, defining the **target population** to whom the researcher wishes to generalize his or her results. In our illustrative case, that population might be hospital inpa-

tients who are treated with intravenous antibiotics for any of a variety of infections (e.g., pneumonia, urosepsis) and then discharged home with a prescription for oral antibiotics. The **source population** is the population from which the researcher actually recruits the study participants: in the case example, inpatients at the resident's hospital who are treated for the infections of interest.

Next, the researcher needs to establish **inclusion criteria** to more sharply define the **study sample**, keeping both sci-

CHAPTER OBJECTIVES

After reading this chapter, you should be able to:
- explain the difference between a target population and a study sample and the relevance of this distinction to answering a research question
- identify potential sources of selection bias
- describe the importance of an adequate sample and the factors that enter into a sample size calculation
- apply strategies to enhance recruitment and limit losses to follow-up

Conducting

KEY TERMS

Exclusion criteria	Internal validity	Study sample
External validity	Losses to follow-up	Target population
Generalizability	Selection bias	
Inclusion criteria	Source population	

entific and logistic considerations in mind. Hulley and colleagues[1] describe these as the specific demographic, clinical, geographic and temporal characteristics that are both relevant to the research question and logistically feasible to include. In the case example, the resident would need to specify the period during which the participants will be recruited, such as a single month or season. He will need to decide whether he is interested in patients with *any* condition requiring antibiotic treatment, or only in those with one or more specified conditions. He will need criteria for establishing the presence of infection (e.g., culture vs clinical diagnosis). Other patient characteristics will also need to be specified. For example, will all age groups be eligible? What about patients who are not capable of giving informed consent because of dementia or mental illness?

In contrast, **exclusion criteria** are intended to rule out individuals who, although they may fulfill inclusion criteria, possess characteristics that are unsuitable on demographic, clinical or geographic grounds. Thus, patients who are likely to be lost to follow-up (see later discussion), or cannot provide good-quality information, or are at risk for adverse events if they follow study procedures, might be excluded. For example, the resident in our example might opt to exclude institutionalized patients from the study on the grounds that, although they may have an infection requiring inpatient treatment (e.g. aspiration pneumonia), they may for logistical reasons be unlikely to adhere to study procedures and to attend follow-up appointments.

Narrowly defining a study population improves the **internal validity** of a research project: that is, the less diverse the sample, the more readily we can attribute an observed effect to the variables and population under study. For example, the resident in our example could choose to focus on women over the age of 65 years with urosepsis. There is a good chance, if the study is free from other sources of bias and demonstrates a strong effect of resident follow-up on adherence, that this effect will hold true for other women with these infections in that particular setting. However, such a narrow definition will reduce the **external validity**, or **generalizability**, of the findings to other groups (e.g., men, children, younger women) or to patients with other infections (e.g., pneumonia).

The care taken in defining the research question, target population, source population and eligibility criteria will help to optimize the generalizability of a study's findings. The goal is to ensure that the sample of participants that is ultimately selected reflects the population of interest, to whom the study's results are intended to be applied.

Screening for study participants

Reliable and comprehensive screening procedures for sample selection—i.e., mechanisms for identifying eligible patients—are critically important to any study that seeks to recruit participants for the purpose of data collection. If screening procedures are inconsistent or prone to error, the conduct and completion of the study can be seriously compromised, if not doomed to failure. If patients with a specific characteristic are preferentially included or excluded, the resultant **selection bias** can jeopardize the study's external validity and hence its generalizability. Ideal approaches generally involve the elimination of human factors, such as relying on members of the health care team to alert the research group to potentially eligible patients who might be recruited for the study. Ideally, procedures that incorporate some kind of electronic health record are best suited to the systematic identification of potentially eligible study subjects.

In our case example, a daily review of all admissions and diagnoses would help the resident identify patients who might be approached for recruitment as they enter the pre-discharge phase of their hospital stay. In settings that lack an electronic health record, it is worthwhile to design a process map that describes the movement of relevant patients through the health care system, with an eye to identifying opportune moments to initiate recruitment, along with key personnel to do so. Appropriate prompts can take the form of strategically placed reminder posters or colourful material appended to patient charts to encourage health care providers to contact the research team, alerting them to the potentially eligible patients and allowing them to explore inclusion and exclusion criteria with the relevant parties.

Identifying the participants

Even with well-thought-out study population definitions and inclusion/exclusion criteria, recruitment can still be prone to selection bias. If this occurs, your study sample might not truly represent your target population. Suppose, for example, that you decide to recruit patients from the clinical teaching unit in your hospital, which serves French- and English-speaking populations. If you are not fully fluent in French, you may have difficulty recruiting French-speaking patients and, as a result, will end up with a preponderance of English-speaking patients in your study sample. This is of concern only if there is a possibility that the impact of the intervention (i.e., follow-up with a treating team member) will differ between French- and English-speaking patients. If this is the case, you should involve a colleague with strong French-language skills to assist with recruitment.

In a similar vein, one strategy that can help reduce selection bias is to recruit patients consecutively in order to mimimize factors that might influence the make-up of the selected group. For example, patients discharged on evenings and weekends may differ from other patients in that they require a family member to escort them home outside of regular work hours, thus reflecting a more fragile health status. In our case example, the procedural and logistic implications of consecutive recruitment would include visiting the hospital ward daily to determine who is being discharged on antibiotics and then approaching these patients to invite them to participate in the study.

You will need to keep a log of acceptances and rejections so that you can ultimately determine whether the patients who were enrolled in your study differ substantively from those who were not. Significant differences will threaten the external validity or generalizability of your results. Generally speaking, people who agree to participate in scientific studies (i.e., volunteers) differ in some respects from the general population. The goal is to limit potential differences as much as possible and to be aware of them when they do exist so that your findings can be interpreted appropriately.

Recruitment

To increase the likelihood that potential candidates will agree to participate, make your study procedures as simple and consistent as possible. For example, patients might be more likely to agree to a telephone follow-up interview than to an in-person interview. Equally important, however, are your interpersonal skills. A kind, warm and courteous manner can go a long way toward encouraging interest in your study and a willingness to participate. Although you might not want to explicitly state your underlying hypothesis, patients may be more receptive to a study designed to improve patient care in general, although you must take care to indicate on the consent form that participating in the study will have no impact on the quality of care received.

As important as it is to maintain cordial relationships with potential participants, your interactions with the health care team—including nurses, clerical staff, patient assistants, residents, medical students and attending physicians—are also crucial. Good relationships can determine whether these individuals become key allies in study recruitment or impede the process. Moreover, many Research Ethics Boards require that a potential study participant be informed by a member of the health care team that he or she will be approached to participate in a research study and that a verbal approval be obtained before they are approached.

The difficulty inherent in recruiting participants through physicians and clinic staff is highlighted by Butt and colleagues,[2] who demonstrate how, in a community-based trial targeting postmenopausal women, fewer than 4% of participants were recruited through physician recruiters and the most successful method of recruitment was newspaper advertisement. However, this approach would not be appropriate for all research scenarios, including our illustrative case. Thus, in a study that requires recruitment from a patient care setting, strong working relationships and simple reminders are critical.

Other strategies that can enhance recruitment and discourage loss to follow-up include payments to participants to cover costs such as transportation and parking, and lotteries with small prizes (e.g., movie tickets, gift certificates) for staff who facilitate recruitment, provided that these strategies are permitted by the local Research Ethics Board. In our example, however, given that the resident will be assessing whether follow-up with a treating team member enhances adherence to antibiotic therapy, it may be problematic to cover transportation costs, given that the visit is part of the intervention: reimbursement for parking does not reflect real-world practice and could thus introduce bias.

Losses to follow-up: another potential source of selection bias

The shorter the period between recruitment and follow-up, the easier it will be to avoid losses to follow-up. When we "lose" patients, we cannot be confident about the associations that we identify among the remaining patients, since those lost to follow-up might have systematically different outcomes than participants who remain in the study until the end. For example, in a placebo-controlled trial assessing the impact of a drug to treat heart failure, medication side-effects might lead to more drop-outs from the treatment arm than the placebo arm. This can lead to the faulty conclusion that the study drug was as well tolerated as placebo, when in fact the differential loss to follow-up introduces a bias that makes the experimental drug's profile appear more favourable than it really is.

In our case example, the resident could plan to assess antibiotic adherence through a telephone-based interview.

Participants contacted within a few days of the estimated date of antibiotic therapy completion will be more likely to remember the resident, to answer his questions, and to provide accurate information than participants contacted, say, three months later. The resident will therefore have to track participants and their timelines meticulously, to ensure that information is obtained in a timely fashion. Spreadsheets and built-in time alerts may be useful in this regard. In a rigorous study, any loss to follow-up should be the result of a genuine inability on the part of the patient to comply with or tolerate the intervention (although this is probably a bona fide outcome rather than simply loss to follow-up) as opposed to poorly planned or executed study procedures.

In studies with longer follow-up periods, it may be wise to maintain contact with participants regularly by phone or through newsletters. As discussed with reference to recruitment, some institutions permit researchers to encourage ongoing participation through incentives such as lotteries for small prizes (e.g., gift certificates for books or movies) for those who complete follow-up procedures. Another useful strategy can be to obtain contact information not only for the participant but also for two or three friends or family members, to increase the likelihood of being able to locate participants who move during the study so that the applicable study outcomes might be determined.

How many subjects will you need?

After the careful work of identifying the correct source population for your study, the next step is to calculate what the ideal sample size would be (see ch. 25). At this point, consultation with a statistician will be useful. You will need to be well prepared for this meeting, as the statistician will require some very specific information to be of help. In our case example, he or she would need to know, based on the resident's literature review, an estimate of the minimally important difference in antibiotic compliance rates attributable to the intervention, the acceptable error around the estimate, and the number of additional variables the resident would need to examine as well as the desired study power that would establish the probability of a Type II error (failing to demonstrate a difference when one exists) as well as the alpha level, which is an estimate of the probability of a Type I error (demonstrating a difference by chance when there is no significant difference).

The results of your sample size calculation might send you back to the drawing board. Your actual study design

and study participants will be dictated not only by considerations of what the ideal study design would be, but also by what kind of study is feasible to conduct while still answering your question—or, if necessary, an alternative question that you also consider to be important. Specifically, logistical or feasibility issues such as your operating budget, the number of eligible participants available and the time frame are critically important. Given that the time frame for trainee projects is generally short and the budget limited (or non-existent), practicality is the order of the day.

Let us suppose that your discussions with a statistician suggest that you will require 40 patients in each group to answer your research question, or 80 patients in total. Your institution has some funds for resident research projects, and so you have approximately $2000 to use. You assess the situation and realize that a clinical trial will be possible only if you are able to dedicate at least two years to the project, taking into account the time required for ethics approval, recruitment and data collection, data entry, analysis, and manuscript writing. A more likely scenario is that you will have been able to piece together a three-month period during which you will collect the data.

In this situation, a cohort study may be possible, albeit challenging. You estimate that approximately 20 patients are discharged on antibiotic therapy on the medical teaching ward at your base hospital each month. If they are all accepted to be in your study, you would still be short at least 20 patients. Your options are to include another hospital, which will involve travel or finding a collaborator at that hospital, or to include another type of hospital ward. In any case, you will need to balance logistical and methodological factors as you come up with a plan that is both practical and has the capacity to answer your research question.

Conclusion

To some degree, in conducting a research project as a trainee, you are fulfilling two roles: that of a researcher, and that of a research coordinator. Researchers identify the relevant research questions, design the study, obtain the necessary funding, analyze the results, write the manuscripts and present the findings. Research coordinators actually execute the study (albeit under the researcher's supervision) with respect to recruitment and study promotion, data collection and data entry. The opportunity to fulfill both roles provides key insights that can make you a better researcher in the long term and will certainly increase your awareness of the complexities of study execution, particularly with respect to the identification, recruitment and retention of participants. This experience will provide you with valuable insights when, as a health care professional, you evaluate the evidence base relevant to the care of patients. ■

CASE POSTSCRIPT

The resident combines forces with some of his colleagues and, with guidance from a willing and capable supervisor, embarks on a randomized controlled trial to address his research question. The inclusion criteria are admission for community-acquired pneumonia for individuals living independently who are 18 years of age or older. Potential participants who are dependent on alcohol or illicit drugs are excluded. Outcomes of follow-up at the teaching clinic within 2 weeks after hospital discharge are compared with those of "usual care" and follow-up with the patient's own physician. The research team assesses adherence through telephone interviews and by means of pharmacy dispensing records (the participants having consented to the research team contacting their pharmacist). The research team discovers that roughly 75% of patients report completing their antibiotic regimen as prescribed and that there are no important differences between groups.

REFERENCES

1. Hulley SB, Cummings SR, Browner WS, Grady DG, Newman TB. *Designing clinical research*. 3rd ed. Philadelphia: Wolters Kluwer Health/Lippincott Williams & Wilkins; 2007.

2. Butt DA, Lock M, Harvey BJ. Effective and cost-effective clinical trial recruitment strategies for postmenopausal women in a community-based, primary care setting. *Contemp Clin Trials*. 2010;31(5):447–56.

ADDITIONAL RESOURCES

Hulley SB. *Designing clinical research*. 3rd ed. Philadelphia: Wolters Kluwer Health/Lippincott Williams & Wilkins; 2007. Chapter 3, Choosing the study subjects: specification, sampling, and recruitment; p. 27–36.

Kleinbaum DG, Sullivan KM, Barker ND. *A pocket guide to epidemiology*. New York: Springer Science+Business Media; 2007. Chapter 8, Were subjects chosen badly? Selection bias. p. 127–38.

- These two references provide helpful guidance on the selection of study samples.

SUMMARY CHECKLIST

- ❑ Determine your study's target population.
- ❑ Determine the source population.
- ❑ Establish the inclusion and exclusion criteria for your study sample.
- ❑ Draw up a budget for the study.
- ❑ Establish your recruitment targets.
- ❑ Determine your time frame for recruitment.
- ❑ Frame strategies to use to maximize recruitment.
- ❑ Frame strategies to use to minimize loss to follow-up.

Conducting

21
Pilot studies

Bart J. Harvey, MD, PhD, MEd, FACPM, FRCPC

ILLUSTRATIVE CASE

While preparing the protocol for a full-scale randomized clinical trial to assess the effectiveness of gabapentin for the treatment of menopausal hot flashes, a Family Medicine physician-researcher wonders what efforts would be required to recruit the necessary number of consenting participants. When she raises this question at a departmental research meeting, one of her colleagues suggests she consider conducting a pilot study so that she might gain some experience and insight regarding this and other aspects of the proposed study. She thinks this is a great idea and asks her colleague if he would assist her.

■ **Pilot studies are "pre-studies"** designed and carried out in preparation for a more expensive full study; they are a separate and external[1] "dress rehearsal."[2] Pilot studies are intended to provide researchers with an opportunity to test (**trial run**, or try out) one or more aspects of the anticipated full study's proposed protocol. They allow investigators to more economically identify any potential **barriers** and any areas requiring revision in the proposed protocol that, if left uncorrected, could impede the successful completion of the anticipated full study. In fact, findings from a pilot study sometimes demonstrate that the planned full study is, as proposed, is not feasible (as a result, pilot studies are sometimes referred to as **feasibility studies**).

Simon[3] highlights that pilot studies are particularly useful to assess those aspects of a proposed full study that are "novel, untested, complex, or innovative." In this light, Hinds and Gattuso[4] point out that pilot studies are not always necessary, especially when the researcher already possesses sufficient experience using the proposed methods in a comparable population and an analogous setting. Morse[5,6] argues that pilot studies are not applicable in quali-

tative research because the theoretical scheme of a qualitative study continues to be developed throughout its conduct and analysis (see also ch. 16). Further, Watson and colleagues[7] point out that a qualitative study conducted to inform the development of a questionnaire or any other aspect of a future quantitative study should not be described as a pilot study, because it "clearly generate[s] findings that have value in their own right." With these considerations in mind, the remainder of this chapter addresses the use of pilot studies in quantitative research.

CHAPTER OBJECTIVES

After reading this chapter, you should be able to:

- discuss the range of purposes for conducting pilot studies and identify when a pilot study would (and would not) be indicated;
- discuss how pilot studies are designed and conducted; and
- discuss issues related to the planning and conduct of pilot studies, such as ethics review, obtaining funding and reporting pilot study findings.

Conducting

KEY TERMS		
Acceptability	Pre-studies	Safety
Barriers	Preliminary estimate	Scientific design
Feasibility studies	Processes	Suitability
Operation	Resources	Trial run

A pilot study is not carried out to answer the research question motivating the ultimate full study but, instead, is conducted to address scientific or operational issues and to identify the need for any revisions in the study procedures and protocol. Accordingly, a pilot study is distinctly different from, and this term should not be used to describe, a small study that simply has an inadequate sample size.[2,8] A pilot study yields insights into the **scientific design** and **operation** of the anticipated full study, but not into outcome measures relevant to the research question of the anticipated full study, because its findings are almost invariably gathered from an underpowered number of pilot participants.[1,4,9]

Various authors[1–19] have described a wide range of purposes that pilot studies can serve. However, before we discuss these, it is important to note several study designs that can be confused with pilot studies. These are "exploratory" studies,[3,11,20] "proof of concept" studies[21,22] "adaptive trials"[23,24] "internal pilots"[25,26] and "process evaluations."[27–29] Unlike pilot studies, these types of studies are intended to identify or measure an effect, and not to trial a proposed protocol for an anticipated full study. Exploratory studies are typically used to generate hypotheses that may potentially be pursued in future research.[3,11,20] Proof-of-concept studies are conducted to provide a preliminary assessment of a proposed intervention to estimate the magnitude of its potential effect and determine whether further, more rigorous, study is warranted.[21,22] Adaptive and internal pilot studies are planned assessments made in the midst of a full study to inform possible mid-study adjustments, usually of the sample size needed to achieve a sought-after statistical power.[23–26] Process evaluations, which often employ methods similar to those used in pilot studies, are carried out in conjunction with, and not prior to, a full study to provide supplementary information and insights to inform the interpretation of the study's results, particularly those potentially influenced by the delivery and receipt of the intervention under study.[27–29] Of course, as Power and colleagues[29] point out, even full studies employing a process evaluation can benefit from a planning pilot/feasibility study. It should also be noted that a pilot study can be nested within a full study to provide, for example, insights regarding other potential future full studies. (An example is the work by Klymko and colleagues.[30])

The purposes of pilot studies

Pilot studies serve a wide range of purposes, which can be categorized into at least six main areas:

1. To test and assess one or more of the processes that will be required to successfully complete the proposed main study.
2. To evaluate the **safety**, **acceptability** and **suitability** of any of the aspects of the proposed main study.
3. To test and assess the proposed and potential outcome measures.
4. To estimate the **resources** (e.g., funding, staff, time) needed to successfully complete the proposed main study.
5. To provide evidence of the feasibility and worth of the proposed full study.
6. To provide data (e.g., a **preliminary estimate** the outcome measure) to assist in planning of the proposed main study (e.g., to calculate the needed sample size).

Each of these purposes will be addressed in turn in the following sections.

Testing and assessing the proposed study processes and procedures

Perhaps the most common purpose of a pilot study is to provide an opportunity to test and assess one or more of the **processes** being considered for the anticipated full study, such as:

- identifying and recruiting a sufficient number and diversity of eligible study participants (as well as applying exclusion criteria);
- if applicable, acquiring, preparing and administering the drug or other intervention (and, if applicable, the placebo or other comparator) to be studied;
- assessing the degree to which participants receive (and accept) any applicable treatment or other intervention (i.e., adherence);
- assessing the degree to which participants receive any competing treatment or other intervention (i.e., co-intervention and contamination);
- enabling study personnel, including co-investigators, to gain familiarity in working with one another and applying the procedures outlined in the proposed study protocol;
- if applicable, identifying, recruiting and monitoring additional study sites;

Conducting

- obtaining, using, maintaining and storing any instruments and other equipment needed, particularly those necessary to make study measurements;
- choosing between two or more possible data collection methods (e.g., interview vs self-administered survey);
- assessing the feasibility, accuracy and completeness of data collection and entry (and, if applicable, the ability to match and combine data from different sources); and
- analyzing the data, including the development and assessment of the pilot study results tables.

These assessments should be conducted explicitly and systematically, such that each question to be addressed by the pilot study is clearly identified and articulated in the pilot study plan. Thabane and colleagues[14] recommend that researchers specify "success criteria" before launching a pilot study. However, even with a priori identification of success criteria, pilot studies should be considered to be primarily descriptive; accordingly, investigators should be alert for and take every opportunity to observe, document and assess, in as much detail as possible, each step taken and process used during the pilot study.

Although many of the pilot study assessments will result in quantitative measures—such as recruitment rates, percentage of ineligible participants and average number of questionnaire items not completed by respondents—investigators should also consider gathering qualitative feedback, insights and advice from study participants, staff and co-investigators to gain as complete an understanding as possible of the proposed study's operation and functioning. For example, if asked, people who decline to participate in the study might explain that the excessively long enrolment questionnaire or the frequency of follow-up visits deterred them from participating. Similarly, staff might suggest that preparing follow-up visit materials in advance would improve efficiency and reduce the time demands on each participant.

As Lancaster and colleagues[1] suggest, some study processes are of sufficient importance to warrant particular attention in a pilot study. These include:

- identifying, recruiting, obtaining consent from, and retaining study participants;
- the use of data collection instruments, including questionnaires; and
- if applicable, the randomization and allocation of participants into study groups.

These three elements are discussed in the subsections below.

Identifying, recruiting, gaining consent from, and retaining study participants. As Ross and colleagues[31] highlight, recruiting a sufficient number of study participants presents many challenges, and recruitment problems are a frequent reason for underpowered and failed studies. The identification and recruitment of participants into a study should therefore always be carefully planned and piloted. Even though the final sample size required for the anticipated full study might not be known during the pilot study, it is important to determine whether a suitably diverse group of eligible participants can be identified and recruited through available venues. A pilot study also provides an opportunity to test the procedures to be used to approach potential participants and obtain their consent to enter the study. Experience gained through a pilot study should better enable researchers to estimate the amount of time needed and the ability to recruit an adequate number of eligible participants. The pilot study also provides an opportunity for investigators to assess and receive feedback about the proposed consent form and any informational materials given to potential participants about the study. Pilot studies can also be used to estimate the proportion of recruited participants who will fail to comply with any of the study requirements, including the proportion of those recruited who will withdraw before the end of the study as well as their reasons for doing so.

However, because pilot studies provide only estimates, recruitment rates, like all other aspects of a study, should be regularly monitored through the course of the full study (see also ch. 23). The importance of ongoing study monitoring is illustrated by the experience of Butt and colleagues,[32] who piloted a proposed recruitment strategy and found that the required number of participants could be identified and recruited within the time frame of the proposed full study. However, early in the course of their full study it became clear that the expected recruitment rate was not being achieved. As a result, supplementary recruitment methods, which required the acquisition of additional funding, had to be identified and implemented, which ultimately enabled the study to be successfully completed with the required number of participants.

Specific types of studies, such as surveys, medical record reviews and administrative data studies, pose unique "recruitment" challenges that should be considered and piloted before the proposed main study is implemented.

Conducting

Although these study designs are addressed in chapters 11, 12 and 13, respectively, several aspects are highlighted here.

Surveys, particularly those administered "remotely" through the postal system or the Internet, require the identification of an appropriate list of eligible recipients (i.e., a "sampling frame"). This may require researchers to gain permission from one or more organizations that possess such a list (e.g., membership or enrolment lists). In addition, a suitably inviting introductory communication and survey instrument is usually necessary so that an acceptable response rate can be achieved. A pilot study provides an important opportunity to test these and other components of the proposed full survey. In addition, pilot testing provides an initial estimate of the full survey's anticipated response rate.

Like surveys, medical record reviews and administrative data studies often require researchers to obtain permission to gain access to the necessary data records. In this regard, pilot studies provide an important opportunity to explore important aspects of the proposed study, such as the processes that will need to be followed, the time required to obtain the needed medical records, the cost of retrieving these records, and the feasibility of locating all requested medical records. Payment may also be required to gain access to administrative data and, in many cases, to gain the assistance of specialized staff at the agency holding the needed data. Because these specialized staff are frequently in short supply and very busy, a request for their involvement is often required weeks or even months in advance.

Testing data collection instruments (including questionnaires). Another important aspect of any study is the manner in which the required data are collected from and about each study participant. Pilot studies provide an important opportunity to test these processes, especially when different staff will be collecting the data or when the participants themselves will provide the data on self-administered surveys or other forms. As Lancaster and colleagues[1] outline, piloting provides an important opportunity to ensure that data collection instruments are comprehensible and appropriate, and that data items are well defined, understandable and presented in a consistent manner. Further, Simon[3,33] suggests that pilot studies enable the researcher to explore practical matters, such as whether there is enough room on the data collection form for all the data received and whether any questions tend to elicit no answer, multiple answers, qualified answers, or unanticipated answers. However, Lancaster and colleagues[1] stress that pilot studies, because of their relatively small sample sizes, are generally not an appropriate means to assess the validity and reliability of study instruments (see also ch. 10).

Testing randomization, blinding and concealed allocation procedures for a study. As discussed in chapter 9, two critical components of randomized trials are the appropriate randomization and concealed allocation of participants into study groups. Much of the strength of randomized trials is derived from the comparability of the groups being studied, but this is highly dependent on an appropriate randomization process being carried out to assign participants to study groups.[34] However, the utility of randomization is highly dependent on allocation concealment procedures that keep investigators, health care providers and participants unaware of upcoming assignments so that the group that any participant is assigned to cannot be manipulated.[35] Pilot studies provide an opportunity for investigators to test the proposed procedures for randomization and allocation concealment. Investigators can also pilot and assess any blinding of participants, health care providers or assessors that is being considered for the anticipated full study. Blinding, like randomization and allocation concealment, strengthens the methodological rigour of a randomized trial,[36] and so it is important to take the opportunity to pre-test, during a pilot study, the adequacy of these processes, including the effectiveness of the placebo and its similarity to the intervention.

Assessing the safety, acceptability and suitability of the study and its components

Pilot studies also enable an assessment of the acceptability of the proposed full study and its various components to relevant stakeholder groups, such as potential participants, patients, parents, research collaborators, health care providers, institutional managers and community leaders. This assessment is particularly important for any treatment or other interventions being studied.[11] For example, investigators may wish to assess what proportion of eligible participants consent to receive the proposed intervention and, in the case of randomized trials, the comparison intervention (often a placebo). Pilot studies also allow investigators the opportunity to seek feedback from eligible individuals who decline to participate so that modifications to improve study recruitment might be identified.

A pilot study also provides an opportunity to gather information about the safety of the proposed intervention. For example, a pilot study conducted by Bressler and colleagues[37,38] led to the cancellation of the corresponding full study because the pilot results suggested that the treatment under study would not be beneficial and could possibly be harmful.

Pilot studies also enable investigators to determine the acceptability of other aspects of the full study's proposed protocol, such as the kind and amount of data collected from and about participants, the frequency and length of study visits, and the intrusiveness of outcome and other study measures. If any of these are found to effect participant drop-out rates, investigators will usually identify and implement study modifications and further pilot test these before initiating the revised full study.

Gardner and colleagues,[13] Hinds and Gattuso[4] and Jairath and collaborators[39] also discuss and highlight the value of pilot studies in assessing the administrative environment as well as the staff orientation and education required to successfully conduct the proposed full study. Difficulties in any of these areas can adversely affect any aspect of a study, including access to organizational resources and the identification and recruitment of a sufficient number of study participants.

Identifying, testing and assessing proposed and potential outcome measures

Several authors[1,10,40] have discussed the role that pilot studies can play in identifying, testing and assessing proposed and potential outcome measures. Although this can be designed as a specific pilot study objective, it may arise by serendipity. For example, Beebe[40] describes how, while her pilot study accomplished traditional objectives regarding the feasibility of a proposed full study of a walking program's effect on the well-being of individuals with schizophrenia, alternative outcome measures, such as increased flexibility, increased energy and reduced psychiatric symptoms were also identified by pilot study participants during exit interviews.

In contrast, Arnold and colleagues[10] describe several pilot studies that specifically included objectives to assess proposed study outcome measures and, in some cases, the mechanisms believed to be responsible. Feeley and colleagues[12] and Lancaster and colleagues[1] also discuss the potential importance of pilot studies in assessing the suitability of proposed outcome measures.

Identifying and estimating the required resources

Pilot studies also provide an opportunity to identify and estimate the resources necessary to successfully carry out the proposed full study—both those that are anticipated, such as study staff and needed supplies, and those not foreseen by the investigators. For example, Beebe's pilot study[40] identified the need to provide suitable footwear for study participants. The resource estimates that result from pilot studies can inform the budget requests that accompany research funding applications.

Providing evidence of the feasibility and worthiness of the proposed full study

Several authors[4,11,13,15,16,39] have highlighted the fact that pilot study results can provide valuable evidence of the feasibility and worthiness of a proposed study. Being able to describe findings from a pilot study can be particularly useful, and is often required, in funding applications. Moreover, the completion of a pilot study provides evidence that the study team possesses the necessary skills and expertise to successfully carry out the proposed study. Some authors[13,15] have suggested that this benefit is enhanced when the results of the pilot study are published in the peer-reviewed literature. (See the later discussion of publication issues.) The successful completion of a pilot study and the experience it provides can also be instrumental in convincing others, such as institutional administrators and those who might potentially recruit potential participants, of the study's potential and feasibility.[17]

Providing data estimates to inform the design of the main study

One of the commonly described reasons for conducting a pilot study is to provide estimates to inform planning of the proposed full study. These often include measures of central tendency (e.g., mean or percentage) and variability (e.g., standard deviation) of the outcome measure(s) to assist in the estimation of the sample size needed for the anticipated full study. However, because the number of individuals included in a pilot study is usually (and appropriately) small, the resulting estimates are generally quite imprecise. As a result, several authors[10,41–44] have stressed that estimates arising from pilot studies should be treated very conservatively. Because of the resulting imprecision of the estimates, several authors[41–44] have recommended that best- and worst-case scenarios should be considered when using pilot study estimates to calculate the sample size needed for the corre-

Conducting

sponding full study. For example, Browne[42] points out that the small size of pilot studies often results in underestimates of the variance to be used to inform the calculation of the full study's sample size, which would lead to an underpowered sample size for the full study. To guard against this potential underestimation, Browne[42] has recommended that the upper limit of the 80% confidence interval of the pilot study variance should be used to err on the side of overestimating the underlying variability of the data.

Leon and colleagues[9] and Kraemer and coauthors[41] describe the use of pilot studies to provide an estimate of the anticipated size of effect/difference. However, they warn that, given the relatively small size (and resulting imprecision) of pilot study estimates, these can also be very misleading, capable of both under- and overestimating the actual effect size. Similarly, they suggest that 95% confidence intervals be calculated so that the full range of values consistent with the pilot study's result can be fully and explicitly appreciated. Further, Leon and colleagues[9] stress that an agreed-upon clinically meaningful difference—and not the result determined imprecisely from the pilot study—should be used to calculate the sample size needed for the full study. Lenth[45] also provides valuable advice about how to reasonably estimate the sample sizes needed for full studies.

Recognizing the imprecision of estimates resulting from pilot studies, other authors stress the need to be circumspect; as Lancaster and colleagues note, "the analysis of a pilot study should be mainly descriptive or should focus on confidence interval estimation" and "results from hypothesis testing should be treated as preliminary and interpreted with caution."[1 (p 311)]

Practical considerations in the conduct of a pilot study

As is the case with any other study design, pilot studies pose practical challenges. These include determining the sample size, obtaining approval from a Research Ethics Board, and obtaining funding to support the work. Specific issues concerning publication should be taken into account by researchers contemplating a pilot study. Finally—and importantly—one should be aware of the issues arising from the use of data from pilot studies in the full proposed study and the inclusion of pilot-study participants in the full proposed study. Each of these practical considerations will be considered briefly in the following sections.

Determining the sample size of a pilot study

Although the sample size necessary for a full study is usually calculated to achieve a prespecified statistical study power, determining the sample size needed for a pilot study is less straightforward. However, the determination of sample size for both types of studies should be guided by the same general rationale: to enable the study to achieve its objectives.[10] In this regard, full studies are designed to enable a sufficiently precise measure of the outcome of interest. As discussed earlier, the objective of pilot studies is usually to provide experience and insight concerning scientific and operational aspects of the anticipated full study. As a result, pilot studies require a sample size that will enable their objectives to be achieved. In this regard, several authors[3,9,12,39,43] have provided advice to consider when selecting the sample size for a pilot study.

Leon and colleagues[9] emphasize that "the pragmatics of recruitment and the necessities for examining feasibility" should guide the sample size of a pilot study. Jairath and colleagues[39] also point out that the sample size may be guided by a "predefined time frame for data collection or an arbitrarily selected proportion of the parent study sample size." Hertzog[43] suggests that the width of resulting confidence intervals should be considered when deciding on the sample size of a pilot study so that suitable estimates regarding the anticipated full study can be determined. Although Feeley and colleagues[12] remark that usual sample sizes for pilot studies are between 10 and 40, they also stress that additional factors such as human and financial resources, timelines and the proposed full study objectives should also be taken into account. Further, Simon[3] suggests that researchers consider not only the number of pilot study participants but also their diversity, so that they reasonably represent those expected to be recruited into the anticipated full study.

Although any estimate of sample size for a pilot study is just that—an estimate—investigators should endeavour to recruit the number of participants they will need to meet their pilot study's objectives. For efficiency's sake, however, the ultimate number of pilot participants should be only a fraction of the number anticipated to be required for the full study. In addition, if researchers are able to conduct a large pilot study without external funding, potential funders approached for the full study may question whether their support is really required.

Conducting

Ethics approval for pilot studies

Like all studies involving human participants, pilot studies require Research Ethics Board (REB) approval. The proposal submitted for REB review should include a clear outline of the objectives of the pilot study and the type of information it is intended to provide, along with a description of and rationale for the anticipated full study.[3] Thabane and colleagues[14] point out that pilot studies are not specifically addressed in any of the commonly cited research ethics guidelines. In addition, they highlight the importance of disclosing to potential participants that the study is a pilot and not the full "substantive" study. To address this, they propose a sample wording for a pilot study consent form.[14] A further consideration is that, although it is not clear whether pilot studies conducted in advance of an anticipated clinical trial require registration, researchers should seek relevant advice before initiating a pilot study to ensure that their full study will remain eligible for publication in a peer-reviewed journal.

The availability of funding for pilot studies

Although guidance about seeking and obtaining funding for research studies is addressed in detail in chapter 19, it should be emphasized that funding to support the conduct of pilot studies is often available from research funding agencies and other organizations, such as the Canadian Institutes for Health Research, the Alberta Heritage Foundation for Medical Research and Physician Services Incorporated. Investigators are encouraged to contact their local research administration office and to consult relevant funding agencies to determine what funding might be available to support the conduct of their pilot study.

Reporting and publishing pilot studies

Whether the results of pilot studies merit publication in the peer-reviewed literature continues to be a controversial topic debated by a variety of authors.[2,5–8,11–15,40] Some[2,7,14] have highlighted the importance of drawing a clear distinction between small, underpowered, hypothesis-testing studies incorrectly termed "pilot studies," and genuine pilot studies that have as their primary objective the testing and assessment of various scientific and operational aspects of an anticipated full study.

The general consensus concerning the publishing of pilot studies is that there are certain circumstances in which their publication is not only appropriate but should be encouraged. Morse[5] asserts that journal articles of any kind should be published only if they communicate something

new that is also substantive, correct, and expected to be of interest to others. Further, several authors[2,7,11] have proposed specific guidelines for the publication of pilot studies. For example, Watson and colleagues[7] suggest that pilot studies may not be suitable for publication because they are not primarily intended to generate generalizable results. However, they and others[2,11,12] point out that it may be appropriate to publish pilot studies for certain purposes, such as to inform the research community of the kinds of research questions being explored and to bring operational issues and barriers to the attention of interested investigators who might benefit from this information.[11–13,15,41]

In this context, the primary focus of such a publication should be the objectives that motivated the pilot study, and not those of the anticipated full study.[2,7,15] Although the results arising from the pilot study that are relevant to the full study's objectives (i.e., applicable hypothesis testing) could be presented in a pilot study publication, these should not be the main focus of such a publication but should be complementary to the pilot study findings that are pertinent to the feasibility, acceptability and other operational objectives addressed by the pilot study.[1,2,15] It should be noted that many pilot study publications include a review of the relevant literature; this feature might make these submissions more attractive to journal editors.

Watson and colleagues[7] and Morse,[5] however, highlight the limited amount of space available in peer-reviewed publications and stress that any pilot studies that are published should add value to the existing literature. Further, it is important that pilot studies be clearly identified as such when they are published, especially to avoid potential confusion if a publication describing the anticipated full study does not follow.[12] Some authors[7,15] have also warned that the publication of a pilot study may affect the chances of the anticipated full study being published, as the latter may be deemed a duplicate or redundant publication. Lancaster[1] and Becker[15] also warn of the potential for published pilot study results to be inappropriately included in systematic reviews and meta-analyses.

Thabane and colleagues[14] have adapted the CONSORT guidelines to develop a checklist of items for authors to consider when reporting the results of a pilot study.

Can pilot study participants and their data be included in the full study?

Several authors[1,9,11,16,33] have discussed the issue of whether the data from participants in a pilot study should be includ-

Conducting

ed in the subsequent full study. Some[9,11] point out that it would be inappropriate to include the pilot study participants and their data if the methods of the full study are modified in light of the pilot study: because these two groups would have participated in studies with differing protocols, the resulting data would not be comparable. Further, Lancaster and co-authors[1] argue that, even if the methods are largely left unchanged, because the decision to proceed with the full study is often dependent on the pilot study results, the pilot study participants should not be included because of the risk of selection bias and the increased likelihood of Type I error (i.e., a false-positive full study result).

Conclusion

Pilot studies provide an important opportunity for researchers to test out various scientific and operational aspects of a proposed full study. The information and experience gained through pilot studies can not only enhance the likelihood of the anticipated study's success, but can also provide valuable evidence to funders and other decision-makers of the feasibility and soundness of the proposed study. ∎

CASE POSTSCRIPT

The Family Medicine physician-researcher works with her colleague to design and carry out a pilot study to estimate how long it would take to recruit the number of consenting participants necessary for the proposed full-scale randomized clinical trial. Although she and her colleague are able to successfully recruit the required four study participants per week in the full study, the other practitioners who agree to recruit participants are much less successful, each recruiting an average of less than one participant per month. As a result, she and her colleague revise the study's recruitment strategies to include running advertisements in local newspapers, thus enabling the clinical trial to be completed successfully.

REFERENCES

1. Lancaster GA, Dodd S, Williamson PR. Design and analysis of pilot studies: recommendations for good practice. *J Eval Clin Pract.* 2004;10(2):307–12.

2. Brooks D, Stratford P. Pilot studies and their suitability for publication in physiotherapy Canada. *Physiother Can.* 2009;61(2):66–7.

3. Simon S. Pilot study. Updated 2008 July 14. Available from: www.childrensmercy.org/stats/plan/pilot.asp (accessed 2011 Aug 4).

4. Hinds PS, Gattuso JS. From pilot work to a major study in cancer nursing research. *Cancer Nurs.* 1991;14(3):132–5.

5. Morse JM. Appropriate use of pilot studies. *J Nurs Scholarsh.* 2001;33(4):307.

6. Morse JM. The pertinence of pilot studies. *Qual Health Res.* 1997;7(3):323–4.

7. Watson R, Atkinson I, Rose K. Pilot studies: to publish or not? *J Clin Nurs.* 2007;16(4):619–20.

8. Perry SE. Appropriate use of pilot studies. *J Nurs Scholarsh.* 2001;33(2):107.

9. Leon AC, Davis LL, Kraemer HC. The role and interpretation of pilot studies in clinical research. *J Psychiatr Res.* 2011;45(5):626–9.

10. Arnold DM, Burns KE, Adhikari NK, Kho ME, Meade MO, Cook D, et al. The design and interpretation of pilot trials in clinical research in critical care. *Crit Care Med.* 2009;37(1 Suppl):S69–S74.

11. Connelly LM. Pilot studies. *Medsurg Nurs.* 2008;17(6):411–2.

12. Feeley N, Cossette S, Côté J, Héon M, Stremler R, Martorella G, et al. The importance of piloting an RCT intervention. *Can J Nurs Res.* 2009;41(2):85–99.

13. Gardner G, Gardner A, MacLellan L, Osborne S. Reconceptualising the objectives of a pilot study for clinical research. *Int J Nurs Stud.* 2003;40(7):719–24.

Conducting

14. Thabane L, Ma J, Chu R, Cheng J, Ismaila A, Rios LP, et al. A tutorial on pilot studies: the what, why and how. *BMC Med Res Methodol*. 2010;10:1.

15. Becker PT. Publishing pilot intervention studies. *Res Nurs Health*. 2008;31(1):1–3.

16. van Teijlingen E, Hundley V. The importance of pilot studies. *Nurs Stand*. 2002;16(40):33–6.

17. van Teijlingen ER, Rennie AM, Hundley V, Graham W. The importance of conducting and reporting pilot studies: the example of the Scottish Births Survey. *J Adv Nurs*. 2001;34(3):289–95.

18. Prescott PA, Soeken KL. The potential uses of pilot work. *Nurs Res*. 1989;38(1):60–2.

19. Grady D, Hulley SB. Implementing the study and quality control. In: Hulley SB, Cummings SR, Browner WS, Grady DG, Newman TB. *Designing clinical research*. 3rd ed. Philadelphia (PA): Lippincott Williams & Wilkins; 2007. p 271–89.

20. Stewart PW. Small and/or pilot studies: GCRC protocols which propose "pilot studies." 2004. Available from: www.cincinnatichildrens.org/research/cores/gcrc/protocols/Small_or_Pilot_Studies.htm (accessed 2011 Aug 4).

21. Lawrence Gould A. Timing of futility analyses for "proof of concept" trials. *Stat Med*. 2005;24(12):1815–35.

22. Smith MK, Jones I, Morris MF, Grieve AP, Tan K. Implementation of a Bayesian adaptive design in a proof of concept study. *Pharm Stat*. 2006;5(1):39–50.

23. Coffey CS, Kairalla JA. Adaptive clinical trials: progress and challenges. *Drugs R D*. 2008;9(4):229–42.

24. Wang M, Wu YC, Tsai GF. A regulatory view of adaptive trial design. *J Formos Med Assoc*. 2008;107(12 Suppl):3–8.

25. Friede T, Kieser M. Sample size recalculation in internal pilot study designs: a review. *Biom J*. 2006;48(4):537–55.

26. Lachenbruch PA, Wittes J. Some aspects of the application of internal pilot studies. *Biom J*. 2006;48(4):556–7.

27. Oakley A, Strange V, Bonell C, Allen E, Stephenson J; RIPPLE Study Team. Process evaluation in randomised controlled trials of complex interventions. *BMJ*. 2006;332(7538):413–16.

28. Campbell NC, Murray E, Darbyshire J, Emery J, Farmer A, Griffiths F, et al. Designing and evaluating complex interventions to improve health care. *BMJ*. 2007;334(7591):455–9.

29. Power R, Langhaug LF, Nyamurera T, Wilson D, Bassett MT, Cowan FM. Developing complex interventions for rigorous evaluation—a case study from rural Zimbabwe. *Health Educ Res*. 2004; 19(5):570–5.

30. Klymko KW, Artinian NT, Washington OG, Lichtenberg PA, Vander Wal JS. Effect of impaired cognition on hypertension outcomes in older urban African Americans. *Medsurg Nurs*. 2008;17(6):405–10.

31. Ross S, Grant A, Counsell C, Gillespie W, Russell I, Prescott R. Barriers to participation in randomised controlled trials: a systematic review. *J Clin Epidemiol*. 1999;52(12):1143–56.

32. Butt DA, Lock M, Harvey BJ. Effective and cost-effective clinical trial recruitment strategies for postmenopausal women in a community-based, primary care setting. *Contemp Clin Trials*. 2010;31(5):447–56.

33. Simon S. Design and analysis of pilot studies. Revised 2009 July 8. Available from: www.childrensmercy.org/stats/weblog2004/PilotStudy.asp

34. Schulz KF, Grimes DA. Generation of allocation sequences in randomised trials: chance, not choice. *Lancet*. 2002;359(9305):515–9.

35. Schulz KF, Grimes DA. Allocation concealment in randomised trials: defending against deciphering. *Lancet*. 2002;359(9306):614–8.

36. Schulz KF, Grimes DA. Blinding in randomised trials: hiding who got what. *Lancet*. 2002;359(9307):696–700.

37. Bressler NM, Maguire MG, Murphy PL, Alexander J, Margherio R, Schachat AP, et al. Macular scatter ("grid") laser treatment of poorly demarcated subfoveal choroidal neovascularization in age-related macular degeneration. Results of a randomized pilot trial. *Arch Ophthalmol*. 1996;114(12):1456–64.

38. Ferris FL 3rd, Murphy RP. The peril of the pilot study. *Arch Ophthalmol*. 1996;114(12):1506–7.

39. Jairath N, Hogerney M, Parsons C. The role of the pilot study: a case illustration from cardiac nursing research. *Appl Nurs Res*. 2000;13(2):92–6.

40. Beebe LH. What can we learn from pilot studies? *Perspect Psychiatr Care*. 2007;43(4):213–8.

Conducting

41 Kraemer HC, Mintz J, Noda A, Tinklenberg J, Yesavage JA. Caution regarding the use of pilot studies to guide power calculations for study proposals. *Arch Gen Psychiatry*. 2006;63(5):484–9.

42. Browne RH. On the use of a pilot sample for sample size determination. *Stat Med*. 1995;14(17):1933–40.

43. Hertzog MA. Considerations in determining sample size for pilot studies. *Res Nurs Health*. 2008;31(2):180–91.

44. Vickers AJ. Underpowering in randomized trials reporting a sample size calculation. *J Clin Epidemiol*. 2003;56(8):717–20.

45. Lenth RV. Some practical guidelines for effective sample size determination. *Am Stat*. 2001;55(3):187–93.

ADDITIONAL RESOURCES

Feeley N, Cossette S, Côté J, Héon M, Stremler R, Martorella G, et al. The importance of piloting an RCT intervention. *Can J Nurs Res*. 2009;41(2):85–99.

Gardner G, Gardner A, MacLellan L, Osborne S. Reconceptualising the objectives of a pilot study for clinical research. *Int J Nurs Stud*. 2003;40(7):719–24.

Hinds PS, Gattuso JS. From pilot work to a major study in cancer nursing research. *Cancer Nurs*. 1991;14(3):132–5.

* These two articles provide informative examples of actual pilot studies.

Lancaster GA, Dodd S, Williamson PR. Design and analysis of pilot studies: recommendations for good practice. *J Eval Clin Pract*. 2004;10(2):307–12.

Prescott PA, Soeken KL. The potential uses of pilot work. *Nurs Res*. 1989;38(1):60–2.

* These four articles provide particularly detailed and informative discussions about pilot studies.

Thabane L, Ma J, Chu R, Cheng J, Ismaila A, Rios LP, et al. A tutorial on pilot studies: the what, why and how. *BMC Med Res Methodol*. 2010;10):1.

Conducting

SUMMARY CHECKLIST

☐ Thinking about your proposed full study, list the possible benefits of conducting a pilot study.
☐ If you did a pilot study, list the elements of your protocol that you would assess and how you would do so.
  Be sure to consider, where applicable, the following:
  — participant recruitment
  — testing data collection and instruments
  — randomization, blinding, and concealed allocation
  — safety
  — performance of outcome measures
  — sample size calculation
  — resource requirements
  — overall feasibility of a larger study
  — overall worthiness of a larger study
☐ List any decisions to be made as the result of a pilot.

22
Data collection and data management

A. Curtis Lee, PhD

ILLUSTRATIVE CASE

A resident in Otolaryngology has designed a needs assessment survey to evaluate curricular changes in her training program. After taking the steps to refine her study goals and the questionnaire design, she implements her survey but finds that the response rate is very low. To make matters worse, many of the survey responses are incomplete and she is having difficulty interpreting her data. She's not sure what to do next, and wonders what she should do differently when she attempts her next research project.

■ **Data collection is a fundamental** component of the research process. This chapter offers guidance on optimizing data collection so that you can get the most out of the information you gather. Data collection forms that are well planned, structured and organized can make the process easier, enhance the quality of the data you collect, and make subsequent steps such as the analysis and interpretation of results more reliable, more valid and more readily achieved. Although many issues concerning data collection will have been addressed in your study protocol and ethics application, when you get down to the details of designing a data collection tool it is helpful to bear certain practical considerations in mind.

Data collection forms

Data collection forms can be as diverse as the research purposes they serve. For example, a form can be designed to guide observations of patients, or the assessment of trainees vis-à-vis recommended practice. Specific types of information from patient records and case files can be organized through data collection forms. Online and paper-based surveys are other examples of data collection tools. Whatever the type of tool that is used, careful organization and design will foster effective data collection and prepare information for subsequent analysis.

The purpose of a data collection tool is to obtain a sample of data that truly reflects what is being measured; therefore, its design must be valid, reliable and practical. In the context of data collection, **validity** refers to the assurance that the data collected will comprehensively and accurately represent what is being measured. **Reliability** ensures that the data are consistent and the resulting conclusions reproducible. **Practicality** is also essential to success: ease and efficiency of use and the ability to analyze the resulting data must be factored into the design.

CHAPTER OBJECTIVES

After reading this chapter, you should be able to:
- describe key steps in developing data collection tools that will enable you to collect reliable and valid information that can be thoroughly and appropriately analyzed (see also ch. 10);
- discuss the importance of well-organized data collection for the successful completion of a research project;
- apply practical, common-sense tips in creating effective data collection tools; and
- describe the basics of preparing data for analysis.

Conducting

KEY TERMS		
Data cleaning	Framing	Relevance
Data element	Likert scales	Reliability
Double entry	Practicality	Validity
Face validity	Questionnaires	

Conducting

General considerations

Contextualizing your data collection

Your data collection form must be developed and/or adapted to fit your research question and methodology. Consider the type of information that you need and its source. For example, if your study involves a survey that is to be distributed to a variety of patients, the form will need to be feasible for the average person to use. Conversely, if your data collection tool is intended for use only within a research team (such as form to extract data from medical records), you may want to focus your efforts on optimizing functionality with respect to data extraction rather than on simplifying the wording and polishing the visual presentation. To take another example, if your study requires the collection of extensive qualitative data, such as those collected in a structured interview, you will need a form that is quite different from one intended for purely numerical data entry. If you are using an established tool, consider the specific context of your study and adapt the form as necessary. It is rare for an existing tool to be suitable for a research project without adaptation and further assessment of its reliability and validity in the proposed study environment.

If a predesigned form is chosen to be used, seek copyright clearance and ensure that proper attribution is made to the creator or distributor of the form. Although many data collection instruments can be found on the Internet, many are proprietary and may have licensing costs associated with their use.

Identification of respondents

Each completed data form or record should be assigned a unique identification code that allows the researcher, if necessary, to trace each response to its source (an individual or group). Identification numbers can also be created to classify participants (e.g., control group or treatment group), identify the session or time of assessment, and so on. By helping to preserve the anonymity of the respondents, the use of identification numbers not only protects the confidentiality of responses but also reduces the potential for bias in the analyses.

Collecting demographic information

Demographic information is pertinent to the generalizability of findings and to subgroup analysis. Consider what information is necessary to collect and, as appropriate, make responses to these questions mandatory. For exam

ple, if a study is comparing residents in their first year of residency with those in their fifth year, it would be essential to collect year-of-training data from each respondent.

When you collect demographic data, ask only for information that is pertinent to your research question and that will actually be used in the analysis. Create a table outlining the data that you hope to collect, and reassess whether all data to be collected are necessary. Eliminate those questions that do not contribute to the purpose of the study. Including irrelevant questions of a private or sensitive nature in a survey is not only unethical but is likely to increase the rate of non-responses to particular items or of refusals to complete or submit the form. A further reason to be judicious in the range of questions posed is expediency: balance the temptation to ask questions that "might" be used against the practicality of simplifying and reducing the effort required for effective data collection.

Consider privacy legislation and ensure that your methods of data collection and storage adhere to the confidentiality standards set out in your protocol and approved by your Research Ethics Board.

Designing a data collection form

The design of your data form or survey instrument—its structure, organization, format and visual presentation—can assist data collection by making it easy to follow and enhancing the clarity of individual items. A well-planned design can also facilitate the interpretation of the results by making the data easy to classify and retrieve. For example, a well-designed interview form is a communication tool that lends clarity and structure to the interaction, helping the researcher to pose questions that are direct, well focused and unambiguous. Similarly, an effective self-administered **questionnaire** should be clear and to the point: the appearance of the instrument should not be distracting or its organization confusing. The organization of the instrument should be logical, helping to focus the participant's attention and to ensure that the type of information that is being asked for is clear. Finally, the form should enable answers to be recorded in a manner that facilitates the data extraction and analysis.

To ensure that your data collection form will result in data that are clear, useful and require minimal correction or elimination (**data cleaning**), keep the following factors in mind:

1. Purpose

- **Relevance.** Each **data element** requested on a data collection form should have a legitimate bearing on the research question. Those who fill out the form should understand why they are being asked the question and how it contributes to the research project's goals.
- **Framing.** Items included on the data collection form should be framed in such a manner that it is clear to respondents what they are being asked to do, or what kind of information is being sought.

2. Clarity

- **Simplicity.** Each item should have a single focus: ask one question at a time. Complex questions often lead to ambiguous or complex responses that are difficult to interpret or abstract. For example, "double-barrelled" questions (i.e., those that ask two questions at once) should be avoided. See chapter 10 for further discussion of item design.
- **Plain language.** Use complete sentences, simple sentence structures, and familiar words.
- **Freedom from ambiguity.** Phrase questions in a manner that enables only one, easily understood, interpretation of what is being asked.
- **Precision.** Response fields should be designed to enable those who complete the form to record responses that accurately reflect their intended meaning. For example, respondents who have no opinion on a particular issue should be able to record "no opinion" rather than being forced into selecting an answer that implies agreement or disagreement.
- **Comprehensiveness.** Questions should account for all possible choices. For example, if you are asking trainees to choose their area of specialization from a list, all specialties and subspecialties must be accounted for on the list.
- The options in a list of choices must be mutually exclusive and logically organized.
- A common method of ensuring comprehensiveness when asking questions is the use of the option "Other." Although this allows for great flexibility, it also presents challenges for analysis. For example, if you ask participants to indicate their favourite food and the majority of responses are included in the "other" category, the analysis will be much more complex than the analysis of choices from a simple,

comprehensive list. This said, however, the analysis would be more accurate with a comprehensive list of "forced choices" as long as the list matched expected choices.

3. Organization

- **Instructions.** When designing a form, ensure that brief, adequate and clear instructions are provided and can be easily accessed.
- **Grouping of questions.** Use headings to group items logically and to facilitate smooth transitions from section to section. Use "skip" questions to enable respondents to avoid sections that are not applicable to them.
- **Order of questions.** When creating a questionnaire, ask the interesting and crucial questions first to capture the interest of the respondent. Some designers prefer to collect simple information such as demographics first while others prefer to ask the demographics questions last in order to gradually close the survey. However, if critical information is included in the demographics, it is best to ask these questions first. In addition, sensitive questions are usually left until the latter portions of a questionnaire to minimize the chance that respondents will give up on the questionnaire when little of it has been completed.

4. Format

To make your data collection form look professional and optimize the design of the form to record data, consider the following recommendations:

- Use a legible typeface in a size that will be easy for all users to read.
- Use space to define and separate the questions.
- If the data form is presented directly to the study participants, avoid splitting questions over a page break.
- Use page numbers and/or provide a guide to indicate the percentage of the survey or questionnaire that is left to complete (or, in a print document, the current page and total number of pages). This is especially important if the study participants are filling out the data collection form themselves.
- Use bold and italic judiciously to provide clarity and emphasize important details.
- Use bold and italic judiciously to provide clarity and emphasize important details.

Conducting

- Use tables sparingly but effectively to guide responses. For example, when asking a series of related Likert type questions, group them in a table format. Do not use too many tables, however, as they will crowd the data collection tool.
- Consider using colour-coded paper to help organize your data collection. For example, highlight important or mandatory questions with a different colour than the less important questions.

Question formats

Whenever possible, avoid open-ended questions on your data collection form (see also ch. 10). Questions with selected responses (such as multiple-choice questions, drop-down selection boxes or **Likert scales**) rather than open-ended questions are easier to answer, and the responses are easier to categorize, code and analyze. Analyzing frequency counts of a limited number of specific selections is simple and unambiguous.

Likert scales provide respondents with a limited number of ordered responses to indicate their answer to a posed question, such as their current state of health (e.g., excellent, very good, good, fair, poor) or their current level of pain (e.g., none, mild, moderate, severe). They might also be used to enable respondents to indicate their level of agreement with a posed statement (e.g., strongly agree, agree, disagree, strongly disagree). Other common anchors used with Likert scales pertain to the respondent's perceptions of importance or frequency in relation to a statement or series of statements. For example, "Rate our level of satisfaction with the following statement. I like buffalo wings: strongly agree, agree, disagree, strongly disagree." When using Likert scales, researchers often need to determine whether it is better to offer the option of a mid-range or neutral answer or to force the respondent to choose between a positive and negative response. For example, a typical Likert item would likely have a respondent "strongly disagree," "disagree," "neither agree nor disagree," "agree" or "strongly agree" with a statement. If the researcher would like the respondent to have only four options, "neither agree nor disagree" would not be included. To reduce the variability of interpretation, scales should have no more than five options.[1]

If your research project builds on current research, or if you anticipate that you will want to compare your results with those of previous research, using the same wording of questions and response options as in the previous research will help to enable this direct comparison. For example, if you administered a survey two years ago and wanted to track changes from year to year, you may want to ask the same question, worded in the same way, and do a direct comparision. If wording changes are made to the question, on the other hand, you will be unable to determine whether any changes in the responses reflect the participants' interpretation of the revised phrasing of the question, or actual changes in behaviour over time. Many useful question scales have been used in past research and are available in the literature; these should be identified and assessed before you decide to create questions *de novo*.

Finalizing the data collection form

Once a draft of the data collection form is created, it should be reviewed thoroughly from the following perspectives:

- **Face validity**. The data form, survey or questionnaire should look professional and contain no spelling, grammatical or formatting errors. It should seem evident to anyone filling it out that it is indeed appropriate for the stated purpose of the research.
- **Relevance.** Each question in the form should relate to the research goals and contribute to answering the research question(s) posed in the project proposal.
- **Clarity.** Ask a knowledgeable colleague who is not directly associated with the project to review the form to test whether his or her interpretations of the questions are in line with your intention. An approach that can be helpful in identifying unclear or potentially minsterpreted questions is to have the reviewer talk out loud as he or she works through the draft survey instrument. After examining the form, your reviewer should also understand the purpose of the study and the process required of the participants, and should have a clear understanding of all items and their contributions to the research project.

After you have received feedback from one or more knowledgeable colleagues, your draft instrument could then be reviewed by being administered in one or more pilot projects in which sample data are collected from suitable respondents (see ch. 21).

From data collection to analysis

As you create your data collection form, anticipate how the data will need to be prepared for analysis. Quantitative data are analyzed using programs such as Microsoft Excel, SPSS and other statistical analysis packages. Microsoft Excel tends to be the simplest tool for data entry and is sufficient for most basic research projects. Several user manuals are available, and Excel's online learning resources are very helpful.[a] Because the data requirements for a particular project can be quite specialized, only a few general tips on using Excel will be described here.

To illustrate the use of Excel for data collection and management, consider the resident in our case example, who is evaluating curricular changes. She created and distributed a questionnaire and used it to collect information pertaining to assessments within the curriculum. The spreadsheet in Table 22.1 shows some of her data. Note that in spreadsheets of this kind it is typically best to organize the data using one row per respondent and to assign each individual item to be analyzed to its own column. In the sample case, the researcher has 10 respondents, allocated to rows 3 to 12. Each question is given a different column. A sample of four questions is shown in the figure.

Each column should contain consistently labelled information, and a glossary or standard list of terms that will be accepted on the input form should be used to ensure consistent data input. For example, if you are collecting information about Canadian universities, all Canadian universities should be listed as possible options in a consistent manner, such that responses that are not included on that list would be rejected by the input form. In Excel, using drop-down lists for selections of this kind is recommended. In our case example, Excel is able to count the number of "Yes" and "No" responses because they have been entered consistently. Note that the formula in cell F22 (=countif(E3:E12,"Yes") counts the number of "Yes" responses in column E, rows 3 to 12, to the question "Do you prefer the new curriculum?" If a "Y" were entered rather than "Yes" it would not be counted: hence the need for consistency.

If dates are used, use a consistent, unambiguous format such as 05-Jul-2010 or YYYYMMDD. If you are analyzing frequencies, ensure that all submitted responses fit into fixed categories. Numeric data should be entered as numbers, not with words, to enable addition and other computation within the spreadsheet. Some common descriptive statistics are included in the spreadsheet example in Table 22.1.

Once the data are entered, they should be reviewed and data cleaning should be done. In addition to reviewing each questionnaire as soon as possible after it is received, simple descriptive statitistics should be completed on the entire data set so that inconsistent or unreasonable values might be identified. Data cleaning is the detailed process of reviewing collected data to identify any incorrect and/or inconsistent entries in preparation for the analysis; if obviously invalid responses are found, they need to be either corrected or eliminated prior to analysis. For example, if a group of medical residents are asked for their ages, and a value of "8 years old" appears in the resulting data set, this invalid value should, if possible, be corrected or removed prior to analysis. Incorrect or inconsistent data items can potentially be corrected by rechecking the original data entry form (to correct a data entry error) or even by returning to the respondent to clarify, correct or confirm the response.

Data entry errors can be assessed by having the data (or at least a portion of it) independently entered by two different people (**double entry**) and the two sets of entries compared. It is also recommended to verify a sample of data by randomly selecting as many data as possible within the Excel file and comparing them with the original data source (e.g., the original, completed questionnaires).

A copy of the raw data should be kept and a back-up copy should be made before the process of data cleaning begins.

Conclusion

In most health research projects a considerable amount of time and effort is directed toward developing the research question and ensuring that the research proposal receives ethical approval. A reasonable amount of effort will also be required on the design and organization of data collection tools to ensure that these initial efforts result in data that can lead to successful research outcomes, and to ensure that an instrument acceptable to the ethics review committee will be submitted with your application for ethics approval. Carefully designed data forms can enhance the quality of your findings: by standardizing data collection, they can make the analysis and interpretation of results more reliable, more valid, and more readily achieved. ∎

---

a   See http://office.microsoft.com/en-us/excel-help/

■ **Table 22.1: Example of a spreadsheet used for data management**

	A	B	C	D	E	F
1	**Evaluation of the curriculum changes (Survey questions 5 and 6)**					
2			On average, how many assessments were you able to make using the OLD training program?	On average, how many assessments were you able to make using the NEW training program?	Do you prefer the new curriculum?	When did you start using the new curriculum?
3	Respondent 1		5	8	Yes	15-Sept-10
4	Respondent 2		4	7	Yes	16-Aug-10
5	Respondent 3		3	8	Yes	17-Sep-10
6	Respondent 4		4	8	Yes	09-Jul-10
7	Respondent 5		10	9	No	19-Jul-10
8	Respondent 6		9	8	No	01-Sep-10
9	Respondent 7		6	8	Yes	23-Jul-10
10	Respondent 8		1	6	No	10-Oct-10
11	Respondent 9		5	8	Yes	23-Aug-10
12	Respondent 10		6	7	Yes	10-Oct-10
13						
14	Average		5.3	7.7	<- =AVERAGE(D3:D12)	
15	Minimum		1	6	<- =MIN(D3:D12)	
16	Maximum		10	9	<- =MAX(D3:D12)	
17	Std Dev		2.67	0.82	<- =STDEV(D3:D12)	
18	Median		5	8	<- =MEDIAN(D3:D12)	
19	Skew		0.43	-0.81	<- =SKEW(D3:D12)	
20	Kurtosis		0.18	1.24	<- =KURT(D3:D12)	
21						
22	Correlation		.70	<- =CORREL (C3:C12,D3:D12)	# Yes = 7	<- =COUNTIF (E3:E12,"Yes")
23	*t* test		0.01	<- =TTEST (C3:C12,D3:D12,2,2)	# No = 3	<- =COUNTIF (E3:E12,"No")

Conducting

REFERENCE

1. Wasek PA. Practical considerations in designing data collection forms. *Inf Control Hosp Epidemiol.* 1990;11(7):384–9.

ADDITIONAL RESOURCES

Dillman DA, Smyth JD, Melani Christian L. *Internet, mail and mixed-mode surveys: the tailored design method.* 3rd ed. Hoboken (NJ): John Wiley; 2009.
   • The best resource for designing surveys and creating forms for research.

Jamieson S. Likert scales: how to (ab)use them. *Med Educ.* 2004;38(12):1217–18.
   • Provides examples of scales and practical methods of improving the use of Likert scales.

Wasek PA. Practical considerations in designing data collection forms. *Inf Control Hosp Epidemiol.* 1990;11(7):384–9.
   • A good guide to designing forms.

http://people.usd.edu/~bwjames/tut/excel/
   • An online tutorial helpful for beginners in Excel.

www.baycongroup.com/el0.htm
   • An online resource for Excel users.

Conducting

EXERCISE: ASSESSING YOUR DATA COLLECTION FORM

Consider the following questions:

1. If all the questions on your data collection form are answered, will you have the information you need to answer all of your research questions?

2. Would someone not involved in your study interpret your questions in the way you intend?

3. Will your data collection form be clear to all users (e.g., interviewers, data abstractors, and study participants)?

4. Can your data collection form be practically implemented? How long does it take to fill out? Are participants likely to complete the entire form? How much work will it take to extract data from the form? Have you tested all of these aspects in one or more pilot administrations, using a group of suitable respondents?

SUMMARY CHECKLIST

- ❏ Consider your research protocol, identify all of the data that you will need to collect, and determine how you will collect it.
- ❏ Identify how many data collection instruments you will need.
- ❏ Select, adapt or design each instrument, keeping in mind best practices and the elements needed to create an effective tool.
- ❏ Revisit the context and protocols of your study. Decide how the instruments will be administered, by whom, and when. Revise as needed!
- ❏ Pilot your instruments and protocol. Revise again as needed.
- ❏ Finalize your forms prior to ethics review.
- ❏ Manage your data in a relevant spreadsheet suitable for analysis.
- ❏ Clean your data.
- ❏ Ensure your data are always kept safe and secure.

Conducting

23
Managing and monitoring a study

Stacy Ackroyd-Stolarz, MSc, PhD

ILLUSTRATIVE CASE

During an intense, month-long research rotation, a resident develops a study protocol and prepares a submission to his institution's Research Ethics Board. Developing the protocol takes far more work than he had anticipated, but after some minor clarifications it receives full approval. Now he's ready to do the study, but his rotations and call schedule for the next four months allow little or no time for it. He is being encouraged to present his findings at the departmental Research Day, but he doesn't know how he will manage to finish the study by then. He begins to wonder why physicians bother doing research.

■ **Earlier chapters in this guide** described the essential first steps in planning a research study, including finding a research supervisor (ch. 3,) formulating an "operational" research question (ch. 6), determining which methodological approach to take (ch. 9) and developing a study protocol (ch. 17). However, the day-to-day conduct of a study also needs careful planning. The practical aspects of how a study is carried out can have a significant impact on its overall quality and scientific rigour. This chapter provides an overview of study management and of the various responsibilities that it entails.

Responsibilities of study management

When you assume the role of **principal investigator**, the overall conduct of the study becomes your responsibility, from assembling the study team to fulfilling post-study obligations such as ensuring the secure storage of data and proper study closure with the **Research Ethics Board**. Essentially, these duties involve the key functions of oversight, monitoring and communication, as follows:[1,2]

- **Oversight of:**
  — study team
  — study conduct
- **Monitoring of:**
  — patient enrolment, allocation and follow-up
  — financial expenditures
  — data quality and security
  — adherence to study protocol and to timeline

CHAPTER OBJECTIVES

After reading this chapter, you should be able to:
- describe the responsibilities of a principal investigator;
- discuss the distinction between designing and conducting a research study;
- describe key considerations in managing resources, including time, for research;
- discuss the importance of, and processes for, monitoring the progress of a research study;
- summarize issues related to data management and security; and
- identify online resources for new investigators

Conducting

KEY TERMS			
Authorship	Monitoring	Recruitment	Study identifiers
Communication	Oversight	Research Ethics Board	Study team
Data security	Personnel	Research coordinator	Threats to internal validity
Funding	Personal identifiers	Research diary	Time management
Information technology	Principal investigator	Statistician	

- **Communication with:**
  - — study team (including preceptor)
  - — study participants (where applicable)
  - — Research Ethics Board
  - — program director
  - — relevant institutional departments

These responsibilities can be challenging during a busy training program, but you can take practical steps to make them more manageable. The following sections describe various aspects of research management that are important to consider as you gear up for your project. The sample project checklist provided at the end of the chapter lists the main tasks and functions for which you will be responsible, either directly or through the supervision of others on the team. Also provided are a template for keeping track of expenditures and a sample project timetable.

Keeping it manageable

One of the most important resources that you will need to manage during the course of your research project is time—that of others, and your own. Developing a project that is feasible to complete during the allotted time during your training may mean tackling something smaller in scope than you (or your preceptor) had initially imagined. However, the lessons learned in a small study are just as valuable as those gained from a large one, since the process and tasks are similar. Whether you undertake a health record review, a survey, or a randomized controlled trial, you will have to develop a study protocol and will benefit from the experience of preparing a submission to a Research Ethics Board. (Increasingly, institutions require that even small studies involving health record reviews undergo ethics review.) Regardless of the scale of your study, you will have to get it up and running, monitor it on a regular basis, and ensure that follow-up (if required) is carried out and that the analyses are complete.

Your first foray into health research has a better chance of being a positive experience if you can complete your project during training. Many a trainee has had every intention of finishing a study once he or she starts practice, only to find that work demands make it impossible to give the project the attention it deserves. This means that either the preceptor has to finish the project, or that it is never completed—a result that is not only frustrating for everyone involved but that also means that patients enrolled in the study may have been needlessly exposed to risk. Moreover,

if you have a positive experience with research during your training, you will probably be much more interested in incorporating research into your professional career (see ch. 32)—and an important component of that positive experience is tackling a project that can be realized within a reasonable time.

Expecting the unexpected

Although it may seem obvious that a study protocol must be followed as written, the reality is that unexpected situations almost invariably arise in the conduct of a study that make it difficult, if not impossible, to adhere to the protocol in every detail. In some cases, an amendment to the protocol will be necessary. Consider the following examples:

- You have designed a study that involves a series of monthly follow-up interviews with patients that take an average of 30 minutes to complete. After collecting data for a couple of months, you realize that a majority of study participants are withdrawing from the study after the first follow-up interview.
- You want to conduct a survey of fourth-year residents in Internal Medicine across Canada. The Research Ethics Board has approved the study, but in view of the personal nature of the questions has requested that you seek written informed consent from each participant.
- In a study involving review of electronic health records, the time it takes to extract the data is 45 minutes longer per record than originally assumed. With 500 records to review, you're going to run out of funding to pay the reviewers.

Each of these examples has potential solutions. Although some problems should be prevented during the protocol development phase (e.g., the situation in the first example could have been avoided by pilot testing the follow-up questions and interview schedule), there must be a defensible scientific and ethical rationale for any protocol amendments or changes in study methods, and these must be documented. Moreover, any changes must be approved by your Research Ethics Board before they are implemented.

Working effectively with your study team

A **study team** typically includes investigators and study staff (e.g., a **research coordinator**). Other **personnel**, such as human resources managers, database analysts and tech-

Conducting

nicians, might not be part of the scientific team, but are important to the overall operation of the study. In all training programs there are people who can help you with your research project. Although you must retain oversight and primary responsibility for your study, it is both reasonable and wise to seek assistance from others. Help is available from many sources, including senior trainees, research coordinators, **statisticians**, **information technology** (IT) personnel, health records technicians, and your preceptor, Research Director and Program Director. Most people involved in research are more than willing to take the time to answer questions or direct you to another resource. Finding out about the expertise available in your department, faculty and institution will save you time.

It is important to consider the nature of your relationship with each person who is assisting you. For example, the team might include a medical student working as a volunteer to help with data collection in order to get some research experience, or perhaps you have sufficient funding to hire a research assistant. In either situation, it is important to: (1) define responsibilities; (2) agree on remuneration, if any; (3) monitor the quality and quantity of the person's work on a regular basis; (4) provide constructive feedback; and (5) be available to answer questions related to your study.

Statisticians are an invaluable resource during the development of your protocol for such tasks as calculating an adequate sample size. They can advise you on appropriate statistical analyses and on the particulars of data collection to ensure that you are collecting the right information to enable a meaningful analysis. In some situations, statisticians are involved as consultants who provide advice at the beginning of the study and conduct analyses at the end. Usually this is done on a contractual basis, with professional fees ranging from $50 to $150 per hour. Your department or preceptor may have some discretionary funds to cover these costs. In other situations, a statistician becomes involved as a member of the research team and contributes his or her services as part of the role of co-investigator. Statisticians sometimes have a graduate student conduct analyses under supervision. You can also directly contact graduate programs in statistics, public health, psychology or other disciplines at your university to find graduate students who might be interested in assisting you with the study analyses. In any case, it is important to involve a statistician early in the development of the study rather than waiting until you have collected all of the data. This will not only make the most efficient use of your time (and that of the statistician), but will also ensure that the data are in a usable format and of sufficient quality to be analyzed.

The key to a successful research project involving a team of people is routine and effective **communication**. Even if you are doing most of the work on your project, it is still important to keep in touch with others to let them know how things are progressing. A brief email on a weekly or monthly basis is often all that is needed. For studies involving larger teams, regular face-to-face meetings are an excellent strategy for building a more effective team. Using a consistent format and routine timing of any study-related updates or meetings will often save you time by avoiding potential miscommunication. You will also be responsible for ensuring timely correspondence with certain departments in your institution, such as Research Finance for funded studies or IT for studies involving institutional data. In addition, you will need to ensure that team members are able to contact you at any time during the study if they have questions or no longer wish to participate.

Another important study-related task is negotiating **authorship** of any published results. It is always best to have this discussion early so that expectations are clear and consistent. There are excellent references describing guidelines and other considerations for authorship.[3,4] The International Committee of Medical Journal Editors recommends that authorship be "based on 1) substantial contributions to conception, design, acquisition of data, or analysis and interpretation of data; 2) drafting the article or revising it critically for important intellectual content; and 3) final approval of the version to be published."[3] Decisions about the order of authorship on a final paper may change over time to reflect the relative contribution of each investigator during the conduct of the study and preparation of the manuscript.

Keeping data secure

Chapter 22 of this guide provides excellent information on data management from the perspective of facilitating high-quality and reliable analyses. In your role as PI you will also be responsible for patient confidentiality and **data security**, and will need to ensure that everyone associated with the study adheres to the requirements of your Research Ethics Board with respect to data acquisition and storage. Stringent requirements for ensuring data security have evolved in recent years in tandem with an increasing sensitivity to issues surrounding privacy and patient confidentiality.[5] When personal information that can identify individual patients (e.g., a health insurance number) is contained in an institutional database, it is common practice to remove these personal identifiers and create a unique study identification number or code for each patient record extracted from the database for the purpose of research. The code for matching the **study identifier** with the **personal identifier** must be stored in a separate, secure place. It is generally prohibited to remove data collection forms or electronic data that contain participant information from an institution. You are responsible for ensuring that all study-related correspondence and data are archived according to these requirements.

Managing the study finances

Many excellent resident research projects are completed using existing departmental resources and do not require additional **funding**. Some departments or faculties provide seed funding for trainee research projects. Check with your Program Director or Research Director and preceptor to see if funding might be available for your project. There are also a number of institutional, provincial or national funding opportunities for which you may be eligible (ch. 19). The Research Services office at your university and/or hospital will likely have information on these funding agencies.

Awards for research projects generally do not go directly to an investigator, but are managed through an institution such as a hospital or university. It will be important for you to familiarize yourself with the specific requirements of each funding agency you plan to approach. For example, some funding agencies will allow an organization to keep any unspent monies. Others require unspent monies to be returned. If you are successful at securing funding for your research project, it is important that you check with your department about the processes for establishing and monitoring a research account. Often a departmental administrator will be able to assist you with setting up an account and monitoring monthly statements, but you must retain oversight (see Table 23.1).

Managing time

Training is a demanding phase of your career, not least with respect to time management. Even if your longer-term career aspirations do not include research, the experience in **time management** that you will gain during your first research project will serve you well in the future.

It is very common to run into unanticipated delays in research projects. Some of these—such as a prolonged review time by your Research Ethics Board—will be out of your control. Others will be entirely within your control, but not necessarily any easier to manage. Always factor in time for delays, even if you can't anticipate exactly what those delays might be. One strategy to prevent eleventh-hour panic is to create a timetable for your project early on. This will help you to break tasks into manageable parts and to plan around the clinical and educational demands of your training program. You may be able to use the timetable to negotiate protected time for research at critical points during the project (see Table 23.2).

Monitoring protocol compliance and study progress

Once your study is up and running, it is important to monitor its progress on a regular basis to identify problems, ensure that the protocol is being implemented correctly, and ensure that the study can be completed in the time allotted and with the resources available. Monitoring can be simplified by establishing a routine that doesn't necessarily require a lot of your time. The frequency and intensity of monitoring will likely need to be higher at the beginning of the study so that unanticipated problems are spotted early. Your monitoring will cover quantitative aspects such as the number of enrolments, surveys completed or health records reviewed, but will also need to include an assessment of the quality of the data collected (e.g., laboratory results, completeness of surveys, etc.). For example, in studies involving participant **recruitment**, you will need to monitor the number of patients enrolled per week or month to ensure that the rate is keeping pace with your target. If you need to recruit 200 participants in one year but by the end of the first month have only enrolled 5, then you will need to re-evaluate your recruitment strategies, the study period and/or sample size considerations. Similarly, you will need to monitor the dropout or lost to follow-up rate for enrolled patients. In studies involving surveys, the response rate needs ongoing monitoring, as does the response to individual questions (to detect problems of non-response).

Every study faces potential **threats to internal validity**, such as selection bias, maturation (normal changes over time), repeated testing, regression toward the mean, and changes to the measurement instrument. Most often, these potential threats are dealt with in the design of a study or are controlled for during the analyses. Although a separate chap-

Conducting

■ **Table 23.1: Sample line items for study budget**

BUDGET ITEM	COST		
	PROJECTED	ACTUAL	VARIANCE
Wages (and benefits)			
Administration			
Information Technology			
Research assistant/coordinator			
Other types of compensation			
Consulting fees			
Research participant honoraria			
Statistical consultation			
Transcription services			
Supplies and general expenses			
Stationery			
Mailing			
Long distance and fax costs for data collection			
Photocopying			
Printer cartridges			
Courier			
Software			
Equipment			
Telephone			
Computer			
Printer			
Dissemination expenses			
Travel			
Mileage			
Per diem for meals			
Flight			
Accommodation			
Other			
Poster production			
Manuscript preparation			
Review by professional copyeditor			
Other costs			
Development of website for ongoing dissemination			
Costs for lab tests, diagnostic imaging etc.			
Total expenses			
In-kind or other contributions			
TOTAL COSTS			

Conducting

■ Table 23.2: Sample timetable for a two-year study

Conducting

YEAR ONE

Phase	July	Aug	Sept	Oct	Nov	Dec	Jan	Feb	Mar	Apr	May	June
Pre-study	Identify topic and preceptor; Develop protocol; Consult with statistician (if applicable); Identify potential funding sources; Develop study timetable		Prepare REB submission	Submit to REB	Revisions as per REB	B R E A K	Meet with study investigators to establish roles and responsibilities; Establish routine study-related communication (format/timing); Determine specific study procedures					
Start-up									Hire and train study staff; Set up research account	Start data collection; Develop and initiate monitoring regimen	Data collection; Monitoring: • recruitment (includes response rate for surveys) • adherence to protocol • data quality • consistency of clinical and lab procedures and/or assessments by multiple assessors • confidentiality • study budget; Routine contact with: • study team • preceptor • REB (as needed) • participants (as needed)	

YEAR TWO

Phase	July	Aug	Sept	Oct	Nov	Dec	Jan	Feb	Mar	Apr	May	June
Ongoing	Data collection; Monitoring: • recruitment (includes response rate for surveys) • adherence to protocol • data quality • consistency of clinical and lab procedures and/or assessments by multiple assessors • confidentiality • study budget; Routine contact with: • study team • preceptor • REB (as needed) • participants (as needed); Submit request for annual approval to REB				Data analysis	B R E A K	Prepare abstract for presentation in January; Synthesize results and review with preceptor; Start manuscript; Complete follow-up for participants			Present study; Familiarize preceptor with study documentation; Work with study team to prepare documents for archiving; Revise manuscript and prepare for submission	Submit study closure to REB and archive documents(or make arrangements to have it done)	

ter could be devoted to these concepts, they are raised in this section to highlight how the day-to-day decisions or events that occur during the implementation of a study can adversely affect its internal validity. The following examples describe different situations that could pose a potential threat.

- **Selection.** Although you designed your study with rigorous inclusion and exclusion criteria to minimize selection bias, you discover on follow-up that several enrolled patients failed to mention pre-existing medical conditions that should have excluded them from participating.
- **Instrumentation.** You have enrolled 60 patients with asthma from a family practice to participate in a home-based intervention for self-management that will take place over 12 months. The protocol requires that patients monitor their respiratory function on a daily basis using standardized, calibrated spirometers. As the study proceeds, 6 of the study patients (10%) have problems with their spirometers, which must be replaced. Unfortunately, similar spirometers are no longer available because the hospital has switched suppliers; they must be replaced with models from a different company.
- **History.** You are conducting a survey of residents' perceptions of the impact of working hours on patient safety in the hospital, using a sample of residents from all residency programs from 2 consecutive years. Near the end of the first year, a patient dies in hospital because of a medication error that is attributed to an order given by a resident post-call. The family involves the media and the incident attracts considerable public attention.
- **Repeated measures.** You are involved in a medical education research study examining retention of procedural skills. The protocol involves re-testing

psychomotor performance of the procedure and a multiple-choice questionnaire designed to examine the cognitive aspects of the procedure. This is done on a monthly basis for one year.

It is important to document any decisions or events that might pose a threat to the internal validity of your study and to actively consider their potential impact as you interpret your results. One valuable tool to help with this is a **research diary**. Virtually every investigator runs into unforeseen circumstances that may necessitate a change—some minor, others more significant. For instance, a change might be made to a data collection form or the timing of a follow-up interview might have to be altered to increase the yield of completed interviews. In the weeks and months that follow, it is often difficult to recall the rationale or exact circumstances for a given change. By documenting all changes, along with the methodological insights that you gain as the project moves along, you will have a record of the process and a rationale for each specific change. When the time comes to write a manuscript or respond to detailed questions from an editor, the diary you have kept will be surprisingly helpful.

Conclusion

As a health care professional, you are poised to ask salient questions that have the potential to lead to improvements in patient care. A well-planned and well-executed research study can help you to answer those questions. Hands-on involvement in your own study will provide not only insight into the challenges of conducting research, but also the thrill of creating new knowledge or understanding old problems in new ways. ∎

Conducting

CASE POSTSCRIPT

When the resident creates a timetable, he is struck by how much needs to be done to complete the study in the time he has available. He also realizes that the project seems less daunting and easier to schedule if he breaks it down into a series of smaller tasks. He speaks to his senior resident, who tells him about the excellent support she has received from the Research Coordinator in the department, especially with regard to documentation for the Research Ethics Board and the archiving of study records. His preceptor gives him the name of a statistician, who subsequently helps him with data analyses. The resident is able to present the final study results at his departmental Research Day. He is even more surprised to realize that his project has given him a new appreciation of the way in which research influences his thinking about clinical practice.

REFERENCES

1. Hulley SB, Cummings SR, Browner WS, Grady DG, Newman TB. *Designing clinical research: an epidemiologic approach*. 3rd ed. Philadelphia (PA): Lippincott Williams & Wilkins; 2007.

2. Wolf DC, Katz S, Safdi MA, Sandler RS, Lewis JD. Site organization and management. *Inflamm Bowel Dis*. 2005;11 Suppl 1:S29–33.

3. International Committee of Medical Journal Editors. *Uniform requirements for manuscripts submitted to biomedical journals: ethical considerations in the conduct and reporting of research: authorship and contribution*. Philadelphia: The Committee; 2009. Available from: www.icmje.org/ethical_1author.html

4. Tsao CI, Roberts LW. Authorship in scholarly manuscripts: practical considerations for resident and early career physicians. *Acad Psychiatry*. 2009;33(1):76–9.

5. Canadian Institutes of Health Research. *CIHR Best Practices for Protecting Privacy in Health Research*. Ottawa (ON): The Institutes; 2005. Available from: www.cihr-irsc.gc.ca/e/documents/et_pbp_nov05_sept2005_e.pdf

ADDITIONAL RESOURCES

Canadian Institutes of Health Research. CIHR knowledge translation publications. Available from: www.cihr.ca/e/29484.html

- This link provides a list of resources on knowledge translation activities relevant to CIHR. This has become an increasingly important consideration for funding agencies.

Canadian Institutes of Health Research. *Research in ethics: web-based tutorials* [Internet]. Available from: www.cihr.ca/e/30489.html

- This link provides a list of web-based resources on research ethics, including a link to an online tutorial for the *Tri-Council Policy Statement: Ethical Conduct for Research Involving Humans* (TCPS). This tutorial has seven sections that can be completed at your own pace. You can receive a certificate of completion once you have finished the tutorial. It takes approximately two hours to complete.

McInnes R, Andrews B, Rachubinski. *Guidebook for new principal investigators: advice on applying for a grant, writing papers, setting up a research team and managing your time*. Ottawa: Canadian Institutes of Health Research. Institute of Genetics. Available from: www.cihr-irsc.gc.ca/e/27491.html

- This guidebook is designed for health researchers, including basic and clinical scientists. It provides guidance on grant writing, managing a research team or laboratory, writing papers and time management. This is a useful and easy-to-read resource, particularly for those interested in pursuing further research.

EXERCISE: QUESTIONS TO CONSIDER

1. Develop a timetable for your research study. Build in additional time (at least 25%) for inevitable delays.

2. Talk to trainees nearing the end of their training to get their input on dealing with unexpected challenges, suggestions for useful research resources at your institution, and time-management strategies.

3. Talk to your Program Director and Research Director and to research personnel in your department to learn more about the resources available to help you with your research project.

SUMMARY CHECKLIST

Pre-study
- ❏ Develop protocol
- ❏ Consult with statistician (if applicable)
- ❏ Develop study procedures (e.g., data collection form, mechanisms for tracking progress, etc.)
- ❏ Identify potential sources of funds
- ❏ Develop study timetable (plan for delays)
- ❏ Ethics submission and approval
    - ❏ Approval date _____
- ❏ Determine roles and respnsibilities of study team
- ❏ Determine method(s) and timing of routine study-related communications (e.g., bi-weekly updates)

Start-up
- ❏ Hire and train study staff (if applicable)
- ❏ Establish research account (if applicable)
    - ❏ Account number _____
- ❏ Develop and initiate monitoring

Ongoing
Routinely monitor:
- ❏ Recruitment of study participants/response rate for surveys
- ❏ Adherence to protocol
- ❏ Data quality
- ❏ Consistency of clinical and laboratory procedures and/or assessments by multiple assessors
- ❏ Confidentiality
- ❏ Study budget
- ❏ Other

Maintain relevant correspondence with Research Ethics Board regarding:
- ❏ Request for annual approval
- ❏ Amendments to protocol and/or consent forms
- ❏ Reports of serious adverse avents
- ❏ Study closure

Schedule routine meetings and/or contact with preceptor and study team

Post-study
- ❏ Complete follow-up for participants (e.g., communicate study results)
- ❏ Perform data analysis (with statistician if applicable)
- ❏ Review study documentation with preceptor
- ❏ Archive all study documents as per institutional requirements

Conducting

24
Data analysis: Descriptive statistics

Bart J. Harvey, MD, PhD, MEd, FACPM, FRCPC

ILLUSTRATIVE CASE

A General Internal Medicine resident, completing a rotation at a community health centre, wants to determine what proportion of people served by each of the centre's two practice groups have received the recommended preventive services during the previous two years. After speaking to his field supervisor and deciding to carry out a review using the centre's electronic health record database, he wonders what procedures and techniques will be needed to summarize the data once they are collected.

■ Quantitative health studies address

research questions about people and conditions by collecting and analyzing data obtained by counting, observing and measuring. In chapter 8 we examined the types of data collected in quantitative research. The present chapter is the first of two that introduce and discuss the statistical tools and techniques used to analyze these data. The analytic techniques used in qualitative health studies are presented and discussed in chapter 16.

The statistical techniques used to analyze quantitative data generally fall into two main categories: **descriptive statistics,** which, as the name suggests, enable collected data to be summarized and described; and **hypothesis-testing** or **inferential statistics**, which comprise a diverse set of tests and techniques that enable comparisons and other analyses to be completed. In addition, and related to both of these uses, statistics also enable a determination of the precision with which any measure has been made. In general, the most important role of statistical testing is to assess what role chance may have played in the collected data and the degree to which it might be a plausible explanation for the observed study results.

CHAPTER OBJECTIVES

After reading this chapter, you should be able to:

- list and describe key descriptive statistics (e.g., measures of central tendency and variability) used in health-related quantitative research studies;
- describe the situations and circumstances in which each of these descriptive statistics should and should not be used;
- describe the characteristics of normal and skewed distributions;
- describe the difference and the relationship between a sample and a population;
- explain how each individual sample provides a single estimate of the quantity being estimated and how (and why) the estimates arising from multiple samples are distributed around the "true" (population) value;
- state what is measured by the standard error (SE) and which factors affect its size; and
- define the confidence interval (CI) and describe what information it conveys and how to use it when reporting study results.

Conducting

KEY TERMS

Biological variation	Graphical displays	Outlier	Skewed (non-normal)
Census	Hypothesis-testing (inferential)	Parametric statistical tests	distribution
Central tendency	statistics	Percentile	Standard deviation (SD)
Confidence interval (CI)	Interquartile range (IQR)	Population	Standard error (SE)
Descriptive statistics	Mean	Precision	Variability
Dispersion	Median	Random variation	Variance
Frequency	Mode	Range	
Frequency distribution	Non-parametric statistical tests	Sample	
Gaussian distribution	Normal distribution	Sample size	

This chapter and the next have been written from the perspective of a health researcher, rather than that of a statistician. From a researcher's perspective, statistics should be a means to an end, and not an end in itself. This chapter strives to introduce statistics as a "tool box" from which tests and techniques may be selected and used to complete the needed data analyses. In working with any set of tools, one requires an understanding not only of what the available tools are and how they should be used, but also of which tools should be used for which tasks.

This chapter discusses descriptive statistics, while the next discusses the statistical methods used for hypothesis testing, as well as the concepts of precision and statistical power, and the determination of a study's required **sample size**. However, before beginning, it is important to reiterate a theme that recurs throughout this guide: researchers should ensure that they consult with someone knowledgeable about statistical methods during the planning and design stages of their research projects! Only then can they be confident that they will collect the necessary data, using the right techniques, and then be able to analyze their findings appropriately to obtain a valid answer to their research question.

Descriptive statistics

Making sense of group data (e.g., measurements taken from multiple persons, or multiple measurements taken from the same person) usually requires the use of descriptive statistical techniques that summarize values into a more readily understandable form. Descriptive statistics provide the most basic form of data summarization and should be the starting point of any data analysis. Descriptive statistics summarize data and allow them to be expressed in a few, easily communicated numbers.

As an example, let's consider a cardiac rehabilitation specialist who wishes to assess various characteristics of program participants. One of the health variables she wishes to examine is baseline (pre-exercise) heart rate (in beats per minute, bpm). In a group session attended by 40 program participants, she obtains the following heart rate values:

76, 81, 65, 86, 70, 79, 83, 87, 71, 80, 90, 77, 71, 84, 78, 77, 73, 85, 80, 81, 82, 74, 81, 90, 79, 82, 82, 74, 86, 80, 83, 77, 81, 81, 78, 83, 79, 85, 82, 80

What do you make of these results? Probably not much: it's hard to make sense of a list of numbers, even when there are only 40 of them. Almost all of us need some sort of summary before we can discern patterns within a set of data. The subsequent sections of this chapter will, using mainly this sample data set, describe several graphical and numerical statistical techniques that can be used to describe and summarize data.

Data distributions

Graphical displays are frequently used to summarize and present data. An example is the **frequency distribution** shown in Figure 24.1, which depicts the 40 heart rates obtained at the beginning of the cardiac rehabilitation session.

Figure 24.1
A frequency distribution of participants' heart rates (n = 40)

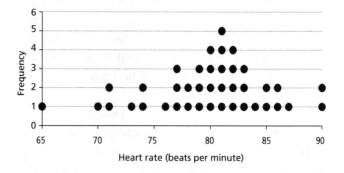

This graphical plot depicts several characteristics of the collected data. For one thing, we can see the **frequency** of individual data values, or how often each value occurs in the data set (e.g., 5 participants had a heart rate of 81 bpm, 4 had a heart rate of 80 bpm, and 4 had a heart rate of 82 bpm).

We can also see that most of the data points fall between 79 and 82 bpm. In statistics, this clustering is called the **central tendency** of the data, which means that the data tend to fall near the central value. We can also see the degree to which the data points are spread. The values range from 65 to 90 bpm, and most cluster between 76 and 87 bpm. This spread of the data points is called the **variability** or **dispersion** of the data.

As illustrated in the next two figures (which are based on different sets of hypothetical data than our main example), we can depict differences in dispersion by graphing the fre-

Conducting

quency distribution of the data. In Figure 24.2, values are tightly clustered around 80 bpm, with few values lower than 75 bpm or higher than 85 bpm. In contrast, Figure 24.3 depicts a wider range of values; the graph includes heart rates lower than 60 bpm and higher than 100 bpm.

Figure 24.2
A "narrow" frequency distribution of participants' heart rates

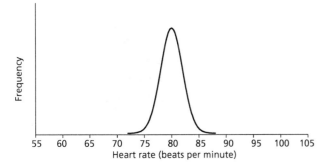

Figure 24.3
A "wide" frequency distribution of participants' heart rates

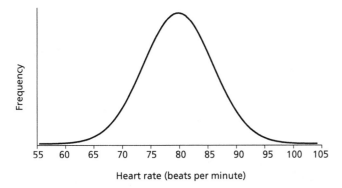

When describing data samples, researchers (and authors) should report both of the following:

- a measure of central tendency
- a measure of variability (also called dispersion or spread)

Measures of central tendency

The centre of a set of data is usually reported as one or more of three descriptive statistics: mean, median, and mode. The best way of describing the centre of a particular set of data depends on how the data points are distributed, as discussed later in this chapter.

The (arithmetic) **mean** (often abbreviated as $\bar{x}$ or as M) is the average value and is calculated by adding all of the individual values and dividing this total by the number

(i.e., count) of values. In our heart rate example, the mean heart rate is 79.8 bpm: the total of the individual values (3193) divided by the number of values (40). Depending on the context, we may round up such a result and report it more simply as 80 bpm. This is often referred to as the arithmetic mean because there are other means (e.g., geometric mean, harmonic mean) that are used in special situations; these are beyond the scope of this chapter.

The **median** (abbreviated Mdn) is the middle value of a sequential (i.e., ordered) set of data, or its 50th **percentile**—the value that divides the distribution into an upper and lower half (i.e., the value at which half of the data points are greater than the median value and half are less). When we have an odd number of sequential data points, the middle value is easy to find; however, when we have an even number of data points, as in our example of 40 heart rates, there is no single middle value. In this case, the median is the average of the two values closest to the middle of the sequential set of data: these two values would be the 20th (80 bpm) and 21st (81 bpm). By averaging these two values, we obtain the median value of our data set: 80.5 bpm.

65 70 71 71 73 74 74 76 77 77 77 78 78 79 79 79 80 80 80 80 81 81 81 81…

The **mode**, which doesn't have an abbreviation, is the most frequently occurring value in a set of data. In this study of heart rates, the mode is 81 bpm, a value reported by 5 participants. The mode is rarely used to describe biomedical data, although it is useful for reporting distributions that have two or more peaks (e.g., a bimodal distribution), each of which is indicated by its mode. Figure 24.4 depicts a bimodal distribution of heart rates, with modes at 60 bpm and 80 bpm.

Figure 24.4
A bimodal distribution of participants' heart rates

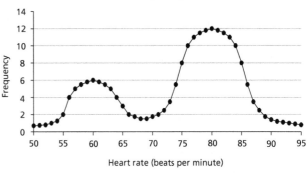

Measures of variability (dispersion)

The variability of the values within a set of data is usually indicated by one or more of three descriptive statistics: range, interquartile range, and standard deviation.

The **range** is the difference between the lowest and highest values in a data set. However, because the range is defined by the two most extreme values, it can sometimes be misleading. For example, if a few individuals in our example had extremely low (and/or high) heart rates, the range would be large, even though only one or two values were responsible. In scientific publications, the range is usually written as an "interval" in which the minimum value is followed by the maximum value, such that the scale of the data is obvious. For example, data values from 10 to 15 have a range of 5, but so do values from 95 to 100. Instead of reporting the range as 5, we provide the minimum and maximum values so that the reader will know where those 5 values are located on the measurement scale.

The **interquartile range** (IQR) is the range between the data's first quartile (25th percentile) and third quartile (75th percentile)—the middle 50% of data values. As the name implies, a data set can be divided into four quartiles, each of which contains one-fourth of the values in a sequential list of data points. The IQR is composed of the two middle quartiles of a given data set. The interquartile range is often reported with the median. As is the case with the range, we usually report the interquartile interval rather than simply the difference between the 25th and 75th percentiles. For example:

Length of hospital stay (days): median, 6; interquartile range, 1 to 22.

This example indicates several characteristics of this distribution, as follows: (1) for at least 25% of the patients the hospital stay was 1 day or less; (2) for at least 25% it was 22 days or longer; (3) for another 25% it was between 1 day and 6 days; and (4) for the remaining 25% it was between 6 and 22 days.

The IQR is preferred to the range because it is less affected by extreme values.

The frequency distribution shown in Figure 24.5 illustrates another way of describing the data set of 40 heart rates in our earlier example. The 40 sequential values can be divided into quartiles containing 10 values each. By counting the data values from the left, we find that the 25th percentile (between the 10th and 11th value) is 77 bpm, and

that the 75th percentile (between the 29th and 30th values) is 83 bpm. As described earlier, we also find that the 50th percentile (the median, between the 20th and 21st data points) is 80.5 bpm.

Figure 24.5
Quartiles of a distribution (n = 40; 1 quartile = 10 data points)

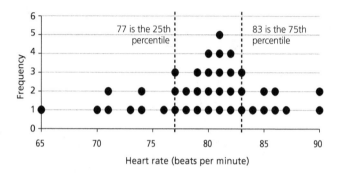

The **standard deviation** (abbreviated as either SD or s) describes the average "distance" between each data point and the mean value of the distribution. We'll illustrate what this means in a moment. The SD (and the mean) should be used and reported only when the data are normally distributed (or nearly so). This will be discussed with an example shortly.

The process used to calculate the standard deviation for a data set such as our sample heart rates can be illustrated with five steps. (Calculating the SD is fairly simple when the number of data values is small, as in our example. However, because health studies can involve hundreds or thousands of participants, it is necessary to use computerized statistical programs (e.g., Stata, SAS, SPSS) or web-based calculators that quickly and accurately process the applicable formulas and calculations.)

1. Calculate the mean by adding the 40 heart rate values and dividing the total by 40 (i.e., 3193 ÷ 40 = 79.825 bpm).
2. Determine the distance of each data value from the mean by subtracting the mean from each of the 40 heart rates (e.g., 90 bpm minus 79.825 = 10.175; 70 bpm minus 79.825 = –9.825).
3. Square each of these 40 calculated differences (distances) from the mean, which converts the negative values to positive values (e.g., $10.175^2 = 103.53$; $–9.825^2 = 96.53$). (Note: If we don't perform this step, then when we add these 40 differences, as we will do in the next step, we will obtain a total of zero

Conducting

because all of the positive differences will be balanced exactly by the negative differences.)

4. Add these 40 squared differences (this yields a number called the sum of square differences) and divide the total by the number of values minus 1 (n − 1, or 39 in this example) to obtain the average squared distance from the mean: 28.1. This number is known as the **variance**. The variance is rarely reported as a numerical value; we use the term to describe the dispersion of data points, as in the sentence, "The two distributions exhibited different variances." (The sum of the squares is divided by n − 1 rather than by n because this slight increase in the average "distance" provides a more accurate estimate of the "underlying" data variability; in this case, of all cardiac rehabilitation participants—not just of the 40 studied here.)

5. Finally, find the square root of the variance (the average squared difference) to determine the standard deviation: 5.3. Calculating the square root compensates for our squaring the differences in step 3 and provides us with a measure of data variability that is in the same units as the actual data: in this example, heart rate in bpm.

As discussed above, the standard deviation indicates the amount of variability within a set of data. In our example, the SD of 5.3 bpm suggests that the data points are, on average, about 5 bpm away from the mean value. The SD can also be used to compare distributions. For example, a distribution of heart rates with an SD of 2.0 would be less dispersed (i.e., narrower) than our distribution, which has an SD of 5.3 (see, for example, Figs 24.2 and 24.3). As we will discuss in the next section, perhaps the greatest value of the SD is the fact that it enables us to determine what proportion of values are included within certain portions of a normal distribution.

Types of distributions

Although many types of data distributions exist, the following sections will discuss in detail only two basic ones: normal and skewed distributions.

Normal distributions

In view of its unique properties and widespread use, it is important to understand the normal (or "bell-shaped") distribution. The **normal distribution** is often called the

Gaussian distribution in recognition of Johann Karl Friedrich Gauss, the German mathematician who rediscovered it in 1820 while graphing the variability in planetary orbits. The bell-shaped curve has several characteristic properties:

1. The mean, median, and mode are equal in value.
2. The frequency distribution is symmetrical about its centre (the mean).
3. As depicted by Figure 24.6 below, the area under the curve can be precisely defined by the mean and standard deviation, as follows:
   - about 68% of the data points fall within plus or minus 1 SD of the mean
   - about 95% of the data points fall within plus or minus 2 SD of the mean
   - about 99.7% of the data points fall within plus or minus 3 SD of the mean

Some biological data fall into normal distributions. For example, blood pressure, heart rate, body temperature, and red or white blood cell counts all tend to be normally distributed.

Figure 24.6
Areas under the curve in a normal distribution

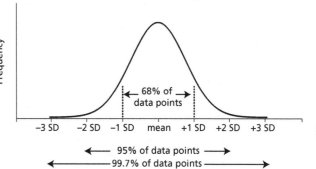

Skewed distributions

In contrast to normal distributions, **skewed distributions** are asymmetrical. This asymmetry entails important considerations in communicating these distributions and in selecting and performing the various descriptive statistical analyses. To illustrate, let's return to our heart rate example. Imagine that, at the next rehab session, 8 participants who had been absent from the previous session in order to compete in a local road race ask to be included in the measurement of heart rates. The heart rates of these additional participants were 48, 55, 60, 63, 64, 65, 66, and 67 bpm.

Figure 24.7 shows the data set for the 48 participants.

The heart rates of most of the additional 8 participants, who are very fit runners, are lower than the heart rates of the original 40 participants. Because each of these 8 additional heart rates is lower than 70 bpm, the lower portion of the original distribution has been further extended (i.e., the distribution is now skewed to the left, in what is called a left-skewed or negatively skewed distribution). Data values so extreme that they don't appear to be part of the rest of the distribution are called outlying values or **outliers**. The skewness of the distribution exerts marked effects on the measures of central tendency and dispersion.

What happens to the mean value when these 8 additional heart rates are added? Will it increase, decrease or remain the same?

If we perform the appropriate calculations, we find that the mean has decreased from 79.8 bpm to 76.7 bpm. Examining the two frequency distributions (Figs 24.7 and 24.8) shows us that the mean of 79.8 bpm reasonably reflects the centre of the original distribution of 40 heart rates; however, because this mean has shifted to the outer edge of the main cluster of heart rates, the revised mean of 76.7 bpm poorly reflects the centre of the extended group, which now includes the road racers.

This shift has occurred because the mean is strongly influenced by extreme values, namely, the 8 additional heart rate values from the more physically fit road racers.

Also, what happens to the median when these 8 additional heart rates are included? Will it increase, decrease or remain the same?

The median is always less sensitive to extreme values than the mean. As a result, adding the 8 additional lower heart rates shifts the value of the median only slightly, from 80.5 bpm to 79.5 bpm. Unlike the corresponding mean of 76.7 bpm, the new median value of 79.5 continues to reasonably reflect the centre of the data, remaining within the main cluster of heart rate values (see Fig. 24.7).

As noted earlier, a skewed distribution will also affect the measures of dispersion. For example, although the standard deviation of the original 40 heart rates is 5.3 bpm, it increases substantially to 8.9 bpm when the 8 additional lower heart rates are included. This increase occurs in part because the higher data values are now farther from the mean, which has decreased by more than 3 bpm. The increase in the SD also occurs in part because many of the additional 8 values have further extended the lower portion of the distribution; as a result, these values are also farther from the mean. These increased distances increase the aver-

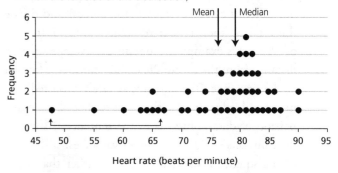

Figure 24.7
A skewed distribution of participants' heart rates (n = 48; the 8 additional heart rates are included within the bracket on the left side of the distribution)

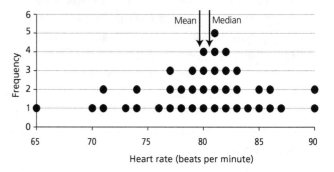

Figure 24.8
A relatively normal distribution of participants' heart rates (n = 40)

age distance of all data points from the mean (and thus increase the value of the SD).

In contrast, as Figure 24.9 illustrates, the interquartile range (IQR), which is based on the rank-ordering of the data and not on the actual values, continues to accurately reflect the actual variability of the data. Notice also that the standard deviation doesn't indicate on which side of the distribution the outliers are found. In contrast, the interquartile range shows that the addition of the 8 marathoners' heart rates has skewed the distribution to the left, and that the 25th percentile has shifted from 77 bpm (3.5 bpm below the median) to 72 bpm (7.5 bpm below the median). However, the distance of the 75th percentile from the median is unchanged: in both distributions, the 75th percentile is 2.5 bpm higher than the median. We would expect that this distance between the median and the 75th percentile would be the same in both sets of data, given that all of the additional 8 heart rates were lower values and no new values were added to the upper portion of the distribution.

Many types of biomedical data fall into skewed distributions. For example, laboratory values for which the clinically normal (i.e., expected) range lies near zero (e.g., serum bilirubin or urinary protein concentrations) generally produce skewed distributions because abnormal values can be

Figure 24.9
Quartiles of a skewed distribution (n = 48; 1 quartile = 12 data points)

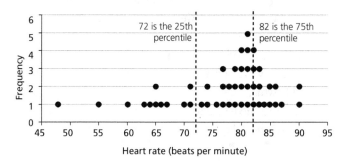

quite high on one side of the distribution but can never be less than zero on the other side. Other examples of health care data that might be expected to produce skewed distributions include birth weight and number of days in a hospital stay.

The mean and the standard deviation should be used only to describe data that are normally distributed (or nearly so). As illustrated by the heart rate example, the more skewed the distribution, the more misleading the mean and SD will be in describing the central tendency and the variability of a set of data. In fact, the use of these two statistics, by definition, implies that the distribution is generally bell-shaped and is centred at the mean, 68% of the data values being within plus or minus 1 SD from the mean, 95% within plus or minus 2 SDs from the mean, and more than 99% within plus or minus 3 SDs from the mean. A review of the frequency distribution (Fig. 24.9) presented above shows that the distribution of 48 heart rates, including those of the road racers, is not normal/bell-shaped. Skewed distributions such as this one are best described by the median and the interquartile range. Because most biological data are not normally distributed, the median and interquartile range should appear more commonly in the biomedical literature than the mean and standard deviation.

Recognizing skewed distributions. As stated earlier, it is important to recognize skewed (non-normal) distributions. One way of doing so is to visually inspect a graphical plot of the data. Unfortunately, research publications usually do not provide this; instead, they provide only measures of central tendency and variability. However, by understanding the meaning conveyed by these measures, we can determine whether a distribution is normal or skewed.

In skewed distributions, the mean and the median will differ from one another, because the mean is drawn in the direction of the skew. Unfortunately, even when distributions are obviously skewed, many research publications do not appropriately provide median values and are even less likely to include the interquartile range. In such circumstances, the distribution of the values implied by the reported mean and standard deviation can still be quite informative, especially when certain values are implausible (or even impossible).

For example, let's imagine that a report indicates that the mean size of a particular type of tumour (n = 20) at the time of diagnosis is 40.1 mm, with a standard deviation of 42.0 mm. Are these descriptive statistics consistent with a normal, or a skewed, distribution of values?

The distribution must be skewed. If it were a normal distribution, we would expect that 68% of the data points would be within plus or minus 1 standard deviation of the mean (i.e., 34% of the data points would fall within an area 1 SD above the mean, and 34% would fall within an area 1 SD below the mean). In this example, however, subtracting the SD (42.0 mm) from the mean (40.1 mm) yields an impossible tumour diameter of −1.9 mm! Therefore, this distribution must be positively skewed, with some large tumours pulling the mean to the right. In such a case, we would expect that the median tumour size would be less than the reported mean tumour size (40.1 mm). Looking below at the actual list of tumour sizes (in mm), the median tumour size can be seen to be 17 mm (the average of 16 mm and 18 mm, the 10th and 11th data points):

9 10 11 12 12 13 14 14 15 16 18 21 21 45 55 75 80 95 105 160

In some instances we can also recognize a normal or a skewed distribution simply by considering what is being measured. For example, what kind of distribution would you expect to arise from a community health survey question that asks respondents how many cigarettes they smoked during the previous day?

Because the prevalence of smoking is much lower than 50% in many populations, we should expect that the most frequently reported answer will be zero. If most of the respondents to our survey are non-smokers, then we should expect the distribution of the data to be skewed to the right (positively skewed). Most of the values will be zero, and the

Conducting

positive values will reflect the reported smoking habits of the minority of respondents who are smokers.

Figure 24.10 depicts such a distribution, arising from the responses of 1000 surveyed individuals. In this example, would you expect the mean, or the median, to be larger?

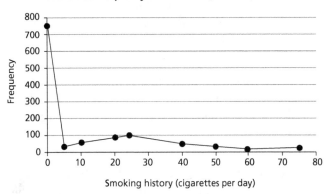

Figure 24.10
A skewed frequency distribution (n = 1000)

In this case, we would expect the mean to be larger than the median. If we are correct in our assumption that more than half of the survey respondents are non-smokers, the median will be zero. The mean will be larger than zero because of the minority of respondents who report having smoked some number of cigarettes during the previous day.

Descriptive statistics, distributions, reporting, and statistical testing

In keeping with the goal of accurate and informative health research reporting, the distribution of the underlying data should guide the selection of the statistics and statistical tests used to summarize and analyze the data. For example, we could describe the initial set of 40 heart rates as follows: "The mean (SD) heart rate was 79.8 (5.3) bpm." In contrast, we would most accurately describe the expanded set of 48 heart rates, which produced a skewed distribution, with the following sentence: "The median heart rate was 79.5 bpm (IQR, 72 to 82 bpm)."

Of course, the original set of 40 heart rates could also be described as follows: "The median heart rate was 80.5 bpm (IQR, 77 to 83 bpm)." However, because the original set of 40 heart rates produced a reasonably normal distribution, it is most appropriately described using the more frequently used mean and standard deviation. Reporting the data by using the mean and the SD should imply that the data are normally distributed (or at least nearly so). However, not all authors adhere to these principles for reporting descriptive statistics,

usually because they don't understand these concepts. Summarizing skewed distributions with the mean and the SD is a very common error associated with statistical reporting in the health research literature. After all, if the mean and standard deviation for the smoking data depicted in Figure 24.10 (6.2 and 12.4, respectively) were reported, this would imply that the data follow a distribution similar to the one shown in Figure 24.11, which they certainly do not! This further emphasizes why the median and interquartile range (0 and 0–5, respectively) should be used instead to describe these data.

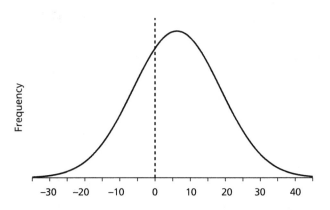

Figure 24.11
A normal distribution (mean = 6.2, SD = 12.4)

The distribution of data also determines which statistical tests should be used for their analysis. **Parametric statistical tests** should be used only to analyze continuous data that are normally distributed (or at least nearly so). For continuous data that are not normally distributed, the corresponding **non-parametric statistical tests** should be used. These types of tests are discussed in more detail in chapter 25.

Descriptive statistics for other types of data

So far, we have discussed descriptive statistical techniques for continuous data (e.g., heart rates). Before we conclude this portion of the chapter, however, we should briefly consider statistical concepts specific to other types of data (e.g., nominal, dichotomous, ordinal, and discrete data). These types of data are also discussed in chapter 8.

Nominal data

Nominal data fall into categories that are named but have no inherent order. These data are usually summarized as

Conducting

simple counts or as proportions or percentages of the entire sample. For example, a study of the frequency of ABO blood types being used for the 415 transfusions administered in a hospital last year might report that 190 (46%) of the 415 were type O, 166 (40%) were type A, 35 (8%) were type B and 24 (6%) were type AB. Graphically, these data can be depicted with a box, dot or pie chart that displays the proportion represented by each nominal category, or with a bar chart that uses bar height to indicate the size of each nominal category (as either a count or percentage). Figure 24.12 depicts these data in a pie chart.

Figure 24.12
A pie chart of ABO blood types used in hospital transfusions

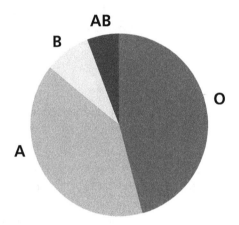

Like nominal data, dichotomous data are usually summarized with simple counts or percentages of each of the two categories. They are often graphically depicted with simple, 2-component box, dot, pie or bar chart.

Ordinal data

Ordinal data fall into inherently ordered categories. As such, although ordinal data may be summarized with the same approaches used for nominal data, they can also be subjected to analyses that take into account the additional information provided by the rank order of the categories.

As an example, let's imagine that a placement site evaluation form contains the following question: "Overall, how would you rate your experience at this placement site?" Trainees answer by selecting an option on a 5-point scale ranging from 1 (poor) to 5 (excellent). Because the ordered categories are numbered, we could summarize the data with the measures of central tendency (e.g., mean, 3.7) and dispersion (SD, 0.4) that are used to describe continuous data. However, doing so carries the implicit assumption that health has been measured on a continuous scale from 1 to 5. Is that a good assumption?

For example, are we sure that the distance between 5 (excellent) and 4 (very good) is the same as the distance between 1 (poor) and 2 (fair)? If not, it may make more sense to describe the data by using the median, as follows: "The median response was 4 (very good) on a 5-point scale ranging from 1 (poor) to 5 (excellent)." Perhaps it would be even better to present these data as categories: "Of the respondents, 30% reported the placement site as excellent, 40% as very good, 15% as good, 9% as fair, and 6% as poor." Graphically, ordinal data can be illustrated with dot, pie or bar charts. Figure 24.13 depicts our example with a bar chart.

Figure 24.13
A bar chart of trainee evaluations of their experience at a placement site

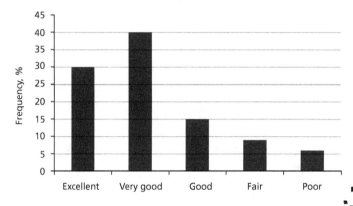

Discrete data

Discrete data are numerical counts (i.e., whole numbers) on a scale with known and equal distances between each value. Examples of discrete data include the number of stairs climbed during a 12-minute exercise test, the number of members in a family, and the number of decayed, missing or filled teeth. Because they represent numeric counts, discrete data are often summarized with measures of central tendency (e.g., mean, median, and mode) and dispersion (range, standard deviation, and interquartile range).

Depending on the range of values, discrete data may be depicted graphically as a frequency distribution or as a bar, dot or pie chart. However, as is true in every circumstance, the choice of summary technique should be guided by the researcher's purpose and the needs of the intended audience. For example, although the length of time in hospital (in days) can be summarized by calculating a mean, a value such as 4.8 might be of limited use to the hospital leadership team who are trying to understand the length of hospital admissions and how they might be shortened. The mean of 4.8 days certainly doesn't accurately represent any specific hospital stay! These data may be more useful for health planning purposes if they are depicted with a chart illustrating that 40% of hospital admissions are less than 2 days long, 45% are 2 to 5 days, 10% are 5 to 14 days, 4% are 14 to 30 days, and 1% are longer than 30 days.

Descriptive statistics summary

Numerical and graphical methods of summarizing data are important because they provide effective means of communicating and identifying patterns in data. In fact, because most of us can't make sense of more than a few items of data at a time, summarizing data with descriptive statistics and graphical techniques enhances our ability to recognize underlying patterns in the data. Furthermore, we must remember that the selection of descriptive statistics that are used to summarize data should be guided by the type and distribution of those data.

However, the summarized data usually describe only a sample of persons, not the entire population of interest. Therefore, statistics obtained from samples should be considered simply as estimates of the true values found in the population. This concept of estimation will be discussed in the next section.

Measuring and interpreting data variability

In the previous section, we discussed how a set of data can be summarized with descriptive statistics such as the mean and the standard deviation or median and interquartile range. However, given the practical problems associated with measuring large populations, it is rarely possible for a data set to include observations from every eligible person of interest. (If every eligible person were included, we would have a **census**.) More realistically, researchers select a **sample** of individuals who, ideally, are representative of the entire population of interest, obtain data from them, and then "generalize" the results from this representative sample to the entire population of interest. Consider that a single taste of wine can sell the bottle because the taste is representative of the entire bottle.

In our heart rate study, for example, we measured the heart rates of a sample of 40 (or 48) participants in a cardiac rehabilitation program and calculated the mean. But this is only the average heart rate of this particular sample. How close is this sample mean to the true mean heart rate of the entire **population** of cardiac rehabilitation program participants?

To begin to answer this question, we must recognize that any given sample is simply one of many possible samples that could have been studied. If we had measured heart rates a day earlier, or a day later, we might have recruited a slightly different sample of cardiac rehabilitation program participants from the same underlying population. Therefore, it makes sense to think of each of these possible samples as simply providing an estimate of the "true" underlying population mean. For example, measurements of the heart rates of 5 other samples of cardiac rehabilitation program participants could have resulted in the following mean heart rates:

80.1 bpm
78.9 bpm
81.0 bpm
79.5 bpm
81.4 bpm

Why should 6 samples produce 6 different, albeit similar, means? The answer is **random** or **biological variation.** We expect that the heart rate of any person will vary from moment to moment and that the variation in heart rate from one person to another will be even larger. Therefore, even under stringent study procedures, the mean heart rate of each sample will vary according to precisely when each person's heart rate is measured and exactly which persons are selected for and participate in the study. Although the mean heart rate of each sample is a reasonable, independent estimate of the "true" underlying population mean, these variations—both within and between the individuals studied—cause sample means to differ from one another.

With this fact in mind, which of these many possible sample means will be closest to the "true" underlying population mean? If we consider that the means of all of these samples differ from one another only because of random (chance) variation, and that the mean of each sample is a reasonable, independent estimate of the "true" underlying population mean, then the "centre" of these many sample means (i.e., the mean of the means) should be the best estimate of the "true" underlying population value. An illustrative frequency distribution (Fig. 24.14), created by plotting multiple independent sample means, is shown below.

This frequency distribution illustrates several concepts. First, this group of sample means is clearly "centred" at 80 bpm. This finding indicates that the means of most of our samples are close to 80 bpm and suggests that 80 bpm is the underlying "true" mean heart rate of the population. Second, this distribution exhibits less variation (i.e., the values are closer to the centre) than does that of any of the individual samples of heart rate distributions (for an example, see Figure 24.15). The reason for this reduced variation is that calculating a mean "averages out" individual extreme values, thereby causing the mean of a sample to be (by definition) less extreme than the individual values within that sample. This fact explains why the means of samples are clustered more closely around the population mean than are the individual heart rates of any given sample around its sample mean.

Figure 24.14
Frequency distribution of sample heart rate means
(the 6 sample means are indicated by arrows)

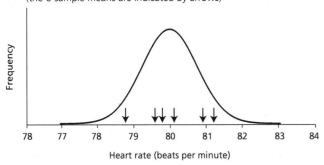

Heart rate (beats per minute)

Figure 24.15
Frequency distribution of participants' heart rates

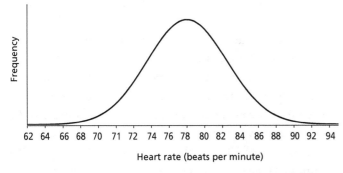

Heart rate (beats per minute)

Standard error

We can estimate the variability among this hypothetical group of sample means just as we determined the standard deviation for a sample of individual measures. Such an estimate of the variability among sample means is called the **standard error** (SE) of the mean. Of course, the SE would not be very useful if we needed to conduct multiple studies to derive an estimate of it. In reality, a single study provides enough information to allow us to estimate the standard error of the mean. To do so, the SD of the sample is divided by the square root of the **sample size**:

$$SE = \frac{SD \text{ of the sample}}{\sqrt{\text{sample size}}}$$

To illustrate, let's consider our heart rate example, in which 40 cardiac rehabilitation program participants had a mean heart rate of 80 bpm with an standard deviation of 5.3 bpm. What is the estimated SE for this sample? To begin, we must determine the square root of the sample size. Using a calculator with the square root function, we find that the square root of 40 is 6.3. Dividing 6.3 into 5.3 bpm, the SD of the sample, yields a result of 0.8 bpm, the estimated SE of the population. This example further illustrates that we should expect much less variability among sample means (i.e., the SE) than among the individual data values in any single sample (i.e., the SD).

Like the standard deviation, the standard error provides an estimate of variability—in this case, the variability expected among the means obtained from various samples. And, as is true for the SD, perhaps the greatest value of the SE is the fact that it enables us to determine the proportion of sample mean values that will be expected to fall within certain portions of the normal distribution (e.g., 68% of all possible sample mean values will occur within plus or minus 1 SE of the "true" [population] mean value).

One way of expressing the **precision** with which a mean has been estimated is to report the mean and the corresponding standard error, as follows: "The estimated mean (SE) heart rate of the population is 80 (0.8) bpm." However, in the health sciences, the SE is not the preferred way of reporting the precision of an estimate (although it is commonly used as a descriptive statistic in basic science journals). Journals and health scientists prefer that authors report the mean plus or minus approximately 2 SEs; this interval is called the 95% confidence interval (CI).

Confidence intervals

The characteristics of the normal distribution allow us to determine **confidence intervals.** Like the individual data points in a sample, 95% of all possible sample means will fall within approximately 2 SEs (or more precisely, 1.96 SEs) on either side of the true mean (see Figure 24.16). Therefore, the range encompassed by 1.96 SEs above and below the mean of any individual sample has a 95% probability of including the "true" (population) mean (i.e., the mean of the means). That is to say, only sample means that lie at the extreme ends of the hypothetical normal distribution of multiple sample means would be more than 1.96

Conducting

SEs away from the "true" mean. This interval, which captures the true mean with a probability of 95%, is known as a 95% confidence interval. (Probability is a continuous numerical quantity, ranging from zero to 100%, indicating the chance that an event will occur; it is determined by dividing the number of times an event is observed by the total number of times the event could have occurred. For example, if out of 10 000 children born in a province, 5100 are boys, then the probability of a boy is 0.51.)

Figure 24.16
Area under the curve of the distribution of sample means

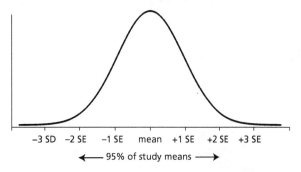

The 95% CI for our heart rate example with 40 participants can be calculated as follows:

$$CI = \text{mean plus or minus } (2 \times SE)$$
$$= 80 \text{ plus or minus } (2 \times 0.8) \text{ bpm}$$
$$= 80 \text{ plus or minus } 1.6 \text{ bpm}$$
$$= 78.4 \text{ to } 81.6 \text{ bpm}$$

Interpreted mathematically, a 95% confidence interval captures the "true" (population) mean 95% of the time. In practical terms, we recognize that the "true" (population) mean might not be exactly equal to the individual sample mean of 80 bpm, but we know there is a high probability (i.e., 95%) that it is no lower than 78.4 bpm and no higher than 81.6 bpm (the 95% CI). Put another way, there is only a 5% probability (chance) that the "true" (population) mean lies outside this interval.

In general, researchers should calculate and provide 95% confidence intervals when reporting estimated treatment effects. For example, imagine that a journal article includes the following statement: "The new drug reduced total cholesterol concentrations by a mean of 20 mg/dL (95% CI 12 to 28 mg/dL)." This sentence suggests that the study drug will probably reduce cholesterol by an average of at least 20 mg/dL but not by more than 28 or less than 12 mg/dL.

Are narrow, or wide, confidence intervals preferable?

Narrow confidence intervals are preferable because they reflect a more precise estimate, given that the width of the CI indicates the range of values consistent with a given estimate. The "homogeneity" of a CI's upper and lower values/limits is also important. A homogeneous CI indicates a consistent result (i.e., the upper and lower values both lead to the same general conclusion), irrespective of the size of the *P* value and the width of the interval.

If narrow CIs indicate a more precise estimate, how can the width of the CI be reduced?

Remember that a 95% confidence interval is calculated as the mean plus or minus 1.96 SE and that the SE is calculated as follows:

$$SE = \frac{\text{SD of the sample}}{\sqrt{\text{sample size}}}$$

The confidence interval reflects the size of the standard error, which in turn reflects the standard deviation and, more importantly, the size of the sample. Therefore, we can reduce the width of the CI by increasing the sample size, because a larger sample will result in a smaller SE.

Finally, the upper and lower bounds of the confidence interval can provide valuable information. For example, let's consider a study report stating that a new type of chemotherapy reduced tumour size by a mean of 20 mm (95% CI, –10 to 50 mm). These results indicate that the chemotherapy is consistent with an average reduction in tumour size of 20 mm, a finding that appears quite promising (i.e., of clinical interest). However, the 95% CI indicates that the chemotherapy is also consistent with an average increase in tumour size of 10 mm (the lower bound of the CI is –10 mm, a change in the opposite direction), as well as with an average decrease in tumour size of 50 mm (i.e., a heterogeneous CI). This study has obtained an imprecise estimate of the chemotherapy's effectiveness, most likely because the sample was too small.

In contrast, another study report indicates that a new medication reduced systolic blood pressure by 2 mm Hg (95% CI, 1 to 3 mm Hg). Although this result suggests that the medication will probably reduce blood pressure, this reduction is unlikely to be larger than an average of 3 mm Hg, a reduction that will generally be perceived to be too small to be of clinical importance. In this example, the results indicate that the study has very precisely measured the effectiveness of the new medication, probably because

Conducting

the sample was very large. It is also possible, in fact, that the sample size for this study was too large, given that it is rarely necessary to make an estimate as precise as this one (i.e., plus or minus 1 mm Hg). When determining the sample size for a study, researchers generally strive to balance the benefit of having a sufficient number of study participants with the risks and costs assumed by each study participant (i.e., researchers should strive to achieve a sample size that is neither too small nor too large, but just right).

Data variability summary

In this section three important concepts have been discussed: standard deviation, standard error of the mean and confidence interval.

Standard deviation is a measure of the variability (dispersion) observed among individual measurements in a sample. Standard error of the mean is a measure of the variability (dispersion) that we might expect among sample means when we estimate population values from sample values.

So, which will be larger, the SD or the SE? Recall how we estimate the standard error of the mean:

$$SE = \frac{SD \text{ of the sample}}{\sqrt{\text{sample size}}}$$

Clearly, the SD must be larger than the SE, because we calculate the SE by dividing the SD by the square root of the sample size. However, watch out for SE being used as a descriptive statistic to imply more precise measurements.

The confidence interval (CI) is another measure of the variability (dispersion) that can be calculated when population values are estimated from sample values. The size of the 95% CI is approximately twice the SE on either side of the estimate. The CI is the preferred value for indicating the precision of an estimate. It approximates the range of values that are consistent with an individual result (i.e., it brackets our best guess of the "true" population estimate).

Conclusion

This chapter provides an overview of the techniques used to summarize quantitative data and to enable readers to become more comfortable and competent carrying out, interpreting and reporting descriptive statistical methods and results. In particular, after reading this chapter you should be better able to critically discern the "story" behind commonly used descriptive statistical procedures and results.

For example, after reading this chapter, you'll be much better equipped to interpret results such as these:

Length of hospital stay (days): mean, 13; median, 6; standard deviation, 12.

You'll have noticed the large difference between the values of the mean and the median and conclude that this difference has occurred because the distribution of data is positively (right) skewed. Your conclusion is further confirmed by the large standard deviation and the impossible negative values that would occur at a point less than two standard deviations below the mean. Of course, this makes perfect sense because you recognize that the variable "length of hospital stay in days" can be measured only by positive values, negative values being impossible.

The next chapter will build on your understanding of descriptive statistics to enable the use of additional statistical tests and techniques to carry out hypothesis testing and determine the sample sizes needed to ensure sufficient statistical power. ■

Conducting

CASE POSTSCRIPT

After consulting his supervisor and the department's statistician, the resident learned that he would need to calculate the 95% confidence intervals for proportions to determine and illustrate sufficiently precisely the proportion of people in the 2 practices who had received the recommended preventive services in the previous 2 years. For example, he found that the proportion of eligible persons who had received the seasonal influenza immunization in the 2 practices was 98/211 (46.4%) and 149/262 (56.9%), respectively. In addition, he was able to determine that the 95% confidence interval for these 2 percentages are 39.6% to 53.4% and 50.6% to 63.0%, respectively.

Acknowledgements

All referenced web-based calculators were located at and accessed from www.statpages.org.

The development of this chapter was informed by: Harvey BJ, Ancker JS, Bairnsfather S, Bukowski JA, Hudson S, Lang TA, et al. *Statistics for medical writers and editors*. Rockville (MD): American Medical Writers Association; 2009.

ADDITIONAL RESOURCES

Glantz SA. *Primer of biostatistics*. 6th ed. New York: McGraw-Hill Medical Publishing Division; 2005.

Lang TA. How to display data in tables and graphs. In: Lang TA. *How to write, publish, and present in the health sciences: a guide for clinicians and laboratory researchers*. Philadelphia: American College of Physicians; 2010. p. 67–100.

- This chapter provides a great overview of the principles and techniques of summarizing data using tables and graphics.

Lang TA, Secic M. *How to report statistics in medicine: annotated guidelines for authors, editors, and reviewers*. 2nd ed. Philadelphia: American College of Physicians; 2006.

- This book is a comprehensive reference discussing how statistics and the results of statistical tests and procedures, including descriptive statistics, should be correctly reported.

Norman GR, Streiner DL. *Biostatistics: the bare essentials*. 3rd ed. Shelton (CT): PMPH USA; 2008.

- These three books are quite comprehensive, while also being readable and understandable (and include informative discussions concerning descriptive statistics).

Norman GR, Streiner DL. *PDQ statistics*. 3rd ed. Shelton (CT): PMPH USA; 2003.

Tufte E. *The visual display of quantitative information*. 2nd ed. Cheshire: Graphics Press 2001.

- This is considered a classic text, written by one of the "gurus" in the field. I recommend reading it cover to cover.

Wainer H. *Visual revelations: graphical tales of fate and deception from Napoleon Bonaparte to Ross Perot*. New York: Springer-Verlag, 1997.

- This is an easy-to-read, comprehensive and informative text by an author who, like Edward Tufte, is "visionary" in the art and science of describing quantitative data.

PRACTICE QUESTIONS

The answers to these questions are provided below.

Descriptive statistics

1. What measure identifies the middle value (the 50th percentile) in a set of data?

2. What measure identifies the lowest and highest values in a set of data?

3. What measure is determined by adding all of the values in a data set and dividing that total by the number of values?

4. What measure identifies the 25th and 75th percentiles in a set of data?

5. What measure identifies the most frequent value in a set of data?

6. What measure is the average distance from the mean value in a set of data?

7. Respondents to a community health survey were asked to report how many cigarettes they had smoked during the previous day. With Figure 24.10 in mind, what measures of central tendency and data variability **best** summarize "number of cigarettes smoked"?

8. In the Women's Health Initiatives Trial, women who were randomly assigned to receive hormone replacement therapy (HRT) had heart dise*ase* more frequently than did women who did not receive HRT. What measures of central tendency and data variability **best** summarize had heart disease?

9. The following statement appeared in a journal article: "Tumour size: mean, 46.7 mm; median, 21.3 mm; SD, 34.3 mm." What measures of central tendency and data variability **best** summarize this result?

10. The following statement appeared in a journal article: "Gland diameter: mean, 18 mm; median, 17 mm; SD, 2 mm." What measures of central tendency and data variability **best** summarize this result?

Measurement variability

1. What measure is an estimate of the amount of variability expected between sample means?

2. What measure approximates the range of expected sample means that is consistent with an individual result (i.e., it brackets our best guess of the "true" population mean)?

3. What measure is an estimate of the variability (dispersion) among a group of individual measurements?

4. Researchers conduct a study to assess the association between age (in years) and the occurrence of osteoporosis (i.e., low bone density) among a sample of 100 women. The mean bone mineral density of this group of women is 0.6 gr/cm^2 with a standard deviation of 0.1 gr/cm^2. What is the standard error of this measurement?

5. For the study described in question 4, what is the 95% confidence interval of this measurement?

6. For the study described in question 4, if the sample size remains unchanged at 100, but the standard deviation is 0.3 gr/cm^2, what is the standard error of this measurement?

7. For the study described in question 4, if the sample size is increased to 400 and the standard deviation is 0.2 gr/cm^2, what is the 95% confidence interval of this measurement?

8. Which of the following confidence intervals is narrowest?

    A. −10 to −2

    B. −5 to 0

    C. −3 to 1

    D. −1 to 2

    E.   2 to 4

9. Which of the following statements is false?

    A. A larger sample size makes the standard error smaller.

    B. A smaller sample size makes the confidence interval wider.

    C. A smaller standard error makes the confidence interval wider.

    D. A larger standard deviation makes the standard error smaller.

    E. A smaller standard deviation makes the confidence interval wider.

Conducting

Answers to practice questions

Descriptive statistics

1. Median
2. Range
3. Mean
4. Interquartile range
5. Mode
6. Standard deviation (or variance)
7. Median and interquartile range (because the large number of expected zero values will cause the distribution to be negatively skewed to the left)
8. Percentages (to present two dichotomous categories)
9. Median and interquartile range (because the data distribution appears to be negatively skewed to the left)
10. Mean and standard deviation (because the data appear to be normally distributed)

Measurement variability

1. Standard error of the mean
2. Confidence interval
3. Standard deviation
4. 0.01 gr/cm² (the standard deviation divided by the square root of the sample size)
5. 0.58 to 0.62 (the mean plus or minus twice the standard error of the mean)
6. 0.03 gr/cm² (the standard deviation divided by the square root of the sample size)
7. 0.58 to 0.62 (the mean plus or minus twice the standard error of the mean)
8. E: 2 to 4, which is only two units wide
9. C: A smaller SE yields a narrower (not a wider) confidence interval (recall, the CI equals the mean plus or minus twice the SE)

SUMMARY CHECKLIST

- ❑ Review your research protocol and the types of data to be collected to identify the descriptive statistics that should be used.
- ❑ Review your draft data analysis with a statistician, methodologist, members of your study team, and your supervisor.
- ❑ Revise as need.

Conducting

25

Data analysis: Hypothesis testing, sample size and study power

Bart J. Harvey, MD, PhD, MEd, FACPM, FRCPC

ILLUSTRATIVE CASE

The General Internal Medicine resident we met in the previous chapter has determined that the proportion of eligible people served by a community health centre's two practice groups who had received seasonal influenza vaccination was 98/211 (46.4%) and 149/262 (56.9%). Now, he'd like to determine whether the two practices actually differ from one another in their ability to deliver this preventive service. He decides to arrange another meeting with the department's statistical consultant to determine how to do this.

■ **Quantitative health studies address** research questions about people and conditions by collecting and analyzing data obtained by counting, observing and measuring. Building on the previous chapter, this chapter introduces and discusses the statistical tools and techniques used to analyze data arising from quantitative health studies. The analytic techniques used in qualitative health studies are presented and discussed in chapter 16.

As noted in the previous chapter on descriptive statistics, the statistical techniques used to analyze quantitative data generally fall into two main categories: descriptive statistics, which, as the name suggests, enable collected data to be summarized and described; and hypothesis-testing or inferential statistics, which comprise a diverse set of statistical tests and techniques that enable comparisons and other analyses to be completed. In addition, and related to both of these uses, statistical methods also enable a determination of the precision with which any measure has been made. In general, the most important role of statistical testing is to assess what role chance may have played in the collected data and the degree to which it might be a plausible explanation for the observed study results.

Like the previous chapter, this chapter has been written from a practical perspective and strives to introduce "statistics" not as an end in itself but as a "tool box" from which the health researcher may select tests, tools and techniques to complete the necessary analytic tasks. It aims to provide the reader with an overview of the statistical tools that are available for hypothesis testing, how they should be used, and which tools should be used for which tasks. It also addresses the concepts of precision and **statistical power** and describes how to determine the **sample size** necessary to provide a specified level of precision and/or study power. However, before beginning, it is important to reiterate a theme that recurs throughout this guide: researchers should

---

CHAPTER OBJECTIVES

After reading this chapter, you should be able to:
- discuss probability and the process of hypothesis testing;
- describe how a study result and the standard error are used to determine the test statistic and the resulting probability (*P*) value;
- define the alpha (α) level and explain how it is used to determine whether a given study result is statistically significant;
- discuss Type I and Type II errors;
- discuss "multiple testing" and its effect on statistical testing;
- explain the difference between statistical significance and clinical importance;
- define statistical power and describe how it is determined, along with the factors that affect a study's power and how they relate to one another;
- discuss the effect of sample size on a study's power, and list the factors to consider when calculating a study's sample size and how they relate to one another; and
- list common statistical tests, both parametric and non-parametric, and discuss the factors used to determine which test should be used under a given circumstance.

Conducting

KEY TERMS

Alpha (α level)	Multiple testing	Sample size
Analysis of variance (ANOVA)	Non-parametric statistical tests	Spearman rank correlation
Beta (β) level	Null hypothesis	Statistical power
Chi-squared (χ^2) test	One-tailed tests	Statistical significance
Correlation	Paired *t* test	Test statistic
Clinical importance	Parametric statistical tests	Two-tailed tests
Confidence interval	Pearson product moment	Type I error
Hypothesis testing	correlation	Type II error
Kruskal-Wallis test	*P* value	Unpaired *t* test
Mann-Whitney *U* test	Regression	Wilcoxon signed-rank test

---

consult with someone knowledgeable about statistical methods during the planning and design stages of their research projects! Only then can they be confident that they will collect the data they need using the right techniques and then be able to analyze their findings in a manner that results in a valid answer to their research question.

It should also be noted that intermediate and advanced methods of data analysis used to assess and adjust for confounding and effect modification are beyond the scope of this chapter; good discussions of these techniques are available, however, in other resources.[1–4]

Statistical hypothesis testing

As discussed in the previous chapter, it is possible to estimate a distribution of sample means in which each value is the mean value of different samples from the same population. For example, Figure 25.1 illustrates the distribution of means that might arise from a series of heart rate studies.

Figure 25.1
Frequency distribution of mean heart rates from several samples

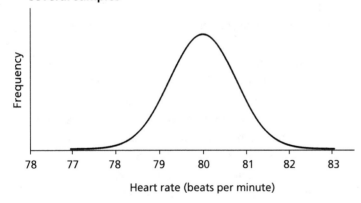

Heart rate (beats per minute)

Given this distribution of mean heart rates, how probable is it that a randomly selected sample of cardiac rehabilitation program participants would have a mean heart rate of 83 beats per minute (bpm)?

Recalling what we know about the normal distribution, we can assume that a sample mean of 83 bpm, although possible, would be very improbable, given that 83 bpm is much higher than nearly all of the mean values in the distribution. In fact, a mean heart rate of 83 bpm is 3.75 (3 ÷ 0.8) SEs (standard errors of the mean) higher than 80 bpm, the mean of the distribution of means (i.e., the mean of the means). As such, the probability of observing a mean this "extreme" by chance is less than 1 time in 1000 (*P* < .001).

In contrast, how probable is it that a randomly selected sample of cardiac rehabilitation program participants would have a mean heart rate of 79 bpm?

As Figure 25.1 shows, this value is located near the centre of the distribution; in fact, it lies slightly more than 1 SE below the mean of the means (i.e., it is among the possible means closest to the centre value as predicted by the properties of the normal distribution). Therefore, the probability that a random sample would have this mean heart rate is quite high (*P* = .21).

Hypothesis testing

As an illustration of how the distribution of sample means can also be used to inform study results, let's consider a hypothetical study conducted to determine whether the heart rates of participants in a cardiac rehabilitation program increase between the beginning and end of a rehab session. To answer this question, we could measure the heart rate of the program participants twice: once when they arrive at a rehab session, and again at the end of the session. The truncated table below illustrates what the resulting data might look like.

Participant	Beginning	End	Difference
1	79	87	+8
2	80	78	–2
3	76	87	+11
–	–	–	–
–	–	–	–
–	–	–	–
40	82	89	+7

We calculate the mean difference or change in heart rate by summing the differences between the 40 pairs of heart rates (given in the fourth column above) and dividing that total by 40, the size of the sample. In this case, imagine that the resulting mean difference is +5 bpm—that is, the heart rate of cardiac rehabilitation program participants is, on average, 5 bpm faster at the end of a rehab session than it was at the beginning.

But is this 5-bpm difference in heart rate the result of the rehab session (i.e., a real difference) or the result of chance?

A common scientific approach allows a question such as this to be explored by looking at the other side of the coin. That is, we start with the assumption that participation in the rehab session has no effect on heart rate—that the heart rate at the beginning is, on average, equal to the heart rate at the end. This assumption constitutes what is called a **null hypothesis**. Our goal will be to determine whether the data allow us to rule out or reject this null hypothesis and thus be fairly sure that the increase in heart rate is indeed attributable to participation in the rehab session and not to chance. This process is referred to as **hypothesis testing**.

We know that heart rates differ from time to time, even if a rehab session is not involved. That is to say, we expect heart rates to be different within or between persons simply because of random and biologic variation. It's possible that we might observe one of these chance variations and mistakenly assume that it was caused by participation in a rehab session. It is important to determine whether an observed result may have arisen by chance so that we can avoid drawing incorrect conclusions, especially when those conclusions will affect people's health. To determine whether chance is responsible, let's ask the following question: If participation in a rehab session truly has no effect on heart rate, how large might the mean heart rate difference be, simply because of random variation alone? On the basis of the concepts that have already been discussed, we know that we can measure the variation among these 40 differences between the beginning and end of a rehab session by calculating the standard deviation (SD). In this case, imag-

ine that we calculated the SD and found that it is 10 bpm. However, it's more important that we know how much the mean heart rate differences might vary from sample to sample, rather than how much the individual heart rate differences might vary within any single sample.

To determine how much the mean differences between the beginning and end of a rehab session heart rates from several samples might vary, we calculate the corresponding standard error (SE) of the mean for these differences. As you recall, the SE can be estimated by dividing the SD (10 bpm) by the square root of the sample size ($\sqrt{40}$ = 6.3). This calculation yields a standard error of 1.6 bpm for this hypothetical example. Recalling the properties of the normal distribution, we know that 68% of sample means will fall within plus or minus 1 SE of the true (population) mean—in this case, within plus or minus 1.6 bpm. The hypothetical distribution of the mean heart rate differences, assuming that there truly is no difference between the values obtained at the beginning and end of rehab sessions, is shown in Figure 25.2.

So, is a 5-bpm difference between the heart rates at the beginning and end of rehab sessions the result of the rehab session (i.e., a real difference) or the result of chance?

Because the SE is 1.6 bpm, the observed mean heart rate difference of 5 bpm for the sample of 40 participants is an improbable result. Why? Figure 25.2 shows that a mean difference of 5 bpm is slightly more than 3 SEs larger than the result that would be expected if there were truly no difference between the heart rates measured at the beginning and end of a rehab session (i.e., the probability of it occurring by chance is less than 1 time in 250).

Figure 25.2

Estimated frequency distribution of mean differences between beginning and end heart rates (SE = 1.6 bpm)

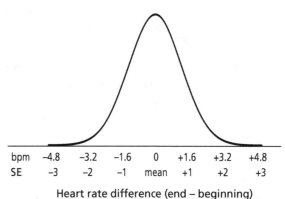

We can explain this improbably large mean heart rate difference in one of two ways:

Conducting

1. The null hypothesis is true (i.e., the rehab session truly has no effect on heart rate), and this improbably high mean difference between stressed and relaxed heart rates (5 bpm), while improbable, has simply occurred by chance.
2. The null hypothesis is not true. We can no longer accept the idea that the heart rates measured at the beginning and end of a rehab session do not differ from one another.

To determine the probability of observing a result as extreme as the one observed, we calculate the number of SEs between the mean heart rate difference under the null hypothesis (0 in this case) and the mean difference that we observed (5). In the example above, the SE is equal to 1.6 bpm, and so we use the following formula:

$$(5.0 - 0) \div 1.6 = 3.125.$$

The result of this calculation is called a **test statistic**. By locating this value in a statistical table (in this case, the t table), which can be found in many statistics books or online,[a] we find that the probability that such an extreme value could occur by chance is approximately 34 in 10 000 (i.e., 0.0034). That is to say, only 0.34% (about one-third of 1%) of the values within this normal distribution are more improbable than the one we observed.

The term commonly used to describe the probability that a value could occur by chance is the **P value**. In the context of our hypothetical example, the P value is the probability of detecting a mean difference between stressed and relaxed heart rates of 5 bpm or more when *there truly is no difference*.

A result is considered to have reached **statistical significance** if the observed result is unlikely to have happened by chance alone. In the example above, we would conclude that the difference between the heart rates of cardiac rehabilitation program participants measured at the beginning and end of a rehab session are statistically significant. That is, it is *unlikely to be explained by chance*.

The *P* value

The P value is the probability that, if the null hypothesis is true (i.e., there truly is no effect), chance alone could have produced a result as extreme or more extreme than the one

observed. In our example, this is the probability that we would observe a mean difference between heart rates measured at the beginning and end of a rehab session of 5 bpm if, in reality, the rehab session has no effect on heart rate. Because it is a probability that can be interpreted as a percentage, the P value will always be a fraction between 0 (no chance of occurring) and 1 (certain to occur). A large P value means that the results could plausibly have occurred by chance (i.e., there is a reasonably high probability that the observed results arose simply by chance). A small P value means that the observed results probably did not occur by chance (although, no matter how small the P value, there will always be a possibility that the results arose by chance).

As a matter of convention, researchers commonly set the **alpha** (α) level (the level at which results will be classified as statistically significant) at .05. A P value must be lower than the alpha level to be declared statistically significant. This means that researchers are willing to accept a 5% chance that they could wrongly conclude that an observed result was real when, in fact, it was due to chance. In other words, if there truly is no real effect, the observed result (or one more extreme) will occur by chance less than 1 time in 20 (5%). (The risk of wrongly concluding that an observed result is real is increased by the number of statistical tests that are conducted—it is 5% for the first test conducted, plus almost an additional 5% for each subsequent test, so when multiple statistical tests are conducted and assessed special care should be taken. These include using an applicable technique to adjust for **multiple testing**, such as Bonferroni's correction or the Holm adjustment.)

It should be stressed that the size of the P value determines *only* whether a result could have occurred by chance if the null hypothesis is true. In fact, one of the most common statistical reporting errors in the literature is to confuse statistical significance—a small P value—with **clinical importance**. The size of the P value does not indicate the importance or unimportance of the results. Statistical significance is not the same as clinical importance. One characteristic of hypothesis testing is that small and clinically trivial differences can be statistically significant if the study sample is large, and that clinically important differences can be missed if the study sample is small. Instead, the clinical importance of a study result should be determined by the observed study "effect" (e.g., the size of the difference between study groups). For example, a decrease of 1 mm Hg in mean systolic blood pressure would generally not be considered clinically important even if the P value associat-

---

a   For example, at http://statpages.org/pdfs.html

Conducting

ed with the result is statistically significant—even as low as .001. When writing about *P* values, researchers should be careful not to lead readers to believe that statistically significant results are automatically clinically important—or vice versa! So, although *P* values should be incorporated into the interpretation of study results, biological plausibility and the clinical importance of the observed result should also be considered.

Our example of hypothesis testing about a difference between heart rates measured at the beginning and end of a rehab session is a simplified version of a **paired *t* test** (also called Student's paired *t* test). This is used because the data are paired: two measurements are taken from the same person at different times, or participants in the study groups are "matched." Other statistical tests use similar approaches to compare observations (collected data) to the results that would be expected under the null hypothesis and then to standardize this difference by dividing it by the applicable measure of variability (e.g., the SE).

Let's consider another set of hypothetical heart-rate data:

Participant	Beginning	End	Difference
1	79	91	12
2	80	71	–9
3	76	87	11
–	–	–	–
–	–	–	–
–	–	–	–
40	88	77	–11

As was true of the original set of data, the mean difference between the heart rates at the beginning and the end of a rehab session for these 40 cardiac rehabilitation program participants is also +5 bpm. However, imagine that, in this sample, the variability of the differences in heart rate is higher, with a standard deviation (SD) of 19 bpm (instead of the SD of 10 bpm in the original data set). This higher SD results in a correspondingly higher SE of 3 bpm (instead of the SE of 1.6 in the original data set). As Figure 25.3 depicts, the distribution of mean heart rate differences for possible samples around the null hypothesis is now more stretched out.

Because the variability in the heart rate differences is higher and the corresponding standard error (SE) of the mean for these differences is larger, the mean heart rate difference of 5 bpm is now within 2 SEs (actually, it is at 1.67

SEs) of the null hypothesis value of zero. As a result, the probability of observing a mean heart rate difference at least this extreme by chance is now 9.6% (*P* = .096). This *P* value suggests that the mean heart rate difference of 5 bpm can now be expected to occur by chance alone approximately 1 time in 10. Therefore, this result (because of its larger SE) is no longer statistically significant when compared with the conventional alpha (α) level of .05.

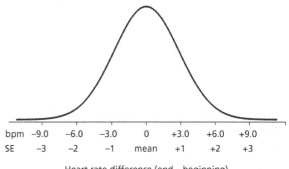

Figure 25.3
Estimated frequency distribution of mean differences between beginning and end heart rates for possible samples (SE = 3.0 bpm)

Heart rate difference (end – beginning)

Other statistical tests

Other statistical tests use methods similar to those illustrated by the examples presented above. All of these tests determine the difference between the observed results and the results that would be expected by chance if the null hypothesis were true (i.e., if there truly was no effect); they then standardize this difference between observed and expected results by dividing it by the applicable measure of variability (e.g., the SE). Researchers select the appropriate statistical test to use by determining the study design (e.g., the number of groups being compared) and the level of measurement of the outcome variables (e.g., nominal, ordinal, discrete or continuous data). A guide for selecting the applicable statistical test—adapted from Glantz[5]—is presented in Table 25.1.

Analysis of variance

Analysis of variance (ANOVA) is used to compare the means obtained from two or more groups, determining whether the variation among the means is greater than might be expected given the amount of variation inherent in the underlying data. However, the result of an ANOVA indicates only whether a statistically significant difference exists; it doesn't indicate which group or groups differ from

Conducting

■ Table 25.1: A guide for selecting the appropriate statistical test

Level of outcome measurement	Type of comparison being carried out				
	Two independent groups	Three or more independent groups	Two matched (dependent) groups	Multiple measures in the same individuals	Association between two variables
Normally distributed continuous data*	Unpaired *t* test	Analysis of variance	Paired *t* test	Repeated-measures analysis of variance	linear regression or Pearson product moment correlation
Nominal	Difference of proportions or chi-squared contingency table analysis	Chi-squared contingency table analysis	McNemar's test		
Ordinal†	Mann-Whitney rank-sum test	Kruskal-Wallis test	Wilcoxon signed-rank test	Friedman statistic	Spearman rank correlation
Survival time	Log-rank test				

Notes:* if the data are not normally distibuted, rank the observations and use the methods for data measured on an ordinal scale.
† Or interval data that are not normally distributed.

the others. For this reason, an ANOVA that has yielded a statistically significant result is usually followed by further tests that, ideally, account for the applicable number of pair-wise comparisons (e.g., Tukey, Newman-Keuls, Holm-adjusted *t* tests) to determine which groups differ from the others beyond what would be expected by chance (i.e., their differences are statistically significant).

Unpaired *t* test

The **unpaired *t* test** is a special case of ANOVA and is used to determine the statistical significance of the difference between the means obtained from two (and only two) independent samples. In contrast, the heart rate examples above involved paired *t* tests because the heart rates are pairs of measurements taken from the same persons, not measurements taken from 2 different groups of participants.

Correlation

Correlation enables the assessment of the relationship between two quantitative measures. The data can be graphically depicted in a scatter plot in which one variable is plotted on each axis. Figure 25.4 plots the number of graduates by year. If a potentially causal relationship were being assessed, the exposure/predictor (i.e., independent) variable would be plotted on the x axis with the outcome (i.e., dependent) variable on the y axis.

The level of association/correlation between the two variables is quantified with a correlation coefficient ranging from –1 to 1: 1 indicates a perfect direct relationship

between the two measures; –1 indicates a perfect inverse/indirect relationship (i.e., as one measure increases, the other decreases); 0 indicates no relationship (i.e., the observed relationship is consistent with what would be expected from random variation); and intermediate values indicating a partial relationship between the two. There are two main types of correlation: parametric and nonparametric. **Pearson product moment correlation** is a parametric method that assesses the actual measured values for each variable, while **Spearman rank correlation**, an example of a non-parametric method, assesses the rank-order of the values for each variable. Pearson product moment correlation assumes that each of the two sets of data being assessed are normally distributed (or nearly so), whereas Spearman rank correlation can be used on continuous or ordinal data that follow any distribution pattern. The correlation coeffi-

Figure 25.4
A scatter plot of the number of graduates per year

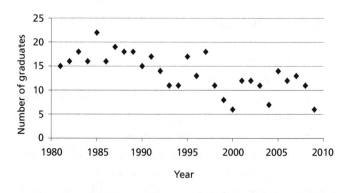

Conducting

cient for the data depicted in Figure 25.4 is –0.70 (by both methods), which indicates an inverse relationship (i.e, the number of graduates is declining over time).

Regression

Regression also enables the relationship between quantitative measures to be assessed. However, unlike correlation, regression should be used only to assess potentially causal relationships between one or more exposure/predictor variables and an outcome variable (e.g., effect of drug dosage on urinary output; effect of age, height and weight on blood pressure). In these circumstances the data can be graphically depicted in a scatter plot with the exposure/predictor (i.e., independent) variable plotted on the x-axis and outcome (i.e., dependent) variable on the y-axis (Figure 25.4). If there is no relationship between the two variables/measures, the resulting scatter plot will approximate a horizontal line. In contrast, the data depicted in Figure 25.4 suggest that the number of graduates is declining over time (with an estimated slope of –0.33 graduates/year). Regression compares the observed data against what would be expected if there were no relationship, by determining the probability of the observed slope differing from zero (i.e., the slope of a horizontal/flat line).

Non-parametric tests

Like Pearson product moment correlation, the *t* tests and ANOVA are examples of **parametric statistical tests** because they are intended for use only with normally distributed (or nearly so) data that can be described by parameters (measurable characteristics) such as group means, SD and variance. However, when study data are not normally distributed, researchers should use alternative **non-parametric statistical tests**. Some examples of nonparametric tests are the **Wilcoxon signed-rank test** (the non-parametric alternative to the paired *t* test), the **Mann-Whitney *U* test** (the non-parametric alternative to the unpaired *t* test), the **Kruskal-Wallis** test (the non-parametric alternative to ANOVA) and the Spearman rank correlation (which, as noted above, is the non-parametric alternative to the Pearson product moment correlation).

Chi-squared (χ^2) test

Probably the most widely recognized non-parametric statistical test is the χ^2 (chi-squared) test of proportions, which is used to assess the statistical significance of results obtained with categorical data. This test determines the dif-

ferences between the expected proportions or categorical counts and the proportions of data obtained from two or more independent samples. It produces a *P* value that assesses the statistical significance of these differences (i.e., the probability that a difference as great as the one observed could have arisen by chance).

Interpreting study results

Let's consider further how statistical methods are used to assist in the interpretation of study results. Imagine that a clinical trial, conducted to assess the efficacy of radiotherapy (a dichotomous indicator variable) to reduce death from breast cancer (a dichotomous outcome variable), provides the following results:

	Alive	Dead	Total
Radiotherapy	24	16	40
No radiotherapy	16	24	40
Total	40	40	80

These results indicate that the death rate in the group receiving radiotherapy was lower (40%; 16/40) than in the comparison group (60%; 24/40). Although these results appear promising, they (like all quantitative study results) can be explained in one or more of three ways. The first explanation, of course, is that the results are real—that in this example radiotherapy does, in fact, lead to a reduced rate of death from breast cancer. However, there is no way to directly measure or otherwise determine the degree to which this explanation accounts for any set of observed quantitative study results. Instead, we must assess this explanation indirectly by first considering two alternative explanations.

The first of these is that the study was flawed, either in its design or in its conduct, and that this resulted in a biased result. For example, if the allocation process was flawed, resulting in a disproportionate number of patients expected to die being allocated to the comparison group, this "selection bias" in how patients were allocated to the two study groups could reasonably explain the apparent efficacy of radiotherapy. To assess the degree to which study errors, biases and confounding might account for the observed results, we would need to use critical appraisal techniques, such as those discussed in chapter 9 and described in the CONSORT (Consolidated Standards of Reporting Trials)

Conducting

Statement.[6] Such details would include, for example, the source of random numbers, how the allocation schedule was kept secret from those who enrolling patients and those who assigning patients to the study groups and, if applicable, the success of blinding patients.

The second alternative explanation is chance—that the observed excess of deaths in the comparison group is simply the result of a larger proportion of study patients who were ultimately destined to die being randomly allocated to that group. Even with the use of scientifically sound and rigorous randomization processes (i.e., all patients have the same chance of being assigned to the treatment or comparison group), the distribution of patients who are ultimately destined to die may, by chance, be imbalanced. As described above, the probability that such an unbalanced allocation may have occurred can be determined by statistical testing. More specifically, applicable statistical tests answer the question, "If there truly is no difference between the groups (i.e., the so-called "null hypothesis"), what is the probability of observing a result at least as extreme as the one observed, simply by chance alone?"

In the example study, if radiotherapy truly has no effect, then we would expect 20 patients in each group to have a recurrence, because the 40 (i.e., 16 + 24) patients with a recurrence would be expected to be evenly divided between the 2 study groups. However, the observed results in our hypothetical study differ from this "expected" amount by 4 patients each. By completing the appropriate statistical test (in this case, a chi-squared test) either by hand or by using suitable computer software,[b] this probability is found to be 0.117, or 11.7%. That is, assuming that the null hypothesis is true (that radiotherapy truly has no effect on the risk of dying), a difference as large as the one observed could have occurred simply by chance more than 1 time in 10 (i.e., P > .1).

It is important to note that P values like this one should almost always be based on a two-tailed hypothesis test. **Two-tailed tests** are used when differences can potentially occur in either direction: to take our example, the death rate could be either higher or lower in the radiotherapy than in the comparison group. Two-tailed tests give the probability for a difference in either direction and so should be used when the direction of a difference is unknown,[7] whereas **one-tailed tests** should be used only in those infrequent instances when the direction of the result is known in advance. When one-tailed tests are used, however, they should be clearly identified as such and their use justified.[7]

As discussed earlier, this probability (i.e., P value) needs to be sufficiently low that chance is considered an improbable explanation for the observed results before researchers conclude that there is an alternative explanation for the observed results—i.e., that the observed results reflect a true effect: in the case of this example, this alternative explanation would be that radiotherapy really does reduce the risk of dying of breast cancer. As noted earlier, this cut-off value, the alpha (α) level, should always be selected by the researchers before the study. The traditional threshold (the α level) for indicating statistical significance is .05. However, using this threshold does not guarantee that these conclusions will be correct. In fact, if we reject the null hypothesis every time we find a P value of .05, we will be wrong 5% of the time: recall that a P value of .05 means that the null hypothesis would produce results at least as extreme 5% of the time. This type of error—of mistakenly concluding that there is an effect when in fact there isn't one—is called a **Type I error.**

On the other hand, researchers can make a different kind of mistake. They can incorrectly conclude that there is *no* effect when in fact there really is one. This mistake is referred to as a **Type II error.**

Researchers can never know for sure whether they've made one of these errors in their studies. But to avoid these potential errors they try to set an α level that represents an acceptable trade-off between the risk of wrongly concluding that there is a real effect when such an effect in fact doesn't exist (a false-positive result) and the risk of failing to detect a real effect when such an effect in fact does exist (a false-negative result).

Although the most frequently chosen α level is .05, there are circumstances in which either a higher α level or a lower α level may be more appropriate, depending on the balance between the consequences associated with false-positive results and those associated with false-negative results. For instance, in the presented example, the researchers might have selected a lower alpha level (e.g., .01) so that they could further reduce the risk of wrongly concluding that the radiotherapy is effective, particularly in light of its potential side-effects, costs and limited availability. However, even if the P value is as low as .01, chance might still be responsible for the observed results (in this case, it is a low probability: 1 chance in 100). As such, the probability of chance being responsible for observed results never goes to

---

b   Such as the web-based calculator at www.statpages.org/ctab2x2.html

zero because it is always *possible* for chance to be responsible for the observed results. However, the key question is how *probable* is it that chance could account for the observed results.

In contrast, a study examining the health benefit of eating fruits and vegetables may benefit from a higher α level (e.g., .10) because the risks associated with failing to detect the benefit of this diet (i.e., a false-negative result) outweigh the risk associated with falsely concluding that such a diet is beneficial (i.e., a false-positive result). It should be noted that Type I and Type II errors have a reciprocal relationship: when the probability of one is decreased, the probability of the other is reduced—hence, there is a "trade-off" between them.

The relationship between a study's result and the underlying "truth" can be illustrated as follows.

	The truth	
The study result	**There is an effect**	**There is no effect**
Looks like an effect	True-positive statistical result	False-positive statistical result (Type I error)
Looks like no effect	False-negative statistical result (Type II error)	True-negative statistical result

Although *P* values reflect the probability that an observed result may occur by chance, they do not indicate how precisely an observed difference or effect has been measured (i.e., the range of values consistent with the study's result). In the previous chapter we discussed the use of **confidence intervals** to identify, at a given probability, the range of values within which the "true" (population) value will be found. In a similar manner, confidence intervals can be used to specify the researcher's confidence (i.e., range of values) in an observed difference or effect.

As an example, recall the study report from the previous chapter that contained the following sentence: "On average, the new drug appears to lower patients' total cholesterol concentration by 12 to 28 mg/dL." This statement is far more informative than a statement such as the following: "The new drug results in a statistically significant reduction in patients' total cholesterol concentration ($P = .01$)." As we discussed in the previous chapter, the confidence interval tells us whether there is an effect and also tells us the plausible magnitude of this effect. In addition, the CI also tells us indirectly about statistical significance: this is because, in a study of differences, a 95% CI that does not include zero is,

by definition, significant at the .05 level. That is, the null value of zero (both groups are the same), will occur by chance less than 5 times in 100.

Although confidence intervals are related to hypothesis testing and *P* values, they focus attention on the health effect; on the estimated size of the effect, or the size of the difference between the groups; and on the precision of the estimate. Reviewing this effect size and the precision with which it is estimated allows us to better determine the clinical importance of the results. As a result, researchers are advised (and even required by many publications) to report a confidence interval to indicate the precision of the estimated effect size. By completing the applicable statistical procedure by hand or by using suitable computer software,[c] the 95% CI in our example can be determined to be –0.02 to 0.40, indicating that the "true" difference in death rates will be within this range with a probability of 95%.

When the *P* value is not statistically significant

In the radiotherapy example, the *P* value was sufficiently large (i.e., .117 or 11.7% or $P > .1$) that we would accept chance as a reasonable explanation for the observed results. So, should we now conclude that radiotherapy is ineffective at reducing the risk of death due to breast cancer? As a first step, let's reconsider the apparent effect of radiotherapy. As we noted above, the results of the study indicate that receiving radiotherapy reduced the rate of death by 20% (40% versus 60%). So, although the observed results were not statistically significant (i.e., the *P* value was not less than the chosen alpha level), they suggest a clinically important effect.

Analogous to the discussion above, an examination of this statistically non-significant result requires the consideration of three possible explanations. The first explanation, of course, is that the observed results are real: that radiotherapy is, in fact, not effective at reducing the rate of death from breast cancer. Again, however, there is no way to *directly* measure or otherwise determine whether this explains the statistically non-significant result. Instead, this determination is made indirectly by assessing each of the two alternative explanations.

The first of these alternative explanations is that the study was flawed, either in its design or in its conduct, resulting in a biased result and in a failure to detect a real difference between the groups. For example, if a larger

c   Such as the calculator at http://statpages.org/ctab2x2.html

Conducting

number of participants in the comparison group were lost to follow-up, reducing the number of deaths being recognized in this group, this "measurement bias" could potentially account for the apparent ineffectiveness of radiotherapy. Again, to assess the degree to which study errors, biases and confounding might account for the apparent lack of effect, we would need to know and critically assess the specific details about the research design and activities, such as those discussed in chapter 9 and described in the CONSORT Statement.[6] In this case, a "best-case/worst-case analysis" (i.e., sensitivity analysis)[8] could be done to estimate the potential impact the differences in the rate of patients lost to follow-up might have had on the observed results.

The second alternative explanation is, once again, chance. But instead of asking, as we did above, what the probability is that the observed results arose by chance, we ask what the probability is that the study failed to detect a result of a given size if such an effect truly existed. This probability is called the **beta (β) level** and is related to statistical power, which is the probability of a study detecting a difference of a given size, if one truly exists. Study power is equal to the complement of the beta level, 1 – beta.

Statistical power, beta (β), Type II error, and confidence intervals

To determine the statistical power of our hypothetical study (i.e., the probability that it would detect an effect of a certain size if it actually exists), we must identify and specify four characteristics of the study: (1) the minimum difference between the groups that would be considered clinically important to detect; (2) the estimated amount of data variability (e.g., standard deviation); (3) the sample size of each study group; and, (4) the alpha (α) level used to declare a statistically significant result (i.e., to conclude there is a difference). With this information, it is possible to estimate a study's statistical power.[d]

This calculation gives a result of 34.4%, meaning that the power of our hypothetical study to detect a 20% difference in death rates using an alpha level of .05 and a total sample of 80 was about 1 in 3. So, what does the statistical power of a study tell us? First, let's consider how high this probability would need to be for us to conclude that the study had sufficient statistical power to detect a reasonable

or desirable difference if one truly existed. Traditionally, researchers consider a study power of 80% to be the minimum required, although higher values are commonly used (e.g., 90% or 95%). As such, this study's statistical power of 34.4% helps to explain why this observed 20% difference in death rates was not statistically "detected." Not enough patients were studied to have a reasonable chance of detecting it. Similarly, the wide (i.e., imprecise) confidence interval presented earlier (i.e., – 2% to 40%) suggests a study that lacked sufficient statistical power. So, how could such a situation have been avoided?

Estimating the sample size for a study

To avoid conducting a study only to find that it has insufficient power, researchers are strongly encouraged—and even expected and morally obligated, so that patients are not put at risk unnecessarily—to specify the desired study power and to calculate the sample size needed to achieve this power when planning the study. In our example, how many patients would have been required to provide sufficient study power? To estimate this number, the applicable statistical calculation could be completed using a suitable statistical procedure.[e] In our example, to have an 80% chance of detecting a 20% difference in the rate of death from breast cancer at an alpha level of .05, the power calculation indicates that each of the 2 groups should have at least 107 patients. As you would expect, this sample size will change if any of the specifications are changed (Table 25.2). For example, to detect a smaller difference in death rates (e.g., 60% versus 50%), at least 407 patients would be needed in each study group. Similarly, the use of an alpha level of 0.01 would require each study group to have at least 154 patients. Further, to achieve a statistical power of 90%, each group would require at least 139 patients.

Alternatively, researchers may choose to determine the sample size needed to ensure a sufficiently precise estimate (i.e., a sufficiently narrow confidence interval). Using a web-based calculator[f] indicates that the difference in death rates could be estimated with a precision of about plus or minus 10% if each group included 200 participants (as compared with the precision of plus or minus 20% [the 95% confidence interval of –2% to 40% noted above] that was possible with 40 individuals in each study group).

---

d   A web-based calculator for comparing two proportions is available at www.stat.uiowa.edu/~rlenth/Power/index.html

e   Such as the web-based sample size calculator available at www.statpages.org/proppowr.html

f   Such as the one available at http://statpages.org/ctab2x2.html

■   **Table 25.2:**   **Variables included in statistical calculations for a comparison of 2 percentages using a chi-squared test and each variable's effect on the desired sample size for each group**

Variable*	Group 1 (%)	Group 2 (%)	Alpha (α)	Power ($1 - \beta$)	Sample size (n)
2-tailed test	60	40	0.05	0.8	107
1-tailed test	60	40	0.05	0.8	86
↓ different	60	**50**	0.05	0.8	407
↓Alpha	60	40	**0.01**	0.8	154
↑ power	60	40	0.05	**0.9**	139

*Values in **bold** have been varied from the first line to show how changes in each variable affect sample size as determined using www.statpages.org/proppowr.html.

Determining the sample size necessary to ensure sufficient estimate precision can also be carried out for the planning of surveys. For example, the resident in our illustrative case should determine how precisely he would like to determine what proportion of patients in each of the practices has received the applicable preventive services. For example, if he wishes to determine how patients will need to be assessed to estimate the percentage of patients who have received colorectal screening in the previous two years with a precision of plus or minus 5% (for the resulting 95% CI), he could use a web-based calculator.[9] If he anticipates that about 50% of patients will have received this preventive service, the calculator shows that studying 50 patients provides a precision of only plus or minus 15% (and only plus or minus 10% if 100 patients are studied); in fact, about 400 patients would be required to attain the sought-after precision of plus or minus 5%.

By applying these principles and procedures, researchers are able to better ensure that their studies have an adequate number of patients and therefore sufficient statistical power (and measurement precision) to detect clinically important differences if they truly exist. In fact, if a proper sample size calculation is completed during the planning of a study and if the required number of subjects is recruited into the study, a calculation of power after the completion of the study should never be needed. As such, post hoc calculations of study power should, ideally, never be necessary. Although the example radiotherapy study compares the differences between two percentages, the same principles and analogous procedures are available for other study situations, such as correlation coefficients, regression slopes and testing the differences in means and rates.

Conclusion

This and the previous chapter were written to provide a better understanding of statistics—not to enable readers to become statisticians, but to become more comfortable and competent designing, conducting, interpreting and reporting statistical methods and results. In particular, having read this chapter you should be better able to discern the "story" behind the most commonly used statistical procedures, tests and results.

For example, you should now be better able to discern the "story" behind a study result such as:

Mean reduction in systolic BP, 10.2 mm Hg; 95% CI, 4.1 to 16.3 mm Hg; $P = .003$

You're now more familiar with P values and 95% confidence intervals and should be able to describe the information they convey about the study's results. You'll recognize that the mean reduction in systolic blood pressure of 10.2 mm Hg is clinically important. However, this conclusion is somewhat tempered by the fact that the lower bound of the 95% CI suggests that the mean reduction in systolic blood pressure may be as small as 4.1 mm Hg. On the other hand, you understand that the mean reduction could be as large as 16.3 mm Hg. Finally, you recognize that the reported P value indicates that the observed results are very unlikely to have occurred by chance (only 3 times in 1000).

Although this and the previous chapter are intended to expand your statistical knowledge and skills, you are encouraged to continue to enhance your statistical capabilities regularly, both to solidify them and to further expand them. After reading these two chapters, readers should be better at understanding, designing, conducting, interpreting, reporting and critiquing analytic methods and results and will have gained more confidence in actively interacting with and, dare I say, questioning others about selecting, interpreting and reporting statistical procedures, tests and results. ■

g   Such as the one at http://statpages.org/confint.html

Conducting

CASE POSTSCRIPT

After consulting his supervisor and the department's statistician, the resident learned that he would need to use the chi-squared test to determine whether the observed proportion of preventive services received differed significantly between the health centre's two practices. After doing so, he found that the proportion of eligible persons who had received the seasonal influenza immunization differed by 10.4% between the two practices: 98/211 (46.4%) as compared with 149/262 (56.8%)—a difference that would have been expected to arise by chance with a probability of .026. He also calculated the 95% confidence interval for the observed difference between these two proportions to be 0.9% to 19.7%.

Acknowledgements

All referenced web-based calculators were located at and accessed from: www.statpages.org

The development of this chapter was informed by: Harvey BJ, Ancker JS, Bairnsfather S, Bukowski JA, Hudson S, Lang TA, et al. *Statistics for medical writers and editors.* Rockville (MD): American Medical Writers Association; 2009.

as well as:

Harvey BJ, Lang TA. Hypothesis testing, study power and sample size. *Chest.* 2010;138(3):734–7.

REFERENCES

1. Glantz SA, Slinker BK. *Primer of applied regression & analysis of variance.* 2nd ed. New York (NY): McGraw-Hill Inc.; 2001.

2. Kleinbaum DG, Kupper LL, Nizam A, Muller KE. *Applied regression analysis and other multivariable methods.* 4th ed. Belmont (CA): Duxbury Press; 2008.

3. Vittinghoff E, Glidden DV, Shiboski SC, McCulloch CE. *Regression methods in biostatistics: linear, logistic, survival, and repeated measures models.* New York (NY): Springer Science+Business Media; 2005.

4. Norman GR, Streiner DL. *Biostatistics: the bare essentials.* 3rd ed. Shelton (CT): PMPH USA; 2008.

5. Glantz SA. *Primer of biostatistics.* 6th ed. New York: McGraw-Hill Medical Publishing Division; 2005. p. 446.

6. Altman DG, Schulz KF, Moher D, Egger M, Davidoff F, Elbourne D, et al. The revised CONSORT statement for reporting randomized trials: explanation and elaboration. *Ann Intern Med.* 2001;134(8):663–94.

7. Lang T. Documenting research in scientific articles: Guidelines for authors. 2. Reporting hypothesis tests. *Chest.* 2007;131(1):317–9.

8. Fletcher RH, Fletcher SW. *Clinical epidemiology: the essentials.* 4th ed. Philadelphia (PA): Lippincott, Williams & Wilkins; 2005. p. 118, 121–2.

ADDITIONAL RESOURCES

Glantz SA. *Primer of biostatistics.* 6th ed. New York: McGraw-Hill Medical Publishing Division; 2005.

Lang TA, Secic M. *How to report statistics in medicine: annotated guidelines for authors, editors, and reviewers.* 2nd ed. Philadelphia: American College of Physicians; 2006.

This book is a comprehensive reference discussing how statistics and the results of statistical tests and procedures, including descriptive statistics, should be correctly reported. Norman GR, Streiner DL. *Biostatistics: the bare essentials.* 3rd ed. Shelton (CT): PMPH USA; 2008.

- These three books are quite comprehensive, while also being readable and understandable.

Norman GR, Streiner DL. PDQ *statistics.* 3rd ed. Shelton (CT): PMPH USA; 2003.

Conducting

PRACTICE QUESTIONS

The answers to these questions are provided below.

1. When reading a journal article, you encounter the following sentence: "Influenza occurred less frequently in the vaccinated group (2%) than in the unvaccinated group (30%; $P = .44$)." What would you conclude about the clinical importance and statistical significance of this result?

2. You have high blood pressure, and you read the following sentence in a journal article: "Our findings ($P < .001$) show that the new drug lowers blood pressure by an average of 1 mmHg." What would you conclude about the clinical importance and statistical significance of this result?

3. As a journal editor, you receive a manuscript that contains the following statement: "The treatment regimen prolonged the time to relapse by an average of 65 months (95% CI, 45 to 85 months)." What would you conclude about the clinical importance and statistical significance of this result?

4. The following statement appeared in a journal article: "The new drug lowered the serum cholesterol concentration by an average of 1 mg/dL (95% CI, −14 to 16 mg/dL)." What would you conclude about the clinical importance and statistical significance of this result?

5. A researcher who conducted a double-blinded, randomized trial of a new intervention for reducing dizzy spells reports that the treatment group experienced an average of 3.4 fewer dizzy spells per week than the comparison group (standard error of the mean, 0.8). What would you conclude about the clinical importance and statistical significance of this result?

6. How is the ability to reject the null hypothesis affected by a reduction in the α level?

7. How is the chance of a Type I error affected by a reduction in the α level?

8. How is the chance of a Type II error affected by a reduction in the α level?

Answers to practice questions

1. Clinically important: there is a 15-fold difference in the rate of influenza.
   Not statistically significant ($P > .05$).
2. Not clinically important: the decrease in blood pressure is only 1 mmHg.
   Statistically significant ($P < .05$).
3. Clinically important: there is a 65-month difference in the time to relapse.
   Statistically significant: because the 95% CI does not include the null hypothesis value of zero, this result would be considered statistically significant (i.e., $P < .05$).
4. Not clinically important: the difference in the cholesterol level is only 1 mg/dL).
   Not statistically significant: because the 95% confidence interval includes the null hypothesis value of zero, this result would be considered not statistically significant (i.e., $P > .05$).
5. Clinically important: an average reduction in dizzy spells of 3.2 per week was achieved.
   Statistically significant: the decrease of 3.2 dizzy spells/week is 4 SEs larger than no effect.
6. Make it more difficult: a lower α level would require a lower P value.
7. Reduced chance of a Type I error: a lower α level would require a lower P value.
8. Increased chance of a Type II error: a lower α level would require a lower P value.

Conducting

SUMMARY CHECKLIST

- ❑ Thinking about your study, write down the hypothesis or hypotheses related to your research question(s).
- ❑ For each hypothesis in your study, select an appropriate statistical test to be included in your analysis. Be sure to justify you choice of tests.
- ❑ Determine what you will do to avoid Type I and Type II errors in your design and analysis.
- ❑ Review your proposed statistical analysis with your supervisor and a statistician. Revise.
- ❑ Estimate the sample size for your study (if applicable).

Conducting

26
Interpreting your research findings

Stephen Choi, MD, FRCPC

ILLUSTRATIVE CASE

A resident in Neurology has just performed a medical record review of all patients with severe head injury treated within the past 3 years at the hospital where she is training. She has formulated the hypothesis that patients with certain clinical variables have different outcomes than patients without those variables. She has also collected data on numerous other patient characteristics. Now, with the help of a biostatistician, she is ready to analyze and interpret her findings and to assess her hypothesis against the results.

■ **The collection of data, their logical** analysis, and the interpretation of that analysis form the essence of research. In quantitative research, data means numbers, and analysis means statistical calculation. There is no question that interpreting your results demands familiarity with the statistical tests that were used to generate them. However, this chapter is not meant to provide an overview of the multitude of statistical tests used in medical research (see chs 24 & 25), but rather to provide you with some guidance on approaching the interpretation of your data. This process is the most intellectually engaging part of doing research. After all the grunt work of collecting your data, you can pause to reflect: "What is the discernible point of my results? What is its importance?" This chapter contrasts **statistical significance** with "real-life" or **clinical importance**, in part by explaining the difference between hypothesis testing and the calculation of confidence intervals. Special consideration is given to observational studies, the category of research most commonly performed by health care trainees. Finally, a guide to presenting an interpretation of your study to others is provided.

Are my results significant? *P* values versus confidence intervals

The ***P* value** is a measure of probability that is used time and again in medical research. Although the reporting of *P* values is ubiquitous, the concept of the *P* value is somewhat circuitous and can take a moment to get your head around at first. It is tied to the idea of the **null hypothesis**, which for the purposes of a typical clinical trial might be defined

CHAPTER OBJECTIVES

After reading this chapter, you should be able to:

- determine whether your results are statistically significant and contrast the information conveyed by *P* values versus confidence intervals
- distinguish between *statistically significant* and *clinically important* results and describe the importance of "negative" studies
- list special considerations to take into account in interpreting data from observational studies
- describe how to prepare the discussion section of your manuscript or conference presentation.

KEY TERMS

Associations	"Negative" studies	Publication bias
Causal relationships	Null hypothesis	Statistical significance
Clinical importance	Observational studies	Subgroup analysis
Confidence intervals	Odds ratio	
Hypothesis testing	*P* value	

Conducting

as the hypothesis "that there is no difference between outcomes as a result of the treatments being compared."[1] It is important to grasp that the calculation of the P value is premised on the assumption that the null hypothesis is true. In other words, if we assume the null hypothesis to be true, then what is the probability that the observed finding occurred simply by chance? The lower the P value, the less likely it is that the finding is attributable to chance, and the more likely that the null hypothesis is false and should be rejected. This process of reasoning and calculation is referred to as **hypothesis testing.**[1]

The P value conventionally used in medical research is .05; that is, a probability value of less than 5% ($P < .05$) is the threshhold below which any result is judged unlikely to have occurred by chance and is thus deemed statistically significant. This cut-off, however, is arbitrary. The meaning of a cut-off of .05 can be put in these terms: assuming the null hypothesis to be true, there is a 1/20 probability that the finding observed was due to chance. If you take a moment to reflect on the definition of the P value, you should come to the conclusion that the absolute number of the P value for any given result *does* matter and that it is actually rather crude to dichotomize a value as either greater or less than .05. Therefore, you should always include the actual P values when reporting your data, and not simply whether a finding was "statistically significant."

This definition of the P value and its applicability to hypothesis testing should also make you question the whole notion of hypothesis testing, since it demands a binary outcome: either accepting or rejecting a null hypothesis. **Confidence intervals**—conventionally calculated as 95% confidence intervals—provide an alternative to this binary analysis by presenting a *range* of plausible values for the parameter being described.[2] This range is constructed to include within it the real value of the parameter. Thus, for a given 95% confidence interval there is a 95% chance that the actual value of the parameter being measured falls within that interval. The width of the confidence interval provides a wealth of information as to how small, and how big, the actual value of the parameter that is being estimated might be. In general, a narrow confidence interval reassures us of the precision of the estimate, whereas a wide confidence interval invites doubt as to that precision. The sample size used in your study will likely be the most important determinant of the width of the confidence interval, since a larger sample size usually means more outcomes of interest and therefore would more closely approximate the range

that would result if one were able, hypothetically, to test the entire population.

Given that the confidence interval does not provide a clear-cut outcome, its interpretation requires some nuance. Here is an example used by Guyatt and colleagues to illustrate this.[3] Let's say that you find an absolute risk reduction for patients that favours treatment A over treatment B with a 95% confidence interval of −1.2 to 12. Because the confidence interval spans 0 (and thus includes the null hypothesis), this is not a statistically significant finding (i.e., $P > .05$). The confidence interval indicates that treatment B might slightly increase risk by 1.2%, but it is just as likely that treatment A might result in a 12% absolute risk reduction. However, the finding here should not be dismissed as "negative" because it is more likely that the real value that lies within the confidence interval is probably somewhere in the middle, i.e., around 5%. The conclusion, therefore, must be that a larger study—which would likely produce a narrower confidence interval—is needed to investigate the question further. Here, the adjective "significant" certainly applies to the results, although by the terms of conventional statistics they are not.

And so, wherever possible, report your results with confidence intervals. Although you may be familiar with seeing confidence intervals around estimates such as risks and odds, they can also be calculated for results such as likelihood ratios, sensitivities and specificities, to name a few. When you are interpreting statistical data, it is absolutely crucial that you enlist the help of a statistician. If you take just one message from this chapter, this should probably be it.

What to do if you do not obtain a statistically significant result

It's important to realize that, after all your hard work, you might not end up with a statistically significant result. Although this can be discouraging to the budding researcher, it is nonetheless a reality of doing research: the null hypothesis might win the day. However, the fact that you did not find a difference is still an important finding that the world can benefit from. It is inadvisable to re-run statistical tests until you find a way to achieve a statistically significant result. In her enlightening work, *How to read a paper*, Trisha Greenhalgh[4] lists 10 ways of "cheating" in the writing-up of statistical results (Textbox 26.1).

It is worth mentioning here the issue of **subgroup analysis** as it relates to points 1 and 9 in the textbox. This refers

Conducting

to the strategy of subdividing your population into smaller groups, typically to determine whether a given subgroup is at particular risk for an outcome. Often, subgroup analyses make good sense (e.g., patients with diabetes in a study of cardiovascular disease), and when this is the case it is optimal to plan for these subgroups *a priori*—that is, at the outset of your study. Subgroup analyses can become problematic, however, when they are conducted *post hoc* (i.e., after all the data have been collected). The reason is that when you create many smaller groups within your population, the likelihood of finding a statistically significant result becomes much higher in those smaller groups because the number of outcomes of interest is usually lower. As such, there is a very good chance that you will obtain a result that, although statistically significant, is actually a false positive finding. Do not be tempted to create subgroups that are not clinically meaningful, with the aim of trolling for *P* values < .05. This dubious practice is quite likely to mislead you and your audience into unfounded conclusions.

Moreover, it seems that medical journal editors are gaining a better appreciation of the importance of publishing what are termed **"negative" studies**—that is, studies that do not demonstrate a statistically significant difference between two parameters or that, to use the language of clinical epidemiology, cannot disprove the null hypothesis. There is no question that publishing studies that demonstrate a new finding are inherently "sexier": they generate more interest in the medical community and more buzz in the media after they are published. The result of this selective publication of "positive" results is to limit the range of valid data that are available: this is referred to as **publication bias**. But "negative" studies are crucial to our understanding of a topic, and are especially relevant to systematic reviews and meta-analyses of the literature, whose results will be distorted if negative studies are systematically excluded. Your negative study, if it is of high quality and includes a sufficiently large sample, might in fact trump another study showing a positive result when the literature is reviewed and summarized. By the same token, there is a sound argument to be made that it is unethical not to publish research findings—whether those findings are statistically significant or not—since a null finding nonetheless contributes to our understanding of the hypothesis being posed in the study. The bottom line is to take heart if you do not obtain a statistically significant result; be honest and don't try to fudge the analysis to obtain one, as the null finding is still important and deserves to be published if your study has been well designed and properly conducted.

TEXTBOX 26.1: TEN WAYS TO CHEAT ON STATISTICAL TEXTS WHEN WRITING UP RESULTS.
ADAPTED FROM GREENHALGH.[4]

1. Abandon your *a priori* plans for data analysis, look for any relationship that gives you a *P* value < .05 and choose to focus your paper on that.
2. If baseline differences between the groups favour the intervention group, remember not to adjust for them.
3. Do not test your data to see if they are normally distributed. If you do, you might get stuck with non-parametric tests.
4. Ignore all withdrawals and non-responders from the analysis.
5. Plot data against each other that don't make intuitive sense in the search for a statistically significant correlation coefficient.
6. Disregard outliers when doing so favours your hypothesis.
7. Omit non-significant results.
8. Perform an interim analysis and alter the length of the planned study time if that results in a statistically significant result.
9. Perform subgroup analyses to search for a relationship where *P* < .05 even though the subgroup is not of interest.
10. If none of your results are statistically significant, try different statistical analyses in the hope of obtaining one that is.

Observational studies

It is highly unlikely that you will have the time, resources or expertise to conduct a multi-centre randomized interventional trial during the course of your training program. Rather, you will likely focus on a study design that introduces you to the whole notion of asking a research question and undertaking a practical process for testing an hypothesis. Because observational studies are generally less complicated than interventional trials, they tend to be more feasible to manage alongside the many other demands of training.

Conducting

Specifically, most health care trainees undertake case-control studies and cohort studies (especially retrospective versions of these) to fulfil the research requirement of their program.

Having a solid grasp of the fundamentals of these study designs before you begin will save you grief later. In particular, understanding both the advantages and limitations of observational studies[5] as well as the important sources of potential bias (i.e., selection, misclassification, confounders)[6] is crucial to interpreting your study results. It is important to keep in mind that observational studies provide us with **associations** rather than **causal relationships**, even though the strength of those associations might support the case for causation. Because the **odds ratio** is one of the most common statistics used to measure the association between an exposure and an outcome,[7] it is important to have a good grasp of what it means. Basically, it is the ratio of the odds of an event occurring in one group (e.g., the experimental group) to the odds of the event occurring in another group (e.g., the control group). In clinical studies, it is common to see odds ratios as the final result of a logistic regression analysis that aims to find variables that seem to be independently associated with the outcome. Finally, although logistic regression and correlation analyses are related methods of finding associations between variables, you need to understand the difference between them.[8,9] Simply put, logistic regression analyses aim to determine the relation between an exposure and an event and, in so doing, support the case for a causal relation (e.g., smoking and lung cancer); correlation, on the other hand, aims to determine the closeness of two variables without making a case for causality (e.g., umbrella use on a rainy day, or evaluation scores on professionalism during residency training and frequency of patient complaints post-training).

Perhaps the greatest mistake to make in interpreting an association is to infer causality when none exists. Andrew Wakefield's report of an association between the MMR vaccine and autism, based on the accounts of the parents of 12 children with autism in 1998, is an example of the potential abuse of inferring causality from a weak association between two variables. Besides this transgression, it appears that Wakefield may—far worse—have actually fabricated his data;[10] this aside, the mere inference of causality in this instance was, unfortunately, enough to entice one of the world's most prestigious medical journals to publish Wakefield's paper. The result has been a profound and long-lasting effect on the public's trust in vaccines and on public health policies surrounding vaccination. Wakefield's paper has since been retracted by *The Lancet*.[11]

Preparing the Interpretation section

Whether you are writing a manuscript for publication or preparing a talk for a conference, synthesizing your data into a meaningful interpretation (or discussion) is fundamental to the success of either. If your research paper were a legal argument, your study protocol and analysis would represent its premises, and the interpretation would present your closing arguments. Here is a simple, fail-proof formula for organizing your interpretation section.

- Summarize the most important results of your study. These may be statistically significant or not.
- Put your results into the context of what is already known in your topic area. This should be the bulk of the interpretation. Do your data contradict existing knowledge, or are they consistent with it? How did your study protocol differ from that of previous investigations, and how should those differences influence the interpretation of your results in light of the existing literature? Carefully situating your study within the context of existing literature should help you to determine what your study adds to the field.
- What are the limitations of your study? This is a crucial section to reflect on and prepare carefully. Every study, including yours, has limitations. Interpreting your data in a cogent way demands that you consider these limitations. Overstepping what the data can actually say is a common pitfall for many junior scientists (e.g., making a claim of causality when an association between a risk variable and outcome is found). It is crucial to consider the effect of missing data and not to shy away from any limitations in your study's conception and design. All of this is to say that it is important to be realistic about your study and its contribution to scientific knowledge. You will not find the cure for cancer in your observational study, but if you have carried out the work carefully, you will surely contribute one small piece of a large puzzle that, just maybe, you will choose to spend the rest of your career helping to solve.
- Finally, conclude with what you feel is the most important finding of your study and point the way to further research that is needed in your topic area.

Conducting

Conclusion

It's important to differentiate a finding that is statistically significant from one that is clinically important. Although hypothesis testing is one way of determining statistical significance, also consider wherever possible the use of confidence intervals as a way of reporting and interpreting your data. As many of you will perform observational studies as your first research endeavour, it is important to understand the tests used to determine associations between variables. As a rule, observational studies do not prove causal relationships, and so it is important to understand the limits of when one can make a case for inferring causality versus association. Finally, it's important to convey your results and interpretation by way of peer-reviewed publication. The steps above will provide you with a useful road map to presenting your argument. ■

CASE POSTSCRIPT

After performing initial statistical testing to look for associations between factors in the clinical presentation and the outcomes of interest, the resident finds no statistically significant associations. However, she had intended *a priori* to examine a large subgroup with a pre-existing comorbidity and found that there was, in fact, an association with respect to this factor in this group of patients. Overall, the null hypothesis was true—but, for an important patient group, the association found should prompt, the resident hopes, future clinical trials specifically for this subgroup of patients.

REFERENCES

1. Guyatt G, Jaeschke R, Heddle N, Cook D, Shannon H, Walter S. Basic statistics for clinicians: 1. Hypothesis testing. *CMAJ.* 1995;152(1):27–32.

2. Gardner MJ, Altman DG. Confidence intervals rather than P values: estimation rather than hypothesis testing. *BMJ.* 1986;292(6522):746–50.

3. Guyatt G, Jaeschke R, Heddle N, Cook D, Shannon H, Walter S. Basic statistics for clinicians: 2. Interpreting study results: confidence intervals. *CMAJ.* 1995;152(2):169–73.

4. Greenhalgh T. *How to read a paper: the basics of evidence-based medicine.* 3rd ed. Oxford: Wiley-Blackwell; 2006.

5. Kestenbaum B. *Epidemiology and biostatistics: an introduction to clinical research.* New York: Springer; 2009.

6. Rothman KJ. *Epidemiology: an introduction.* New York: Oxford University Press; 2002.

7. Jaeschke R, Guyatt G, Shannon H, Walter S, Cook D, Heddle N. Basic statistics for clinicians: 3. Assessing the effects of treatment: measures of association. *CMAJ.* 1995;152(3):351–57.

8. Guyatt G, Haynes B, Sackett D. Analyzing data. In: Haynes RB, Sackett DL, Guyatt GH, Tugwell P, editors. *Clinical epidemiology: how to do clinical practice research.* 3rd ed. Philadelphia: Lippincott Williams & Wilkins; 2006. p. 446–60.

9. Guyatt G, Walter S, Shannon H, Cook D, Jaeschke R, Heddle N. Basic statistics for clinicians: 4. Correlation and regression. *CMAJ.* 1995;152(4):497–504.

10. Deer B. How the case against the MMR vaccine was fixed. *BMJ.* 2011;342:c5347.

11. [Editors of *The Lancet.*] Retraction – Ileal-lymphoid-nodular hyperplasia, non-specific colitis, and pervasive developmental disorder in children. *Lancet* 2010;375(9713):445.

Conducting

ADDITIONAL RESOURCE

Haynes RB, Sackett DL, Guyatt GH, Tugwell P, editors. *Clinical epidemiology: how to do clinical practice research.* 3rd ed. Philadelphia: Lippincott Williams & Wilkins; 2006.

• This seminal work in clinical epidemiology and research should be required reading for anyone who strives to understand how research is done and the fundamental principles of evidence-based medicine.

SUMMARY CHECKLIST

- ❏ Review your results. Do they surprise you? Do any stand out? Do the data answer your questions as planned?
- ❏ Identify the results that were "significant" and those that were not.
- ❏ Write your draft interpretation of the results, summarizing them in the context of the existing related literature and hypotheses.
- ❏ Describe the limitations of your data.
- ❏ Write a conclusion that summarizes the relevance and clinical importance of your findings.

Conducting

27
Writing effective abstracts

Carolyn Brown, ELS

ILLUSTRATIVE CASE

A resident is working on a research project comparing cytologic findings after surgery for various conditions, and she tabulates exciting interim results. She asks to discuss the results with her supervisor, who comments that they would make an excellent poster or oral presentation at the upcoming meeting of the Society of Obstetricians and Gynecologists of Canada (SOGC). The deadline for abstract submissions is in a week! The supervisor directs the resident to the website for the conference, which indicates that the conference accepts abstracts for research in progress. The website also provides a word count and some general guidelines for abstracts for the meeting. The countdown starts for the resident to provide a clear abstract that conveys the importance of her work and that (she hopes!) will be accepted for presentation at the meeting.

■ **Abstracts serve several important** functions that vary according to context. In a poster or oral presentation at a meeting, the abstract communicates the nature and significance of a research project in a compact fashion that is quick for other researchers to read and grasp. Through the presentations and the publication of the abstracts in a program or proceedings, researchers learn about current areas of investigation. Since some meetings accept abstracts of research in progress, meeting abstracts can also serve as preliminary reports. However, several studies have shown that only a portion of meeting abstracts—ranging from 34% to 52%—are followed by the publication of final results in the peer-reviewed literature.[1-5]

When an abstract accompanies a paper submitted to a journal, its function is somewhat different. Most definitions state that the abstract summarizes and condenses the research paper.[6-9] While technically correct, this narrow definition misses one of essential roles of the abstract in a journal publication, which is to help the reader decide whether to read the full paper. A reader looking for an answer to a clinical question or for current research in a particular area needs to glean sufficient information from the

CHAPTER OBJECTIVES

After reading this chapter, you should be able to:

- describe the requirements for abstracts for posters or presentations at meetings, and for abstracts for research papers and other types of publications (such as reviews);
- describe and apply an approach to writing abstracts for meetings and for publication;
- use checklists for what to include in an abstract;
- discuss styles of abstracts;
- make abstracts concise; and
- ensure abstracts can be readily found in electronic searches.

KEY TERMS

Abstract guidelines	Electronic searches	MeSH
Abstract headings	IMRAD structure	Methods
Background	Informative abstracts	Objectives
Conclusion	Interim results	Results
Conference abstracts	Introduction	Structured abstracts
CONSORT checklist	Journal abstracts	Unstructured abstracts
Descriptive abstracts	Keywords	

Reporting

abstract to decide whether it is worth the time in a busy schedule to find and read the paper.[7] The abstract should therefore be able to stand alone,[6] as the first—and, unfortunately, often the only—part of the paper most readers read, apart from the title and author list. There are even documented cases in which readers have made clinical decisions from abstracts (although they shouldn't have) because the full text was unavailable.[10]

In the electronic information age, the abstract is also a means for potential readers to find published articles. Electronic searches of abstracts contained in literature databases such as PubMed (MEDLINE), Web of Knowledge, and Scopus (to name a few) lead readers to articles that they might otherwise be unaware of. An abstract must therefore be written in a way that ensures that the paper is not missed in searches where it would be relevant.

From research to abstract

The best abstracts describe a well-designed and carefully conducted study that addresses an important and interesting problem. A good abstract captures the soundness and significance of a good study; it cannot salvage a poor one.

In preparing a **conference abstract** for the SOGC meeting, our gynecology resident goes back to her original research question. What does the study set out to show? How does it do that? Which interim data are relevant to her hypothesis?[11] Finally, why is the research important? What has she learned from it? All other data or outcomes of the research, no matter how interesting, should be set aside.

Once she has collated from her notes the material that answers these questions, the resident checks the guidelines for abstract submissions on the conference website.[12] Such guidelines may include a word limit, **abstract headings**, a list of acceptable acronyms and other abbreviations, information on whether tables and figures can be included with the abstract submission,[6,9] and so on. Not all conferences accept **interim results**; if you are planning to present a preliminary report, be sure to check the guidelines before submitting.

Many beginning researchers do not realize that **abstract guidelines** are strict and should be followed to the letter. Exceeding the word count by even one word, for example, can result in rejection or truncation of the abstract.[12] Use the word count function in word processing software to determine the length of the abstract. It is also a good idea to read abstracts from previous meetings[9] to get a sense of the required content and style.

Most guidelines state that the abstract should summarize the research study following the **IMRAD structure** of a research manuscript: Introduction, Methods, Results, and Discussion.[6,9,11,12] This can apply even when the actual headings are not required.

The **introduction** supplies the research question or study objective as well as background explaining why the question was studied. (In some styles, **background** and **objectives** are broken out separately.[12]) No more than two or three sentences should be used to cover this section.

The **methods** should clearly indicate the study design, instrument (e.g., survey), laboratory technique, assignment or allocation of human or animal subjects, intervention, and outcomes measured.

The **results** should provide data for the outcomes that address the research question. All results should be supported with appropriate descriptive statistics (e.g., mean difference between groups; odds ratio), a measure of precision of the estimate (e.g., 95% confidence interval), and a clear indication of whether the result is statistically significant.[11] However, it may not be possible to provide such statistics for interim results.

If the meeting guidelines allow results to be presented in a table or graph, this is often an efficient way to summarize findings. Again, tables or graphs should include results for the relevant outcomes only; unless the study had few subjects, a table or graph should not include all data.

The **conclusion** should answer the research question and, as appropriate, explain the importance of the findings in the larger research context. Caution should be exercised in reaching conclusions; these should not go beyond the original research question.

The relevance of the research should be clearly conveyed in the abstract, as this is an important opportunity for the researcher to communicate his or her findings to the conference committee. The conference committee judges the abstracts submitted to determine which will be accepted for the meeting. Reviewers on the committee usually assess abstracts on several factors, including the purpose of the research, its methodological rigour, the inclusion of all elements, and the relevance of the study to the discipline in general and to the conference specifically. Clarity of presentation may also be scored. Reviewers may recommend whether abstracts should be accepted for a poster presentation or an oral presentation (the latter is usually more prestigious), or rejected.

Reporting

To ensure that your abstract is clear and conveys its message, apply all of the usual rules of good writing (see ch. 29):

- Prefer the active voice.[6]
- Use strong, simple verbs, such as "to determine," "studied," "found," "treated."
- Use linking words such as "however," "also," "yet," "furthermore."
- Avoid needless phrases such as "We concluded that …"[6]
- Use terms consistently.
- Write in the past tense[8] (except for background about the research question, which may be in the present tense).
- Avoid acronyms and other abbreviations, as they create a difficult-to-read "alphabet soup."[6,12,13]
- If you do use acronyms and other abbreviations, use only well-established ones if possible (do not coin new ones) or those specified in the conference submission guidelines.
- Define acronyms and other abbreviations the first time they are used (some conference submission guidelines allow exceptions such as HIV and DNA).[6]

You may find that, in an effort to include all important points, you have exceeded the word limit in the first draft of your abstract. The next step is to trim it down. Start by finding ways to say the same thing more succinctly. Examine phrases to see if the meaning would be conveyed just as well if the phrase were dropped. Then, if need be, focus the abstract. Is the research question clearly stated, and are all subsequent items tied back to that question? Is there any extraneous information that does not add to the conclusion?

THE CASE REVISITED

The resident writes an abstract, following the submission guidelines carefully, and being sure to include all information relevant to her research question in the IMRAD structure. She submits the abstract by the deadline, and hears from the selection committee a month later. She has been selected to make an oral presentation! A few months later, the big day arrives. She triple-checks her PowerPoint file and boards a bus to the conference. The conference presentation goes very well. Back at her university, she meets with her supervisor, who encourages her to complete her study and write a paper as soon as possible. That means a challenging month ahead, as she tabulates final data and writes the paper. It's almost ready to submit to the *Journal of Obstetrics and Gynaecology Canada*, when she remembers she needs to add the abstract. She opens the abstract she submitted to the conference, selects it, and hits "copy." Fortunately, just as she is about to switch files and hit "paste," she takes a moment to read it over. She realizes her abstract doesn't follow the same structure as the other abstracts she has read in *JOGC*. And the information is now out of date. In fact, in her paper she has changed the conclusion.

From paper to abstract

Despite their obvious importance, **journal abstracts** are far too often unclear and incomplete.[2,6,14–16] Sometimes this is because the main effort is focused on the paper, and the abstract is written hurriedly, as an afterthought. Sometimes it is because a previous meeting abstract has not been updated. Sometimes the problem is a lack of understanding of the abstract's function, or a lack of objective standards for published abstracts—two issues that many journal editors and research organizations have tried to address.[10,17,18]

The best approach is to write the abstract last, working from the completed paper. Any previous version should be either set aside or substantially revised. This means that time and effort must be devoted to the abstract: It should not be forgotten until just before the deadline![12]

Most journals include instructions for the abstract—word limit, structure, headings, and so on—in their instructions for authors. Be sure to consult these before starting to write or revise. For styles of abstracts that may be specified in instructions for authors, see the next section.

Beginning researchers often make the mistake of trying to boil down their entire manuscript into the abstract. In the case of our gynecology resident, she may have presented data from different categories of patients, from different tissues, and so on. In experiments involving humans, the data can be complicated, relating to several arms of the study, side effects, and patient drop-outs. An abstract cannot present every detail of a complex manuscript. You should also be aware that, although tables and charts may be accepted in conference abstracts, they do not appear in abstracts for published papers.

Reporting

Which details should be included? Again, return to your primary research question and focus on the data that answer the question.

Several journals and research groups have made specific recommendations to ensure that relevant data are not missed or omitted from published abstracts. Table 27.1 shows a checklist from the CONSORT group[10] for the data to include in an abstract of a randomized controlled trial. The aim of this checklist is to provide specific instructions about key elements of a trial that should be included in the abstract. The authors argue that, without a minimum of key information, it is difficult to assess the validity and applicability of a trial.

This checklist may not fit the abstract style specified by your target journal in its instructions to authors, in terms of headings and order of elements. However, it is a useful adjunct to the journal instructions to ensure the information is included, even if it is under a different heading or in a different order.

Table 27.2 provides the abstract headings required by the *Annals of Internal Medicine* for original research, cost-effectiveness studies, and systematic reviews (including meta-analyses). These headings were first recommended in 1987–1990 by proponents of evidence-based medicine to facilitate peer review, help clinical readers find articles that are scientifically sound and applicable, and allow more precise electronic literature searches.[18] For manuscripts destined for journals that do not use these headings, the list simply provides another useful checklist for information to include in abstracts of the types of manuscripts covered.

■ **Table 27.1: CONSORT checklist for abstracts for randomized controlled trials[17]**

Title*	Identification of the study as randomized
Authors	Contact details for the corresponding author
Trial design	Description of the trial design (e.g. parallel, cluster, non-inferiority)
Methods	
Participants	Eligibility criteria for participants and the settings where the data were collected
Interventions	Interventions intended for each group
Objectives	Specific objective or hypothesis
Outcome	Clearly defined primary outcome for this report
Randomization	How participants were allocated to interventions
Blinding (masking)	Whether or not participants, care givers, and those assessing the outcomes were blinded to group assignment
Results	
Numbers randomized	Number of participants randomized to each group
Recruitment	Trial status
Numbers analyzed	Number of participants analysed in each group
Outcomes	For the primary outcome, a result for each group and the estimated effect size and its precision
Harms	Important adverse events or side effects
Conclusions	General interpretation of the results
Trial registration†	Registration number and name of trial register
Funding†	Source of funding

* Although they appear in the CONSORT checklist, the title and authors are not usually included in abstracts for conferences or journals.
† While CONSORT recommends that these items be included in the abstract, many journals publish them with the author affiliations or acknowledgements. Check the style of the journal.

Reporting

■ **Table 27.2:** *Annals of Internal Medicine* **headings for abstracts for three manuscript types**[19]

Original research
    Background
    Objective
    Design
    Setting
    Patients
    Intervention (if any)
    Measurements
    Results
    Limitations
    Conclusions

    If the study is a randomized controlled trial, list where the trial is registered and the trial's unique registration number at the end of the abstract.

Cost-effectiveness studies
    Background
    Objective
    Design
    Data sources
    Target population
    Time horizon
    Perspective
    Interventions
    Outcome measures
    Results of base-case analysis
    Results of sensitivity analysis
    Limitations
    Conclusions

Systematic reviews, including meta-analyses
    Background
    Purpose
    Data sources
    Study selection
    Data extraction
    Data synthesis
    Limitations
    Conclusions

Types of abstracts

Before writing the abstract for a paper, ascertain the type of abstract and the format from the journal's instructions for authors. The following outlines some of the considerations in preparing abstracts of specific types.

Structured and unstructured abstracts. Abstracts for research papers may be **unstructured** (consisting of one continuous paragraph) or **structured** (using bolded or italicized headings that break the text into sections).[6] See examples in Appendix 27.1.

Most abstract structures are based on IMRAD, with some variations. The heading scheme for abstracts in *Annals of Internal Medicine* (Table 27.2) has the most headings of any system currently in use.[19] Many journals require structured abstracts for certain types of manuscripts (research papers, reviews), and unstructured abstracts for other types (editorials, brief reports). When writing a structured abstract with many headings, it is acceptable to write in point form (except that the Results and Discussion often require full sentences), whereas unstructured abstracts should be written in full sentences.

Even if an abstract is unstructured, the text should include all the elements of the IMRAD structure, in the appropriate order. For research paper abstracts, an appropriate checklist such as CONSORT is a valuable tool.

Informative vs descriptive abstracts. Abstract styles can also be categorized as informative or descriptive (sometimes called *indicative*).[7] Most abstracts, especially for research papers, are informative, providing the information on the study design, methods, results, and conclusion in the IMRAD structure, or following one of the alternative heading structures. However, there are certain contexts in which it makes more sense to indicate the article's scope, the principal subjects discussed, and how the topics will be addressed in the article, providing an overview of the paper.[7] This type of abstract is called "descriptive." Descriptive abstracts are used mainly for traditional review articles that present a literature search with clinical conclusions. See examples in Appendix 27.1.

Abstracts for systematic reviews and case reports. Many recent review papers are systematic reviews, in which data from systematically identified and selected research papers are extracted and may even be pooled and analyzed together in a meta-analysis. (See ch. 15.) In this case, an informative abstract provides the methodology and the analysis results. See the heading scheme for systematic reviews in *Annals of Internal Medicine* (Table 27.2) for a good checklist to follow in preparing abstracts for such papers. See examples in Appendix 27.1.

Another type of research paper often prepared by trainees is the case report or case series. Again, the abstract content and style differs. The abstract may be shorter than for original research, and some journals do not include abstracts with such papers at all. If required, the abstract should include the following:[12]

Reporting

- objective
- case summary or case presentation (include patient details)
- discussion (omitted by some journals)
- conclusions

For case series, criteria for the selection of cases, and the number of cases thus selected, should also be indicated. See examples in Appendix 27.1.

Considerations in writing or revising abstracts

Electronic retrieval

To find research papers, researchers search abstracts in electronic databases such as PubMed, Web of Knowledge, and Scopus. Although the best-known databases have professional indexers who apply indexing terms to each abstract, there is a delay in applying terms, and not all databases and search engines (e.g., Google) are indexed. Hence, some publishers now recommend "optimizing" abstracts so that **electronic searches** will find them easily.[20] It is worthwhile to consider which terms a researcher would use to search for articles in the pertinent research area, and ensure that those terms appear in the abstract. For example, our resident's abstract should contain terms about cytologic findings ("cytology") in tissue samples from uterine hyperplasia ("uterus," "hyperplasia"), including malignant cells ("uterine cancer" or "uterine neoplasms").

In medical literature, ensure as well that the relevant medical subject headings (**MeSH**) appear in the abstract (see ch. 7). This can be awkward if the researcher has used a non-MeSH term throughout the research: for example, if the paper refers to Stein-Leventhal syndrome, but the MeSH term for the same entity is polycystic ovary syndrome. In this case, the best course would be to use the MeSH term in the paper; if this is not possible, however, it is good practice to include the MeSH term in brackets after the first mention in the abstract, i.e., "patients with Stein-Leventhal syndrome (polycystic ovary syndrome)." This ensures that savvy searchers, who use MeSH terms, will find the paper.[a]

Keywords

Some journals ask researchers to submit a few **keywords** with their abstract. The usefulness of these keywords is questionable, as abstract databases such as MEDLINE (PubMed) are professionally indexed and do not use author-supplied keywords at all. However, if researchers are asked to supply keywords, they should select three to five terms that capture the broad subject areas of the research, either from a list of keywords supplied by the journal, or from MeSH if the journal does not have a list.

Short versions of abstracts

Some journals request, in addition, an even shorter "abstract" of two or three sentences to appear in the table of contents. Read some of the journal's tables of contents to get a feel for style and elements covered.

Remember to revise

Journal editors often complain that abstracts do not reflect the paper: sometimes information in the abstract differs from the manuscript or does not appear in the manuscript at all. Studies have found high rates of inconsistent data and conclusions between published papers and their abstracts, even in major medical journals.[21–23] This is mainly because researchers simply forget to revise the abstract along with the manuscript.

While the best practice is to write the abstract after finalizing the paper, there may be unanticipated changes to a manuscript before submission but after the abstract is written. If so, the abstract should be verified and revised to ensure it is consistent with the paper, as the focus may have changed during revision. After peer review, the paper may be revised, and, again, the abstract should be verified and revised as well. The final abstract should match the paper not only in terms of data accuracy, but also in terms of its conclusions and tone. For example, if the paper reaches a tentative conclusion in a narrow area, the abstract should not state the conclusion firmly or extend the conclusion beyond what was concluded in the paper.

Reporting

---

a For more about MeSH, see www.nlm.nih.gov/mesh.

CASE POSTSCRIPT

The resident writes a 300-word abstract for her manuscript, a case-control study showing that a significantly higher percentage of surgical samples from a certain benign condition (uterine hyperplasia) contain malignant cells than samples from other benign conditions. She receives constructive peer reviews and revises the manuscript and the abstract accordingly. The paper is accepted and appears a few months later in *JOGC*.

Through this process, the resident has demonstrated she can:

- Read and follow the guidelines on the conference website and the instructions for authors on the journal website for word limit, style of abstract (structured versus unstructured, informative versus indicative), and other requirements.
- Focus on the research question, and data that answer it, in preparing a meeting abstract, the paper, and the abstract for publication.
- Use a checklist as a guide to ensure she has included all the needed elements for the abstract.
- Substantially revise the meeting abstract to accompany the subsequent manuscript, ensuring the abstract is succinct, focused, and consistent with the paper.
- Ensure the abstract contains words that will be searched by researchers retrieving papers in the area.

REFERENCES

1. Scherer RW, Dickersin K, Langenberg P. Full publication of results initially presented in abstracts. A meta-analysis. *JAMA*. 1994;272(2):158–62.

2. Bhandari M, Devereaux PJ, Guyatt GH, Cook DJ, Swiontkowski MF, Sprague S, et al. An observational study of orthopaedic abstracts and subsequent full-text publications. *J Bone Joint Surg Am*. 2002;84-A(4):615–21.

3. De Bellefeuille C, Morrison CA, Tannock IF. The fate of abstracts submitted to a cancer meeting: factors which influence presentation and subsequent publication. *Ann Oncol*. 1992;3(3):187–91.

4. Castillo J, Garcia-Guasch R, Cifuentes I. Fate of abstracts from the Paris 1995 European Society of Anaesthesiologists meeting. *Eur J Anaesthesiol*. 2002;19(12):888–93.

5. Marx WF, Cloft HJ, Do HM, Kallmes DF. The fate of neuroradiologic abstracts presented at national meetings in 1993: rate of subsequent publication in peer-reviewed, indexed journals. *AJNR Am J Neuroradiol*. 1999;20(6):1173–7.

6. Cornett PL. Writing abstracts. In: Witte FM, Dew Taylor N, editors. *Essays for biomedical communicators*. Volume 1 of selected AMWA workshops. Bethesda (MD): American Medical Writers Association; 2001. p. 92–100.

7. Eastman JD, Klein ER. Writing abstracts. In: Minick P, editor. *Biomedical communication: selected AMWA workshops*. Bethesda (MD): American Medical Writers Association; 1994. p. 143–6.

8. Day RA, Gastel B. *How to write and publish a scientific paper*. 6th ed. Westport (CT) and London: Greenwood Press; 2006. p. 52–5.

9. Pierson DJ. How to write an abstract that will be accepted for presentation at a national meeting. *Respir Care*. 2004;49(10):1206–12.

10. Hopewell S, Clarke M, Moher D, Wager E, Middleton P, Altman DG, et al. CONSORT for reporting randomised trials in journal and conference abstracts. *Lancet*. 2008;371(9609):281–3.

11. Alexandrov AV, Hennerici MG. Writing good abstracts. *Cerebrovasc Dis*. 2007;23(4):256–9.

12. Boullata JI, Mancuso CE. A "how-to" guide in preparing abstracts and poster presentations. *Nutr Clin Pract*. 2007;22(6):641–6.

13. Foote M. Some concrete ideas about manuscript abstracts. *Chest*. 2006;129(5):1375–7.

14. Hill CL, Buchbinder R, Osborne R. Quality of reporting of randomized clinical trials in abstracts of the 2005 annual meeting of the American College of Rheumatology. *J Rheumatol*. 2007;34(12):2476–80.

Reporting

15. Krzyzanowska MK, Pintilie M, Brezden-Masley C, Dent R, Tannock IF. Quality of abstracts describing randomized trials in the proceedings of American Society of Clinical Oncology meetings: guidelines for improved reporting. *J Clin Oncol.* 2004;22(10):1993–9.

16. Ubriani R, Smith N, Katz KA. Reporting of study design in titles and abstracts of articles published in clinically oriented dermatology journals. *Br J Dermatol.* 2007;156(3):557–9.

17. Hopewell S, Clarke M, Moher D, Wager E, Middleton P, Altman DG, et al. CONSORT for reporting randomized controlled trials in journal and conference abstracts: explanation and elaboration. *PLoS Med.* 2008;5(1):e20.

18. Haynes RB, Mulrow CD, Huth EJ, Altman DG, Gardner MJ. More informative abstracts revisited. *Ann Intern Med.* 1990;113(1):69–76.

19. Information for Authors. Annals of Internal Medicine. Available from: www.annals.org/site/misc/ifora.xhtml.

20. Wiley-Blackwell. Author services: optimizing your article for search engines. Available from: http://authorservices.wiley.com/bauthor/seo.asp

21. Pitkin RM, Branagan MA, Burmeister LF. Accuracy of data in abstracts of published research articles. *JAMA.* 1999;281(12):1110–1.

22. Pitkin RM, Branagan MA. Can the accuracy of abstracts be improved by providing specific instructions? A randomized controlled trial. *JAMA.* 1998;280(3):267–9.

23. Ward LG, Kendrach MG, Price SO. Accuracy of abstracts for original research articles in pharmacy journals. *Ann Pharmacother.* 2004;38(7–8):1173–7.

EXERCISES

1. Choose abstracts from published randomized controlled trials (see examples in Appendix 27.1 or search for recent articles in your area in PubMed). Analyze these according to the CONSORT extension for abstracts. Are any elements missing? How did the researcher organize the elements? Is each abstract clear, readable, and complete?

2. Have a friend choose a good research paper from your field and remove the abstract. Read the paper and write the abstract. Compare your abstract with the author's. Does your version have any omissions or oversights? Does the author's ?

Reporting

SUMMARY CHECKLIST

❏ Consider where you will be submitting an abstract of your work. Assemble any information you will need about the required structure, word count, etc. Review abstracts that have previously been accepted to guide your composition.

❏ Consider the target audience of your abstract. What will they know about this type of study? What will they care about? What results should you emphasize?

❏ Construct your abstract carefully using best practices.

❏ Send your abstract to your team, supervisors and colleagues for review. Revise and repeat.

❏ Select key words.

❏ Submit.

APPENDIX 27.1: ABSTRACT EXAMPLES

UNSTRUCTURED INFORMATIVE ABSTRACT

Soy and the exercise-induced inflammatory response in postmenopausal women[a]
Beavers KM, Serra MC, Beavers DP, Cooke MB, Willoughby DS

Aging is associated with increasing inflammation and oxidative stress in the body, both of which can have negative health effects. Successful attenuation of such processes with dietary countermeasures has major public health implications. Soy foods, as a source of high-quality protein and isoflavones, may improve such indices, although the effects in healthy postmenopausal women are not well delineated. A single-blind, randomized controlled trial was conducted in 31 postmenopausal women who were assigned to consume 3 servings of soy (n = 16) or dairy (n = 15) milk per day for 4 weeks. Parameters of systemic inflammation (tumor necrosis factor-α (TNF-α), interleukin-1β (IL-1β), and interleukin-6 (IL-6)) and the oxidative defense system (superoxide dismutase (SOD), glutathione peroxidase, cyclooxygenase-2) were measured post supplementation, before and after an eccentric exercise bout performed to elicit an inflammatory response. A significant group-by-time effect for plasma TNF-α was observed ($p = 0.02$), with values in the dairy group increased post supplementation and then decreasing into the postexercise period. Additionally, significant time effects were observed for plasma SOD ($p < 0.0001$) and IL-6 ($p < 0.0001$) in the postexercise period. Overall results from our study do not support the notion that 4 weeks of daily soy milk ingestion can attenuate systemic elevations in markers of inflammation or oxidative defense. However, data do suggest that the downhill-running protocol utilized in this study can be effective in altering systemic markers of inflammation and oxidative defense enzyme activity, and that the ingestion of soy may help prevent fluctuations in plasma TNF-α.

Appl Physiol Nutr Metab. 2010;35(3):261–9

STRUCTURED INFORMATIVE ABSTRACT

Long-term effects of dihydrotestosterone treatment on prostate growth in healthy, middle-aged men without prostate disease: a randomized, placebo-controlled trial[b]
Idan A, Griffiths KA, Harwood T, Seibel MJ, Turner L, Conway AJ, et al.

Background: Benign prostatic hypertrophy increases with age and can result in substantially decreased quality of life for older men. Surgery is often required to control symptoms. It has been hypothesized that long-term administration of a nonamplifiable pure androgen might decrease prostate growth, thereby decreasing or delaying the need for surgical intervention.

Objective: To test the hypothesis that dihydrotestosterone (DHT), a nonamplifiable and nonaromatizable pure androgen, reduces late-life prostate growth in middle-aged men.

Design: Randomized, placebo-controlled, parallel-group trial. (Australian New Zealand Clinical Trials Registry number: ACTRN12605000358640)

Setting: Ambulatory care research center.

Participants: Healthy men (n = 114) older than 50 years without known prostate disease.

Intervention: Transdermal DHT (70 mg) or placebo gel daily for 2 years.

Measurements: Prostate volume was measured by ultrasonography; bone mineral density (BMD) and body composition were measured by dual-energy x-ray absorptiometry; and blood samples and questionnaires were collected every 6 months, with data analyzed by mixed-model analysis for repeated measures.

Results: Over 24 months, there was an increase in total (29% [95% CI, 23% to 34%]) and central (75% [CI, 64% to 86%]; $P < 0.01$) prostate volume and serum prostate-specific antigen level (15% [CI, 6% to 24%]) with time on study, but DHT had no effect ($P > 0.2$). Dihydrotestosterone treatment decreased spinal BMD (1.4% [CI, 0.6% to 2.3%]; $P < 0.001$) at 24 months but not hip BMD ($P > 0.2$) and increased serum aminoterminal propeptide of type I procollagen in the second year of the study compared with placebo. Dihydrotestosterone increased serum DHT levels and its metabolites (5α-androstane-3β,17β-diol and 5α-androstane-3β,17β-diol) and suppressed serum testosterone, estradiol, luteinizing hormone, and follicle-stimulating hormone levels. Dihydrotestosterone increased hemoglobin levels (7% [CI,

Reporting

5% to 9%]), serum creatinine levels (9% [CI, 5% to 11%]), and lean mass (2.4% [CI, 1.6% to 3.1%) but decreased fat mass (5.2% [CI, 2.6% to 7.7%]) ($P <0.001$ for all). Protocol-specific discontinuations due to DHT were asymptomatic increased hematocrit ($n = 8$), which resolved after stopping treatment, and increased prostate-specific antigen levels ($n = 3$; none with prostate cancer) in the DHT group. No serious adverse effects due to DHT occurred.

Limitation: Negative findings on prostate growth cannot exclude adverse effects on the natural history of prostate cancer.

Conclusion: Dihydrotestosterone treatment for 24 months has no beneficial or adverse effect on prostate growth but causes a decrease in spinal but not hip BMD. These findings have important implications for the wider use of nonsteroidal pure androgens in older men.

Primary funding source: BHR Pharma.

Ann Intern Med. 2010;153(10):621–32.

DESCRIPTIVE ABSTRACTS

Meningococcal serogroup C conjugate vaccination in Canada: How far have we progressed? How far do we have to go?[c]
White CP, Scott J

Since routine meningococcal C conjugate vaccination was introduced into Canada in 2002, there have been a large regional variation in the routine programs, changes to the timing of the infant series in some provinces, and wide differences in catch-up programs. As immunization is viewed as a provincial responsibility, less attention has been paid to determining national coverage rates and the direct and indirect effects of the widely varying provincial/territorial vaccination programs on the nation as a whole. Canada's disjointed regional immunization campaigns leave the population at risk of disease for an extended length of time. The United Kingdom has proven that with a pro-active approach to planning, coordination, and implementation of a national immunization program, excellent long-term control of invasive meningococcal disease in a large population could be achieved in as little as one year. A summation of the current meningococcal immunization strategies used in Canada and an estimate of overall vaccine coverage of children and youth is provided.

Can J Public Health. 2010;101(1):12–14

Origami in outer membrane mimetics: correlating the first detailed images of refolded VDAC with over 20 years of biochemical data[d]
Summers WAT, Court DA

Mitochondrial porin forms an aqueous pore in the outer membrane, through which selective passage of small metabolites and ions occurs, thereby regulating both mitochondrial function and cellular respiration. Investigations of the structure and function of porin have been performed with whole mitochondria, membrane vesicles, artificial membranes, and in detergent solutions, resulting in numerous models of porin structure. The mechanisms by which this protein functions are undoubtedly linked to its structure, which remained elusive until 2008, with reports of 3 high-resolution structures of this voltage-dependent, anion-selective channel (VDAC). The barrel structure is relatively simple yet unique: it is arranged as 19 anti-parallel β-strands, with β-strands 1 and 19 aligned parallel to each other to close the barrel. The N-terminal helical component is located within the lumen of the channel, although its precise structure and location in the lumen varies. With the basic barrel structure in hand, the data obtained in attempts to model the structure and understand porin over the past 20 years can be re-evaluated. Herein, using the mammalian VDAC structures as templates, the amassed electrophysiological and biochemical information has been reassessed with respect to the functional mechanisms of VDAC activity, with a focus on voltage-dependent gating.

Biochem Cell Biol. 2010;88(3):425–38

SYSTEMATIC REVIEW

Dietary interventions for fecal occult blood test screening: systematic review of the literature[e]
Konrad G

Objective: To determine whether dietary restrictions enhance the specificity of guaiac-based fecal occult blood tests (FOBTs) when screening for colorectal cancer.

Data sources: PubMed–MEDLINE, the Cumulative Index to Nursing and Allied Health Literature, and Cochrane databases were searched.

Study selection. English-language case series, cohort studies, randomized controlled trials (RCTs), and meta-analyses were selected. Studies that did not include dietary manipulation or the use of guaiac-based FOBTs available in North America were excluded.

---

c Reprinted with kind permission of the Canadian Public Health Association.

d Copyright 2010 Canadian Science Publishing or its licensors. Reproduced with kind permission of the publisher.

e Reproduced with kind permission of the College of Family Physicians of Canada.

Synthesis: Ten case series, 5 cohort studies, 4 RCTs, and 1 meta-analysis were critically appraised. All studies used Hemoccult, Hemoccult II, or Hemoccult SENSA tests. Data from case series involving challenge diets showed no increase in positive FOBT results from high-peroxidase vegetables, but results varied with red-meat challenges depending on the amount of meat consumed and the test used. Case series, cohort studies, and RCTs comparing FOBT results during restricted versus unrestricted diets consistently showed no differences in positive FOBT results.

Conclusion: Most of the evidence evaluating the effect of dietary restrictions on FOBT results is dated and of suboptimal quality. However, 4 RCTs and a meta-analysis of these data do not support dietary restrictions when screening for colorectal cancer. Because patient adherence can be an issue with FOBTs, and dietary restrictions can affect adherence in some populations, it is reasonable to abandon these recommendations without fear of substantially affecting specificity.

Can Fam Physician. 2010;56(3):229–38

CASE REPORT

The diagnostic and therapeutic approach of a primary bilateral leiomyoma of the ovaries: a case report and a literature review[f]

van Esch EM, van Wijngaarden SE, Schaafsma HE, Smeets MJ, Rhemrev JP

Introduction: A primary fibroid (leiomyoma) arising from both ovaries is rare and can be difficult to diagnose as a result of the low incidence and its indistinctive presentation. A literature review on the diagnostic and therapeutic approach of this rare benign tumour is presented. We describe a case of bilateral primary ovarian fibroid with an unusual presentation to illustrate our recommendations for treatment.

Case presentation: A 37-year-old woman was admitted with symptoms of acute severe abdominal pain. She had a history of faint abdominal discomfort. Due to the acute deterioration of the abdominal pain a diagnostic laparoscopy was performed. A tumour arising from both ovaries was seen and a biopsy was taken in order to decide on further therapy. Histology showed a fibroid for which excision by a second laparoscopic intervention was planned. Due to excessive adhesions conversion to laparotomy was necessary.

Conclusion: We recommend that in the case of an abnormal adnexal mass, particularly in women who want to preserve their fertility, frozen section histology be performed laparoscopically. A frozen section diagnostic procedure, instead of a regular biopsy, seems to be a useful tool during an elective diagnostic laparoscopic procedure in order to prevent potential morbidity as a result of possible future laparoscopy or even laparotomy. Previous laparoscopic procedures can cause massive adhesions that could impede a subsequent laparoscopic approach.

Arch Gynecol Obstet. 2010;283(6):1369–71

CASE SERIES

Urological complications of laparoscopic inguinal hernia repair: a case series[g]

Kocot A, Gerharz EW, Riedmiller H

Objectives: To illustrate urological complications of laparoscopic inguinal hernia repair and discuss their management.

Patients: Between April 2002 and February 2004, four men (aged 38–63 years) were treated for serious complications 2 days to 11 years after unilateral (1 patient) or bilateral (3 patients) laparoscopic inguinal hernioplasty.

Results: In all cases (extra and intraperitoneal bladder injury, purulent urocystitis due to mesh-erosion of the bladder, secondary retroperitoneal fibrosis) open revision with complete drainage of the urinary tract was chosen as an efficacious therapeutic strategy.

Conclusions: Awareness of rare complications of laparoscopic inguinal hernia repair may lead to early diagnosis and appropriate management.

Hernia. 2010 Jul 4. [Epub ahead of print]

Reporting

---

f   Reprinted with kind permission of Springer Science + Business Media.

g   Reprinted with kind permission of Springer Science + Business Media.

APPENDIX 27.2: APPLYING CHECKLISTS TO ABSTRACTS

EXAMPLE 1

Health promotion program: a resident well-being study. *Iowa Orthop J* 2009;29:83–7.[h]
Watson DT, Long WJ, Yen D, Pichora DR

Background: Surgical training places unique stresses on residents that can lead to decreased levels of presenteeism. We hypothesized that presenteeism levels could be positively influenced by improving workplace hygiene.

Methods: A cohort of surgical residents was asked to complete the Stanford Presenteeism Scale: Health Status and Employee Productivity (SPS-6) questionnaire before, and one year after the implementation of a workplace health promotion program.

Results: Twenty-six of thirty-three residents responded to the initial survey and reported a mean SPS-6 score of 17.3 ± 4.5, well below population normative value of 24 ± 3 (p < 0.0001). At one-year post intervention 25 of 32 residents responded, reporting a mean SPS-6 score of 18.3 ± 4.6. The mean SPS-6 score improved by 1.2 ± 3.8 (p = 0.35). Sub-group analysis showed a trend toward improved SPS-6 in those who participated in the health promotion program (p = 0.15) and a significant difference when junior residents were compared to seniors (p = 0.034). Overall, results were limited by our small sample size.

Conclusions: Presenteeism scores for surgical residents at our institution are well below population values. Use of validated tools such as the SPS-6 may allow for more objective analysis and decision making when planning for resident education and workload.

Presenteeism: the ability while on the job to produce quality work at maximum productivity.
Decreased presenteeism: a state of decreased productivity and below-normal work quality related to health/workplace distracters.)

Iowa Orthop J. 2009;29:83–7.

CONSORT checklist analysis of this sample abstract

- **Trial design.** Can be inferred; qualitative study with questionnaire before and after intervention. From results, it is unclear whether all survey respondents participated in the intervention.
- **Participants.** Thirty-three residents.
- **Interventions.** Workplace health promotion program; little information on what this involved.
- **Objectives.** Hypothesis clear: improved workplace hygiene could improve presenteeism (which is defined).
- **Outcome.** Primary outcome seems to be change in score on SPS-6, but this is not stated explicitly.
- **Randomization.** Not applicable.
- **Blinding.** Not applicable.
- **Numbers randomized.** Not applicable.
- **Recruitment.** Not applicable.
- **Numbers analyzed.** Number that responded to survey given.
- **Outcomes.** (1) Initial SPS-6 score was significantly lower than normal; (2) the intervention resulted in limited, non-significant improvement in SPS-6 scores; (3) a subgroup change in score showed slightly better but still non-significant improvement; (4) significant difference between junior and senior residents. For each result, the effect size, precision (±) and statistical significance are given.
- **Problems with outcomes.** (1) A subgroup analysis seems to suggest not all participants underwent the intervention, and this does not make sense as the methods indicate testing improvement after intervention, presumably in all participants. (2) "A trend toward improved SPS-6" implies an indication of improvement, but the result is not statistically significant and should not be represented as meaningful. (3) It is unclear what is meant by "a significant difference when junior residents were compared to seniors"—junior residents considered as a subgroup had a significant difference before and after the intervention? Junior residents had a significantly different score from senior residents? Which group showed improvement?
- **Harms.** None presented; qualitative study. Does not state the lack of harm explicitly.
- **Conclusions.** Presenteeism values for this group are low. This is the only significant result. Fails to state that other results were not significant and that the results are therefore negative. Discusses use of validated survey tool; however, this was not an objective of the study.

Reporting

---

h   Reprinted with kind permission of the *Iowa Orthopedic Journal*

EXAMPLE 2

Gender preferences in the choice of a pediatric dental residency program.

da Fonseca MA, Stiers ML

The goal of this study was to investigate whether men and women applying for graduate training in pediatric dentistry placed different emphasis on the same factors and program characteristics upon making their final ranking decision. A questionnaire was mailed to the first-year resident class in the United States in 2005 containing both multiple-choice and open-ended questions covering six sections: 1) candidate's background, 2) the application process, 3) program characteristics, 4) nonclinical factors, 5) clinical factors, and 6) the interview process. In sections three through six, respondents ranked factors and characteristics from "not important" or "no influence" to "critical." The response rate was 69.2 percent (180/260), with approximately 57.8 percent females (104/180) and 61.4 percent non-Hispanic white respondents (110/180). Statistically significant differences between genders were as follows: 1) men were older (29.4 years versus 28.1, $p < 0.05$); 2) men applied to more programs (9.9 vs. 8.1, $p < 0.05$); 3) women preferred programs affiliated with their own dental school ($p = 0.046$); 4) women preferred university-based programs ($p = 0.049$); 5) women preferred programs that offered a high amount of patient care under general anesthesia ($p = 0.040$); and 6) women placed more importance on the salary/stipend amount offered by the programs ($p = 0.045$).

J Dent Educ. 2009;73(9):1102–6.[i]

Annals of Internal Medicine checklist analysis of this example abstract

- **Background.** Does not explain background to study. Is there a concern that more men than women (or vice versa) are applying for certain types of graduate training in pediatric dentistry?
- **Objective.** Clearly stated in first sentence: gender differences in factors and program characteristics in making ranking decisions.
- **Design.** Can be inferred: qualitative study with questionnaire.
- **Setting.** Clear that this is a country-wide survey (United States in 2005).
- **Patients.** Participants were all first-year residents in pediatric dentistry.

- **Intervention.** Survey, with detailed explanation of questions, their format and the ranking system.
- **Measurements.** Not stated, presumably scores on the survey.
- **Results.** Response rate and absolute number of respondents indicated. The ethnic background of the respondents is given, which was not an objective of the study and seems to be irrelevant. Consistent with the objective, only statistically significant differences between gender groups are reported. Actual mean rankings are not given; statistical significance is given. Measure of variability is not applicable, as this is a survey of the entire population, not just a sample.
- **Limitations.** Not stated. Does the ethnic group response rate result mean the survey results should not be generalized to all ethnic groups?
- **Conclusions.** No conclusions are stated. The authors may have thought that these were clear from the results, but there should be a statement about gender differences and their practical significance. This would have followed from the background, which is also missing. The authors may have wished to comment on the borderline statistical significance of some of the results.

Reporting

i   Reprinted with kind permission of Journal of Dental Education. Copyright 2009 by the American Dental Education Association, www.jdentaled.org

Reporting

28
Communicating your research with slide and poster presentations

Jeffrey J. Perry, MD, MSc, CCFP(EM)

ILLUSTRATIVE CASE

A diagnostic imaging resident has completed a research project determining the sensitivity of computed tomography for the diagnosis of subarachnoid hemorrhage. She has submitted her structured abstract to the Canadian Association of Emergency Physicians (CAEP) conference and the Society for Academic Emergency Medicine (SAEM) meeting. The abstract was accepted for an oral presentation by CAEP and as a poster presentation by SAEM. Now the resident needs to create slide and poster presentations that clearly convey the importance, methods, results and potential impact of her work.

■ **You've submitted an abstract of** your research to a specialty conference (see ch. 27), and now you've been invited to present your findings at the meeting. This occasion is a valuable opportunity for you to expand on the synopsis given in your abstract, and a chance to disseminate your findings, network with colleagues with similar interests, and get feedback that can be very useful as you prepare a manuscript for submission to a journal or continue with further research.[1] Oral **slide presentations** are usually limited to 10 minutes, with an additional 5 minutes allotted for questions and the transition between presenters. Most conferences are very strict with these timelines, and so it is important to know how to get your message across efficiently and effectively. The essential ingredients of an effective oral presentation are: (1) organization of content; (2) clarity of slides; and (3) a well-rehearsed presentation.

Poster presentations convey similar information but, of course, in a very different format. Depending on the format of the conference, a poster can be presented one-on-one or to a small group, or it may be displayed without the researcher present to provide additional information. Although this type of presentation is more informal, it is no less challenging than a slide presentation. You will need to attract attention to your poster by making it visually appealing, easy to read from a distance and self-explanatory. If the format of the conference involves small presentations, then a short oral presentation needs to be prepared with only the poster available as a visual aid. Given the amount of work that you have invested in your research, you owe it to yourself to prepare an effective and professional-looking poster.

CHAPTER OBJECTIVES

After reading this chapter, you should be able to:
- describe the important aspects of a research presentation
- describe how to prepare an effective oral slide presentation
- describe how to prepare an effective poster presentation

Reporting

KEY TERMS	
Abstract	Poster presentation
Presentation	PowerPoint
Slide presentation	

Slide presentations

Preparing an effective text

In your text, use a point-form presentation but don't compress the phrasing to the point where the meaning becomes cryptic or ambiguous. Avoid acronyms and other abbreviations as much as possible unless they are standard for your audience (e.g., "ED" will be readily recognized as "emergency department" at an Emergency Medicine conference). Citations are typically not given in the main text, but you can decide to make your key references available in a footnote at the bottom of the slide or in a separate slide at the end; these should be large enough to be read easily.

Structuring your presentation

The basic structure of your slide presentation will essentially mirror the elements of the abstract you submitted to the conference (see ch. 27), as follows: Title, Introduction (background), Objectives (research question), Methods (study design, study population, study procedure(s), outcome measures, analysis, and sample size calculations), Results, and Discussion (limitations and strengths, conclusion).

Title slide. On this slide, give the title of the presentation along with the names of the investigators, the institution coordinating the study, the institutions participating in the study, and the funding agency (if applicable). If this information is plentiful (e.g., there are many co-investigators, or granting agencies), move the information about funding sources to the second slide.

Introduction. Your introduction should consist of two slides. The first slide typically gives some background information about the clinical problem, and the second provides the rationale for the study: that is, *why* it was done. This explanation needs to be clear and concise.

Objectives. This slide should concisely state your research question (i.e., the goal of study and specific objectives/hypotheses).

Methods. You will likely need roughly six slides to describe the study methods. These address the *who* and the *how*. Typically, one slide covers the study design, location(s) and time frame. The next slide or two will describe the study population, including inclusion and exclusion criteria. Then, a separate slide describes the study procedure(s) or

intervention, followed by a slide describing the main outcome(s), a slide on the statistical analyses performed, and, finally, a slide showing sample size calculations and assumptions.

Results. The results of your study should be the focal point of the presentation. Display them in a concise manner that is easy to read and interpret. Make sure that the results are "trimmed down" so that only important results are presented and the audience does not get lost in the details and miss the main findings. The data you include must support your comments in the discussion and conclusion.

Discussion: In this section, you can discuss issues that are pertinent to the research question, how the results compare with those of previous studies, or your interpretation of why the results are what they are (see ch. 26). One strategy is to develop a "story" that ties your findings to existing data. This allows the listener to see how your work adds to the current body of knowledge on your topic. Typically, this concise attempt to develop a hypothesis about the implications of results will be the main thing that the audience remembers.

- *Limitations and strengths.* Present one or two of the main limitations and strengths of your study on one slide; point out the potential impact that any limitations might have on your results.
- *Conclusion.* In your concluding slide, summarize your results and what they mean. This slide should succinctly reiterate the "story" you presented earlier, reminding the audience why your research matters. You may suggest directions for further research here as well, but this should not be the main conclusion.

Preparing your slides

Use the "less is more" principle in designing your slides. Microsoft **PowerPoint** offers many stylization features that, if overused, are more likely to make your audience wonder about how you got a certain cool effect than to keep them focused on your message. To create emphasis, change the minimum number of elements possible to do the job: that is, you don't need to combine bold with italic, underlining, capital letters, a new colour and larger type to draw attention to a word. One or two of these attributes will do. Use one typeface, a limited number of sizes, and a

Reporting

consistent colour palette throughout the presentation. A sans serif[a] typeface such as Arial or Verdana is usually the best choice for small blocks of text meant to be read at a distance. Because some typefaces are more compact than others, the type size you need to achieve legibility will vary; using Arial, for example, you might want a size 28 to 32 font for text and a size 34 to 44 bolded font for titles. Also, choose widely used typefaces that are standard to both Mac and PC operating systems; not all fonts display properly on both platforms. Also remember that "reverse type" (white against black or a dark colour) can look attractive but if overused is difficult to read.

Tables and figures. Use tables and figures where possible to replace text: they can compress a great deal of quantitative data into a small space, facilitate comparisons, and show trends and effects at a glance. A rule of thumb for tables is to display percentages, rather than raw numbers, giving the total number of patients or the relevant denominator (the n) in the column heading

Ensure that your tables and figures are self-explanatory, containing all of the information the viewer needs to understand what they are about and how to interpret them. Keep graphs and other figures as simple as possible and ensure that legends and labels are legible. Three-dimensional renderings and other advanced options offered by Excel for making charts can distract the viewer from your message rather than enhancing it. The judicious use of colour can help to emphasize results or make comparisons, but avoid red and green for these purposes (such as a red line on a green or orange background); up to 10% of men and 1% of women in North America have some degree of red-green colour blindness. Reduce visual "noise" in tables and graphs, for example by using the minimum number of gridlines necessary to guide the eye.[2,3]

It is often helpful to be able to re-use appropriate slides from earlier presentations. This is very easily accomplished by selecting the insert tab in PowerPoint and choosing "Slides from … Other presentation" in the drop-down menu. This will enable you to browse your previous PowerPoint files, select the slides you want and insert them into the new presentation. You can either let them be automatically reformatted to your new presentation format, or keep the original source formatting by selecting "keep source formatting."

Examples of slide formats are given in Figures 28.1–28.6.

Figure 28.1
Example of slide summarizing the study rationale

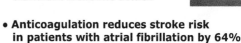

Figure 28.2
Example of slide summarizing the study methods

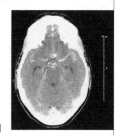

Figure 28.3
Example of slide with figure

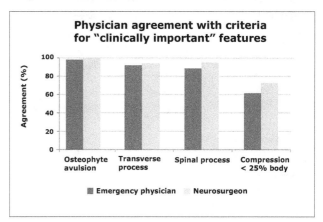

Reporting

---

a   These typefaces are without (French: *sans*) the typically curved terminals (serifs) at the end of strokes, as in T versus T.

Figure 28.4

Example of slide with flow diagram

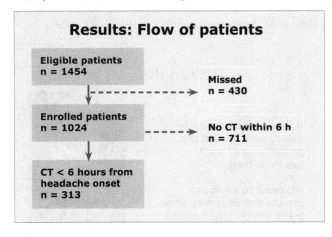

Results: Flow of patients

Eligible patients
n = 1454

Missed
n = 430

Enrolled patients
n = 1024

No CT within 6 h
n = 711

CT < 6 hours from
headache onset
n = 313

Figure 28.5

Example of slide with a table

Cohort characteristics (N = 1024)

Mean age, years (range)	44.5 (16–92)
Female	60.5 %
Worst headache	83.6 %
Vomiting	30.4 %
Transient loss of consciousness	6.4 %
CT < 6 hours	30.6 %
Lumbar puncture	53.7 %

Figure 28.6

Example of slide showing 2 X 2 table

Overall classification performance for 83 cases of subarachnoid hemorrhage (SAH) (N = 1024)

		SAH	
		Yes	No
CT positive	Yes	77	0
	No	6	961

Sensitivity = 92.8% (95% CI: 84.9% to 97.3%)
Specificity = 100.0% (95% CI: 99.6% to 100.0%)

Reporting

Preparing your delivery

Practice your presentation. Although you know the content of your talk, to put it across effectively you need a confident and polished delivery. Remember that you were asked to give this talk because you are knowledgeable—so, don't be intimidated! In anticipation of questions, you might want to insert one to three extra slides at the end of the presentation, giving tables or figures with additional data that time does not permit you to add to the main presentation. If someone asks a question to which these data are relevant, you can then display the appropriate slide and discuss. If you are asked a reasonable question for which you do not have an answer, then say "Good question; I will have to look into this issue further" and move on!

After loading your presentation on the computer provided at the conference, verify that all the slides appear correctly. There can be distortions in some slides depending on the version of PowerPoint you used to make your slides and the version available at the conference. You should always bring your presentation with you on a USB key and/or a laptop computer in case there are technical problems loading your presentation.

There are different techniques for delivering an oral presentation. You may wish to use the notes function in PowerPoint to prompt you; explore the "Presenters Tools" in the software to see what you feel comfortable with. (You will need to make sure that at the presentation venue you will have a laptop computer or a screen in front of you as you give your talk.) Alternatively, you might prefer to read your text to ensure that all important information is included within the brief time allowed. This second method is quite appropriate for a beginner, but the following tips can make it more effective. Memorize your introduction and deliver it in an engaging way while looking directly at your audience. Then, when you advance your slides, all eyes will move away from you and to the slide screen (in the same way a magician uses his wand to distract the audience from what he is really doing), at which point you can refer to your script. Be sure that your script is in a large font, and carry a penlight. (Dimming the room lighting to make the slides more visible can make reading a challenge.) Clearly note all slide changes in the margin of your script; there's nothing worse than delivering an entire talk that is out of sync with the slide projected on the screen. Check to make sure you are speaking about the correct slide after each slide change!

No matter which presentation strategy you choose, make sure that you practise the talk out loud at least five times, and ensure that you have timed the delivery to less than the 10 minutes allocated for the presentation.

Poster presentations

Key content requirements

As with a slide presentation, a poster requires the following sections: Title, Introduction, Objectives, Methods, Results, Discussion, Limitations, and Conclusions.

The title is typically shown at the top of the poster, along with the names of all authors and the organization that coordinated the study. The Introduction should provide one or two brief statements that allow the viewer to understand the rationale for and importance of the study. The Objectives section should provide the specific research aims (i.e. goal and objectives/hypothesis) of the study: it is essential for the viewer to understand what question the study attempted to answer. The Methods need to provide a brief description of how the study was conducted, including the study design, study population, study procedure(s), analysis, and sample size (and how it was determined). The results section should describe the outcomes and findings of the statistical analysis. This section should incorporate tables and figures to present this data. The Discussion section is optional on a poster. So, if it is included, it should be very short and emphasize why the study results are the same as or different from those of similar studies. The Limitations section should point out any weaknesses of the study and what effect they may have on the results. The Conclusion section needs to provide a summary of the significant results and the implications (for clinical practice or research) of these results. References are optional.

Styling your poster presentation

Once you have determined the content and basic structure of your poster presentation, you will need to create a visually appealing format that helps the viewer navigate and understand the content easily. This is always more difficult than it sounds. There are many different layout possibilities for posters, but a few rules of thumb are quite standard. Use "white space" effectively and creatively to make your poster readable and attractive; a presentation that appears too crowded or dense is not appealing to read and might be skipped over. Arrange your text and graphics in columns, working from left to right and top to bottom; a four-column format is typical. Align the edges of the column to form a uniform border on the top, side and bottom margins of the poster for a polished and orderly effect.

The advice given in the section on slide presentations on the effective use of fonts, colour, tables and figures applies to poster presentations. You will need to ensure that the fonts you choose are large and clear enough to be read at a distance of about 10 feet. Keep your text to a minimum, use a point-form style, use graphs and figures where possible instead of text, and ensure that these are self-explanatory. The tables and figures will contain the core information about your results, and may be the only sections of the poster that gain the viewer's attention.[4,5] If photographs are used to illustrate a clinical finding, or for visual appeal, ensure that they are of a sufficiently high enough resolution to retain sharpness once the poster is enlarged. Remember that clinical photographs require the patient's permission to be used in this way, regardless of whether the patient is recognizable.

Figure 28.7 displays an example of a previous poster presentation that captures many of these suggestions.

Making a poster using a PowerPoint slide. A poster can be made easily using a single slide in Microsoft PowerPoint. Before beginning, you will need to know the dimensions of the paper on which the poster will be printed and of the poster board on which it will be mounted. You will need to check the dimensions required by the conference. Select "Page Setup" under the "File" tab in Power Point. Select "Custom" and select the dimensions you need. For most horizontal set-ups, you can safely select 56 inches by 36 inches. Under the "Insert" tab, select "Text Box" to create a frame in which to enter your text; right-click in the box and select "Edit Text," and start typing your text. Use the formatting palette to arrange your text as bulleted lists where needed. The font size should be at least 32 for regular text and approximately 60 for headings. To add pictures and graphics, select "Picture" under the "Insert" tab; various file types (e.g., jpeg, EPS, and PDF) can be imported as picture elements. Ensure that any graphic files you import have a high enough resolution to appear sharp when they are printed at the required size.

Once the poster draft has been created and has all the desired content and illustrations, proofread it carefully, and then ask one or two colleagues to proofread it again. Now that the poster is finalized, have it professionally printed on one page and mount it on your poster board. Professional printing will make the poster more appealing and increase

Reporting

Figure 28.7
Example of a poster presentation

Reporting

Implementation of the Canadian C-Spine Rule by Emergency Department Nurses

Ian Stiell MD; Catherine Clement RN; Jamie Brehaut PhD; Jeremy Grimshaw PhD; Annette O'Connor RN PhD; Jeffrey Perry MD; George Wells PhD; Taryn MacKenzie RN; Christine Beland RN; Pamela Sheehan RN; Barbara Davies RN PhD

Department of Emergency Medicine, University of Ottawa, Ottawa, ON, Canada

Background
- Prolonged immobilization of trauma patients adds to ED congestion and patient discomfort

Objectives
- Evaluate impact and safety of allowing nurses to remove c-spine immobilization of trauma patients
- Implementation of medical directive based on previously validated Canadian C-Spine Rule (CCR)

Methods
- Prospective cohort study in 2 large hospital EDs
- Enrolled alert and stable adult trauma patients who presented with neck pain or were immobilized on an EMS backboard
- ED triage nurses had been trained on the CCR by a CD and hands-on sessions
- RNs had to accurately evaluate 10 patients and 3 interobserver cases, and pass a written test prior to being certified to clear the c-spine
- Evaluated safety and impact from study data forms, imaging records, and 30-day follow-up

Patient Characteristics (N=1,608)

Age (years) [mean ± SD]	42 ± 17
Range (years)	16 - 95
Gender - female (%)	55.5%
Ottawa Hospital Campus (%)	
Civic	48.5%
General	51.5%
Mechanism of injury (%)	
Motor vehicle collision	59.6%
Fall	23.4%
Other	8.1%
Bicycle collision	4.9%
Pedestrian struck	4.0%
Time, injury to arrival ED, hours (median)	1.3
Arrived by ambulance (%)	81.3%
C-spine radiography performed (%)	39.6%
Clinically important c-spine injury (%)	1.0%
Clinically unimportant c-spine injury (%)	0.5%
Developed neurological deficit (%)	0.4%
Stabilizing treatments (%)	1.3%
Internal fixation	0.1%
Halo	0.2%
Brace	0.1%
Rigid collar	0.9%
Time, ED arrival-disposition, hrs (median)	5.2
Admission to hospital (%)	3.9%

Canadian C-Spine Rule Positive Findings in 1,608 Study Patients

Findings from History (%)	
Dangerous mechanism	24.6%
Paresthesias in extremities	14.4%
Simple rear-end MVC	16.8%
Ambulatory at any time	36.0%
Immediate onset of neck pain	40.2%
Findings from Physical Examination (%)	
Sitting position in ED	12.3%
Neck tenderness midline	31.8%
Able to rotate neck	47.8%
C-spine immobilization required	50.3%

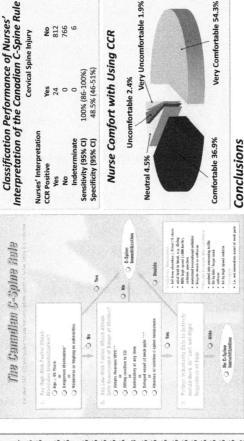

The Canadian C-Spine Rule

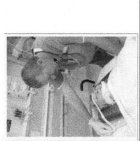
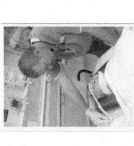

Classification Performance of Nurses' Interpretation of the Canadian C-Spine Rule

Nurses' Interpretation	Cervical Spine Injury	
	Yes	No
CCR Positive		
Yes	24	812
No	0	766
Indeterminate	0	6
Sensitivity (95% CI)	100% (86-100%)	
Specificity (95% CI)	48.5% (46-51%)	

Nurse Comfort with Using CCR
- Very Uncomfortable 1.9%
- Uncomfortable 2.4%
- Neutral 4.5%
- Comfortable 36.9%
- Very Comfortable 54.3%

Interobserver Agreement for Criteria of Canadian C-Spine Rule (N=95)

	Kappa Value	95% CI
Any High Risk Factor		
Age ≥ 65 years	0.71	0.50 - 0.93
Dangerous mechanism	0.72	0.57 - 0.87
Paresthesias	0.52	0.28 - 0.77
Any Low-Risk Factor		
Rearend MVC	0.84	0.66 - 1.00
Upright position	0.77	0.53 - 1.00
Ambulatory	0.73	0.50 - 0.95
Delayed neck pain	0.84	0.66 - 1.00
Midline tenderness	0.40	0.11 - 0.69
Able to Rotate	0.76	0.46 - 1.00
Overall Rule Immobilization	0.70	0.54 - 0.86

Conclusions
- Training and empowering ED triage nurses to clear the c-spine of stable trauma patients is safe and effective
- This use of the CCR should improve patient flow in our crowded EDs, diminish unnecessary patient discomfort, and increase ED nurse decision-making

Acknowledgements
- The wonderful cooperation of the Ottawa Hospital ED nurses

Reference
Stiell IG, Clement CM, O'Connor A, Davies B, Leclair C, Sheehan P, Clavet T, Beland C, MacKenzie T, Wells GA. Multicenter Prospective Validation of the Canadian C-Spine Rule by ED Triage Nurses. CMAJ 2010;Aug 10;182(11):1173-9

its impact. The poster is best printed locally, so that you can ensure it is correct before leaving for your conference. It is optimal to convert your PowerPoint custom file to a high-quality PDF print format, so that nothing will be altered during the printing process. You may also be able to email the file directly to the print shop. The cost of printing varies but is typically $115 to $200 per poster. Group discounts are often possible if multiple posters from your department are being prepared. Once you receive your printed poster, ensure that you have a solid tube to store the poster in without damaging it. Also purchase some Velcro adhesive strips or tabs to stick on the back of the poster so that it can be displayed and subsequently reused without the damage caused by tape or pins. Many poster presenters offer a copy of the poster (a reduced version on legal-sized paper) to those who may be interested in taking away a copy to review the methodology, results or references at a later date.

Presenting your poster

Practise giving an oral summary of your poster. When someone approaches the poster and appears to be interested, ask if you can give them the "two-minute summary." Most people will gladly accept the offer, giving you an opportunity to engage the viewer as you describe your rationale, objectives, methods and results.

Conclusion

Creating a slide or poster presentation for a research meeting can be a very rewarding experience. It allows you to present and disseminate your research, network with colleagues with similar interests and gain valuable feedback that can help you improve your work before submitting a full manuscript for potential peer-reviewed publication. By carefully preparing a clear and concise presentation, you will help your audience understand how the research was conducted, what the results are, and the implications of the findings. ∎

Acknowledgement
I thank Dr. Ian G. Stiell, Chair of the Department of Emergency Medicine, University of Ottawa, for permission to use his work to create Figures 28.3 and 28.7.

REFERENCES

1. Sherbinski LA, Stroup DR. Developing a poster for disseminating research findings. *AANA J.* 1992;60(6):567–72.

2. Tufte ER. *The visual display of quantitative information.* 2nd ed. Cheshire (CT): Graphics Press; 2001.

3. Lang TA. *How to write, publish and present in health sciences: a guide for physicians and laboratory researchers.* Philadelphia (PA): American College of Physicians; 2010.

4. Hardicre J, Devitt P, Coad J. Ten steps to successful poster presentation. *Br J Nurs.* 2007;16(7):398-401.

5. Teaching Support Services, University of Guelph. Effective poster design: a step by step guide. University of Guelph . 2010.

ADDITIONAL RESOURCES

Faulkes Z. DoctorZen.net. Better posters. A resource for improving poster presentations. Blog site. Available from: http://betterposters.blogspot.com

- This lively blog site has regular postings on all aspects of poster presentations.

Faulkes Z. DoctorZen.net. Smart posters. Blog post for 31 Mar 2011. Available from: http://betterposters.blogspot.com/2011/03/smart-posters.html

- A posting from the Doctor Zen blog site about using cellphone-readable QR codes to link your audience to additional information, resources, or a "virtual" presentation of your poster.

Reporting

SUMMARY CHECKLIST

- ❑ Gather all of the information you need to construct your presentation or poster, including any parameters assigned by the conference or forum (e.g. font, slide number, size, etc).
- ❑ Select an appropriate template to use (e.g., one may be provided by your school or department).
- ❑ Create a draft presentation using the general outline of: Title, Introduction, Objectives, Methods, Results, Limitations, Discussion and Conclusion.
- ❑ Review your text to ensure it is an appropriate length. You should aim to use the briefest text that communicates your essential ideas in each section. More than five lines of text on slide is typically crowded, for example.
- ❑ Ensure your fonts are large enough to be read in the room where the slide will be presented.
- ❑ Share your poster or slide set with colleagues for feedback. Revise.
- ❑ Practice your presentation with colleagues and revise on the basis of their feedback.
- ❑ Ensure you list any competing interests that authors may have (such as industry funding).
- ❑ Get your poster printed / submit your slides.

Reporting

29
How to write a health science paper

Grant Innes, MD, FRCPC

ILLUSTRATIVE CASE

Shortly after completing his residency, an emergency physician decides to launch his academic career by conducting his first research study: a 1-year follow-up of patients who had presented to an emergency department with abdominal pain. After convincing his colleagues to fill out data forms for 600 patients, he follows up each case personally by telephone over an 18-month period. He collates the data, painstakingly writes a manuscript and submits it for publication. This takes a mountain of work, but he has no regrets: he has made a major contribution to the medical literature. A Nobel Prize is unlikely, he thinks, but not out of the question. The journal's response arrives two weeks later: an outright rejection. The article is unsalvageable, the editor says. The science is bad and the writing is terrible. The doctor is stunned. As a physician, he has never failed at anything. He had assumed his medical school training qualified him as a scientist and writer.

■ **Publication is a good thing for** health science researchers: it leads to credibility, visibility, prestige and promotion—although not, in any direct way, more money. The objective of this chapter is to guide you through the process of writing a health science research report and to increase your chances of having your work published. Although the specific requirements for research papers vary according to the type—a case report, for example, is structured differently from a systematic review—the following tips will help you to set out on the right path no matter what category of report you are writing.

Ten tips for writing a health science manuscript

1. **Take a writing course.** Medical school did not teach you how to write. Writers train as long as physicians do; hence, many physicians are about as qualified to write manuscripts as writers are to perform invasive

surgical procedures. Journal editors can rapidly judge quality, and one way to have your work rejected is to submit a poorly written manuscript. If you do not have a strong writing background, a medical or scientific writing course is a good investment that will save you tens or even hundreds of hours in manuscript preparation time—not to mention reducing the risk that your submitted manuscripts will be rejected.

CHAPTER OBJECTIVES

After reading this chapter, you should be able to:
- discuss key strategies in approaching the task of writing a research paper
- list the components of an interventional research paper
- describe the submissions and peer review process for biomedical manuscripts
- list general tips for effective writing

Reporting

KEY TERMS

Abstract	Conflict of interest	Limitations	Peer review
Authorship	Copyright	Manuscript preparation	Results
Competing interests	Discussion	Medical record reviews	Systematic reviews
Conclusions	Effective writing	Methods	Tables
Confidentiality	Introduction	Objective statement	Title

Reporting

2. **Identify potential target journals and familiarize yourself with their areas of interest and the types of articles they publish.** Select those that appear to be the best fit for your work, and decide on which one to submit your article to first. Don't send a case report or narrative review to a journal that doesn't publish these. When in doubt, send a query to the editor by email. Ask if the journal would consider publishing an article like the one you plan to write.

3. **Understand your potential readers and what they expect.** Editors want articles that are interesting, important and practice-changing; therefore, strive for brevity, clarity and high impact.

4. **Craft a clear objective statement before you begin writing.** Why are you writing this paper? In a research article, the objective is, ideally, stated explicitly near the end of the Introduction. Review articles and case reports should also have objectives. A clear understanding of the objective is critical: it will help you define the focus of the research and the scope of the article. Every sentence in the manuscript should relate to the objective statement. A clear objective will help you write clearly and succinctly.

5. **Draft as much of the paper as you can before you perform the research.** Research grant applications require a well-defined research question, a comprehensive literature search, a summary of existing knowledge in the research area, a justification for the proposed study, and a detailed description of the methods to be used to address the study hypothesis. You will need to complete these steps even if you are not seeking grant funding. This means that, even before you begin to collect data, you will have drafted the Introduction and Methods, and you will have much of the information necessary for the Discussion. (These components of the research paper will be discussed later in this chapter.) In addition, it is helpful to draft the main data tables *a priori* and to populate them with sham data. This exercise will help you plan the analysis and Discussion, uncover problems or shortfalls you didn't think of, and identify additional data you may need to collect.

6. **Review the Uniform Requirements for Manuscripts Submitted to Biomedical Journals[1] and re-read the author instructions for your target journal.** Ensure that your article is correctly formatted to the journal's requirements. Editors take a dim view of authors who fail to follow simple instructions, and a manuscript that does not conform to a journal's formatting may be rejected outright, or else sent back for repair before the editors will consider it or send it for peer review.

7. **Be brief.** Recognize that, despite your own fascination with the topic, not everyone will find it riveting. Don't compound the problem by being long-winded. Say what you have to say in the fewest words possible.

8. **Do not repeat information in different parts of the manuscript.** Your readers are smart. If they've seen it in the Introduction, they don't need to see it again in the Discussion.

9. **Revise repeatedly.** After finishing a draft of the manuscript, put it aside for a few days and review it again. Is it clear and easy to read? Is it well organized? Does it flow logically? If you didn't understand any part of it, that part is badly written. Revise your paper and read it again. Then revise it once more. Many authors do five to ten revisions before they have a manuscript they feel is ready for submission.

10. **Arrange an internal peer review.** Ask a colleague who is familiar with the publishing process to read your draft and make suggestions before you submit it.

Writing the sections within your manuscript

The guidelines below focus on writing up an interventional trial, but the concepts covered are also very relevant to writing up other kinds of health science studies. The sections that will be discussed in turn are the Title, Abstract, Introduction, Methods, Results and Discussion.

Title

Compose a **Title** that is as concise as possible while giving sufficient information to enable those with an interest in your field to recognize that your paper might be of value to them. This means using specific terminology and giving a clear sense of the question that was addressed. Do not use acronyms and other abbreviations, and ensure that your title contains terms that will make your paper retrievable in a literature search on your topic area. Check the author guidelines for your target journal for any specific requirements; *BMJ*, for example, requires that the study method be indicated in the subtitle of research articles.

Abstract

The **Abstract** collates the main elements of your study, clarifying why it was done (Introduction or Background), how it was done (Methods), what was discovered (Results), how the data answered the research question, and how they should be applied (Discussion or Interpretation).[2] It is arguably the most important component of an article, because it may be the only part that gets read. Many readers will scan an abstract to determine whether to read the article it summarizes. Often, readers who judge the abstract worthy will inappropriately accept the information at face value without reading the rest of the article. Chapter 27 of this guide describes in detail the components of effective abstract writing. Some journals also ask for keywords to publish with the abstract. If this is the case for your target journal, use MeSH terms that cover the main subject areas (see ch. 7).

Introduction

The **Introduction** is the hook that grabs readers' interest. It should convince them that your article is interesting and important—a must read. It should also explain why you did this work, briefly describe the importance of the general research area, specify the knowledge gap that this research will fill, and clarify the research question, study objectives and hypothesis. Introductions should be short and sweet, running to about 300 words. Only the most important references should be cited in this section. A good Introduction has three paragraphs: the first describes the state of knowledge and the scope of the research; the second justifies the need for the study (the knowledge gap being addressed); and the third contains the study's objective statement and hypotheses.[1] If there is a place for long-drawn-out discussions (and there probably isn't), it is in the Discussion section.

The **objective statement**—that is, the statement of your research question (see ch. 6)—warrants special emphasis. Often framed as a question, this statement is the most important sentence in a scientific paper and is a critical part of any research proposal. The objective defines the focus and boundaries of the work, the required methodology, and the format and scope of the write-up. Every concept discussed in the manuscript should be related to it. A clear and focused objective will help you avoid the fatal flaw of rambling off on tangents or presenting extraneous findings. The objective statement also orients readers to what they should expect to find in the body of the article. Both the main and secondary objectives should be clear, and any planned subgroup analyses should be described.

Methods

The **Methods** section describes how the research was done, enabling readers to assess its quality and external validity (i.e., whether the results can be generalized to settings other than the site where the research was performed). The methods should be described clearly enough that another investigator can replicate the work, but should provide only the necessary detail.[1,3,4] If your study employed a complex but previously validated methodology, it might be reasonable to provide less detail here in preference to referring readers to previously published work. Conversely, if your study methods are novel, more extensive detail will be required so that readers can understand (and replicate) what was done.

Subheadings enhance organization and readability. Potential Methods subheadings include Design, Setting, Patients, Intervention, Study Procedures, Outcomes and Data Analysis. You should describe the overall *design,* indicating whether the study was a randomized controlled trial (RCT), a crossover trial, a prospective or retrospective cohort study, a case-control study, a cross-sectional study, a case series, a cost-effectiveness analysis or some other variation (see ch. 9). The *setting* subsection describes where the research was performed, allowing readers to determine whether the results can be generalized to their own practice. Patients and outcomes in inner-city tertiary care centres differ from those in suburban community hospitals, and patients in headache clinics differ from those in emergency departments. Under the *patients* subheading, describe the population sampled (e.g., patients presenting to an emergency department with a primary complaint of chest pain) as well as the inclusion and exclusion criteria used to select study participants.

If applicable, the experimental treatment or *intervention* should be described, as well as the methods for obtaining a comparison group (e.g., randomization, pre-post design). The study protocol or *study procedures* should describe how data were collected. Primary and secondary *outcomes* should be defined, along with the techniques used to collect and measure these. The *data analysis* section should clarify how major variables were analyzed, giving enough detail to enable a knowledgeable reader with access to the original data to verify the reported calculations and statistics. Main outcomes should include estimates of precision, such as 95% confidence intervals and, if a hypothesis is being tested, a *P* value. It is inappropriate, however, to present only *P* values, which tell readers only the likelihood that observed outcome differences occurred by chance, without indicat-

Reporting

ing the precision of the estimate and the range of values consistent with the observed result.[5]

The Methods section should also include a description of the patient consent process, Research Ethics Board approvals and, if applicable, trial registration. If the Methods section is too extensive, the necessary details can be moved into appendices or published in the online version of the journal. In designing a study and writing a manuscript, authors should refer to the appropriate reporting guidelines, such as the CONSORT reporting standard for RCTs.[a4] See Textbox 29.1 for a list of some of the more prominent reporting standards.

TEXTBOX 29.1 GUIDELINES FOR THE REPORTING OF HEALTH SCIENCES RESEARCH

Many evidence-based reporting guidelines have been developed by various working groups. The following list is a sample. Some journals require compliance with certain guidelines; check the instructions for authors of your target journal to be sure. For further information, lists of guidelines and links to the guidelines themselves, see the EQUATOR Network* website at www.equator-network.org/home/.

CONSORT Statement	CONsolidated Standards of Reporting Trials (for randomized controlled trials)
MOOSE	Meta-analysis Of Observational Studies in Epidemiology
PRISMA	Preferred Reporting Items for Systematic reviews and Meta-Analysis (This guideline replaces QUOROM: Quality of Reporting Of Meta-analyses.)
SQUIRE	Standard for Quality Improvement Reporting Excellence
STARD	STAndards for the Reporting of Diagnostic accuracy studies
STROBE	STrengthening the Reporting of OBservational studies in Epidemiology

*EQUATOR: Enhancing the QUality And Transparency Of health Research

---

Results

The **Results** section summarizes the study findings in tables, figures and text. **Tables** are the heart of the Results section, and main findings should be presented in tabular form. Tables and figures should be self-explanatory so that readers do not have to refer back to the text in order to decipher them. However, tables and figures should complement the text, not duplicate it. Before submission, authors should check their tables to ensure that denominators are presented and that calculations and percentages are correct. Surprisingly, manuscripts submitted for publication frequently contain data and calculation errors in the Abstract and the tables. Graphs should be used sparingly: that is, only for important study outcomes and only if they enhance understanding of the data. An essential figure, however, is a study flow diagram to show how the study sample was arrived at; the CONSORT flow diagram, for example, is the standard used to report the number of patients screened, eligible, missed, excluded, included and lost to follow-up in a RCT.[b]

Table 1 in your report should summarize the baseline characteristics of the study population: that is, the relevant attributes of patients in the comparator groups prior to the intervention or exposure of interest. This table typically reports age, sex and other demographic predictors and covariables that could influence patient outcome. For example, in a study of myocardial infarction outcomes, Table 1 might include predictors such as previous coronary artery disease, diabetes, hypertension, dyslipidemia, smoking history, cardiac medications, NYHA (New York Heart Association) classification, vital signs on arrival, and arrival mode. Readers can use Table 1 to determine whether patients in the two groups were similar at baseline and whether they resemble patients in their own setting. In an observational study, Table 1 should include a statistical analysis to show whether the two groups differed significantly with respect to important baseline predictors. Conversely, there is little value in determining P values within Table 1 of a randomized trial: assuming an effective randomization process, any observed baseline differences between groups must have arisen by chance.

Table 2 describes the patients *after* the intervention or exposure, highlighting differences in the primary outcome. Table 2 should display absolute and relative differences, estimates of precision (e.g., 95% confidence intervals) and usually a test of statistical significance. Additional tables are often necessary to illustrate differences in secondary outcomes or to highlight subgroup or post-hoc analyses. Authors should realize that tables and figures consume valuable page space; therefore, journal editors will limit these to the minimum number required to ensure clarity.

The narrative component of the Results section should be written after the tables are populated. It should be concise, presenting only important findings that relate to the

---

a   See www.consort-statement.org/consort-statement/

b   See www.consort-statement.org/consort-statement/flow-diagram

study objective. The text should refer readers to the relevant tables, and all tables and figures should be cited in the text. The text should clarify, highlight or expand upon data presented in the tables, but should not duplicate it.

The first paragraph in the Results section should provide a brief summary of the number and type of patients included in the final study sample, as well as the number excluded and the reasons for exclusion. The second paragraph should describe the primary outcome(s) as they relate to each study objective and hypothesis. Subsequent paragraphs should highlight secondary outcomes and planned subgroup analyses. Each major outcome should be compared descriptively, using the appropriate measures of central tendency, such as means, medians or proportions, and the applicable measures of variability, such as range, variance, standard deviation or interquartile range (see also ch. 24). For key outcomes, an estimate of precision (e.g., confidence interval) is valuable, and a P value is customary for each hypothesis test (see also ch. 25). More complex multivariable analyses or adjustments may be necessary but are beyond the scope of this chapter.

When writing the Results section, it is important to exclude information that is more appropriate for the Methods or Discussion. Authors should also avoid the temptation to present "interesting data" that are unrelated to the study objective, limiting themselves to "just the facts." Opinions and interpretations should be moved to the Discussion.

Discussion

The **Discussion** section should summarize the main findings, explain what the results mean, compare and contrast the findings previously reported in the literature, discuss study strengths and **limitations**, and suggest directions for future research. The Discussion section is the most difficult to write; this is where authors frequently go wrong by losing focus, repeating information presented elsewhere in the manuscript, drawing conclusions that are not justified by the data, or drifting off on tangents that are irrelevant to the study objective. As you draft the Discussion, keep a limit of approximately 750 words in mind. In your first draft, it is helpful to use an outline and subheadings, which can be retained or excluded from the final manuscript as appropriate. The following structure is one possible approach to writing a clear discussion.

The opening paragraph is the power position. It is the only part of the discussion that many readers will read or remember. This paragraph should restate the research ques-

tion, summarize the main study findings, and indicate whether and how they support the hypothesis. This is your chance to state in a few sentences what the take-home message is and why your study is important. The second paragraph should discuss the results in the context of what they add to pre-existing knowledge and how they address the knowledge gap that the study was designed to address. This paragraph or the next should review other important studies that support or refute the main findings. Authors should try to clarify how and why their findings differ from earlier studies and suggest other possible interpretations of the data. Importantly, the Discussion should never introduce data that did not appear first in the Results section.

Take care not to overstate the importance of your findings or to draw inferences that go beyond what the data justify. Moreover, the Discussion section should conclude with a paragraph or two describing the study's strengths and limitations. (Some journals require a separate Limitations section.) The limitations of your study might relate to technical or data-collection problems, potential biases, methodological challenges and external validity. Highlight concerns that might otherwise be apparent only to an investigator who was directly involved in the study. This section should conclude with recommendations for future work in your topic area. For more detail on writing the Discussion section, see chapter 26.

Conclusions

Your **Conclusions** section should be brief, consisting of a couple of sentences or a short paragraph. Don't reiterate arguments presented in the Discussion; instead, state your major findings and how these should be applied. The Conclusions should also highlight appropriate caveats about the generalizability of results, such as specific settings or patient groups to which your conclusions do not apply. It is a critical error to make unqualified conclusions that are not justified by the data. However, simply calling attention to the need for more research is not an adequate conclusion.

Special cases

The following sections describe particular aspects of writing up **medical record reviews** and **systematic reviews**; more detailed information on how to conduct these types of studies are provided in chapters 12 and 15, respectively.

Reporting

Medical record reviews

Medical records are informal descriptions of observations, impressions and hunches. They contain mostly narrative descriptions of people and events, and the translation of these verbal descriptions into hard quantitative data is fraught with error.[6] Schwartz and colleagues[7] demonstrated poor agreement between information derived from the medical record and information gathered directly from the patient. Medical records frequently lack critical data, including chief presenting complaint, historical and physical findings and laboratory results. Errors, inconsistencies and omissions in medical charts are compounded when information is extracted during a scientific investigation. When two abstractors look for the same data in the same medical record, their results often disagree. Common sources of error in medical record reviews include missing charts, missing data, conflicting data, vague or illegible charting, inconsistent transformation of descriptive data into categorical data, and differences in the handling of ambiguous or missing data. In addition, biased abstraction can occur if chart abstractors are aware of the study hypotheses or expectations. To reduce error and increase reliability, studies involving chart review should include the following critical elements:

- a description of inclusion criteria
- definitions of the variables being analyzed
- a description of abstractor training
- the use of standardized abstraction forms
- a description of abstractor monitoring
- a description of abstractor blinding to study hypotheses
- a discussion of inter-rater reliability

Systematic reviews

Traditional narrative review articles, in which the author summarizes published literature in an unstructured document, are subject to several biases, and many journals will no longer consider review articles unless they employ valid systematic review methodology, as described in the PRISMA statement (Preferred Reporting Items for Systematic Reviews and Meta-Analyses).[c] Briefly, these require authors to define a clear research question, to evaluate earlier reviews and justify the need for another one, to develop a systematic search strategy to identify and select primary articles, to apply valid inclusion and exclusion criteria, perform a blinded assessment of source article quality, determine the reliability of this process by measuring the agreement of two evaluators, account for all studies identified, included and excluded, describe the method of combining study results, discuss variation within and between studies, and draw appropriate conclusions. Authors should outline the limitations of their review and suggest areas for future research. The Cochrane Handbook for Systematic Reviews of Interventions is an excellent reference for prospective authors.[8]

Tips on good writing

Remember that you are not a Michael Crichton. You haven't been signed to a five-book deal, and no one is reading your article because they enjoyed the literary style of your previous two. They are reading because your title caught their attention and your abstract convinced them that you had useful information to share. They want this information as quickly and easily as they can get it. Therefore, although good science and a well-organized manuscript are a must, **effective writing** is equally important. No matter how important your topic, readers (including reviewers and editors) are likely to abandon the manuscript if they encounter long, boring or obscure passages.

Good scientific writing is clear and simple. It generally prefers the active to the passive voice, uses strong and precise nouns and verbs, and eliminates all unnecessary words.[9] If you are a typical physician writer, an editor will be able to reduce the word count of your manuscript considerably without eliminating important information, in the process making it clearer and more readable. But substantive editing consumes valuable time, and rejection is a simpler option. It is best for the author to streamline the article before submission. Authors can improve their writing quality by remembering a few important tips, examples of which are given in Textbox 29.2 at the end of the chapter. (Further resources on effective writing are given in Additional Resources.) These tips are as follows:

- Write mostly in the active voice using a subject-verb-object sentence structure. This will help to make your writing clear and succinct.
  — Example: "The scoring system was pilot-tested by the data abstractors." (passive) vs "The data abstractors pilot-tested the scoring system" (active).

c See www.prisma-statement.org/

Reporting

- Use parallel structure by constructing linked phrases and sentences in a similar fashion.
  - Example: "Physicians identified eligible patients; study drugs were given by nurses; radiologists performed image interpretation" (non-parallel) should become "Physicians identified patients; nurses gave study drugs; radiologists interpreted images" (parallel).
- Use logical progressions. When combining ideas, proceed logically from most to least important, largest to the smallest, or first to last.
  - Example: "The study showed more patients with adequate blood pressure control, lower rates of death, and fewer myocardial infarctions in the intervention group" should become "The intervention group had lower rates of death, myocardial infarction and hypertension."
- Eliminate words and phrases that add nothing. Many authors believe that complicated and flowery words add up to better writing. Nothing could be further from the truth. Good writers use a spare style that relies on precise nouns and verbs.[9] If you need to qualify things with an adjective or adverb, this might mean that you have the wrong noun (or verb). To illustrate: athletes don't run quickly; they sprint.
- Minimize the use of abbreviations, especially acronyms (e.g., PAHO) and initialisms (e.g., TIA). Use abbreviations only when they are well established or if it would be cumbersome to spell out a term in full each time it appears in your paper; in the latter case, provide the term in full on first occurrence, e.g., "transient ischemic attack (TIA)."

Formatting your manuscript for submission

Most journals conform to the **manuscript preparation** guidelines laid out in the *Uniform Requirements for Manuscripts Submitted to Biomedical Journals*,[1] and articles that adhere to these guidelines will rarely be rejected on the basis of style or format. Authors should also refer to the specific instructions provided by their target journal. However, the following generally apply: double-space the manuscript, from title page to references, and use a consistent 12-point font. Number pages consecutively, beginning with the title page, and provide a running head.

Do not format the article as you think it might appear in print, with page columns, different typefaces, and figures and tables incorporated into the text. Provide figures and tables at the end of the file or in separate files, as the journal's instructions specify. Many journals prefer that authors use no special referencing software (such as EndNote) and no tracked changes, small caps, superscripts, or special formatting) because these may conflict with journal software.

The manuscript submission package

Most journal submissions should include the following components.[1]

Cover letter. Provide a brief cover letter that describes the study and its findings in a sentence or two, specifies each author's contribution to the work, and confirms that all coauthors have provided their permission to publish the manuscript. Similar work that the authors have published elsewhere, which could be construed as duplicate publication, should be reported to the editor along with a statement of potential conflicts of interest and financial disclosures. If you intend to include previously published materials (such as figures) in your article, you will need to seek permission from the **copyright** holder and to include the appropriate documentation in your cover letter. At a minimum, flag materials for which permissions are needed or pending so that, if your article is accepted, this important task will not be overlooked. Many publishers have streamlined the permissions process through online services such as RightsLink.[d] Because copyright holders may require information about your target journal (e.g., type of distribution, whether the journal is for-profit or non-profit), you may need to consult with the journal editors before completing the permissions process. You will also need to determine who is responsible for covering any associated fees.

Title page. The title page should include the manuscript title, the authors' names, degrees and institutional affiliations, and the name, mailing address, telephone number, fax number and email address of the corresponding author. It should also indicate the number of figures and tables and

Reporting

---

d   Available through the Copyright Clearance Center at www.copyright.com

include a word count for the abstract as well as the main text (excluding abstract, tables and references). Relevant disclaimers should be reported here, along with sources of support in the form of funding, study supplies, drugs or devices. Most journals request a short running head at the bottom of the title page. A conflict-of-interest disclosure page should follow the title page.

Abstract. Structured abstracts of 250–300 words are usually required for original research articles, systematic reviews and meta-analyses. Requirements for case reports differ but typically include a brief unstructured abstract that summarizes the problem or objective, the main points and the conclusions. See chapter 27 for a detailed discussion of abstracts.

Main text. The components of the main text of the article are discussed earlier in this chapter.

Figures and tables. Journal editors often ask that figures and tables be submitted in separate digital files. Most have specifications with respect to the formatting and permissible file types of tables and figures.[e] If you are intending to reproduce or adapt figures, illustrations, tables or other material from another publication, written permission will need to be sought from the publisher or copyright holder to use these items.

Understanding the peer review process

It is important for you to have a basic knowledge of the **peer review** process, which is intensive, time-consuming and often frustrating. The objective of peer review is to have peers as well as scientific and content experts review the submitted work and provide opinions regarding its interest, importance, quality and validity.

Submitted manuscripts are first logged and categorized, and are then assigned to an appropriate senior editor or decision editor on the basis of their content. This editor will reject (or "intercept") a significant proportion of manuscripts immediately after initial screening. Articles that are judged to be potentially suitable for the journal, and of sufficiently high quality, are forwarded for blinded peer review by two or three reviewers selected on the basis of their content expertise, previ-

ous work in the area or methodological expertise. Many journals allow authors to request specific reviewers or to identify reviewers who should not be solicited in light of possible personal or professional conflicts of interest.

Peer reviewers use structured review forms to provide comments on the importance of the work, the quality of the methods, the validity of the findings, the quality of the manuscript and the priority for publication. Most journals invite reviewers to indicate whether the manuscript should be accepted without revision, accepted after specific revisions, revised for resubmission and reconsideration, or rejected outright. Peer reviews help editors gauge the likely interest of the article to readers, and often uncover subtle flaws or concerns in the work, but reviewers do not make publication decisions.

Decision editors collate the peer reviewers' comments and use them to inform their decision about the manuscript. Depending on the size of the journal, this decision may be made at an editorial committee meeting. After the decision, the editor composes a response letter indicating whether the manuscript is accepted, rejected, or requires revision and resubmission. The response letter should summarize important concerns and requested changes to the manuscript. Because not all peer review comments are appropriate, editors should provide some guidance regarding how to respond to these. Many journals provide the actual blinded peer review comments along with the editor's response letter. Editorial response times vary among journals and depend on the type of response. If the manuscript is rejected during its initial screening, authors may receive an email response within days of submission. If the manuscript is forwarded for peer review, response times of 4–12 weeks are typical.

Many manuscripts are rejected outright (see Textbox 29.3 at the end of the chapter), and few are accepted without revision. Most journals have established criteria allowing authors to appeal the rejection decision in cases where they believe there was a fundamental misunderstanding of the data or a potential conflict of interest during the editorial or peer review process. Appeal criteria should be available on the journal's website.

In most cases, authors should hope for a decision letter that requests revision and resubmission. When this happens to you, address all of the queries and revision requests made by the decision editor. If suggested revisions will improve the manuscript, make them without question. If you disagree with any specific change requested, explain

---

e See, for example, the CMAJ guidelines for submitting tables, figures and graphics at www.cmaj.ca/authors/preparing.dtl#tables

your reasons for doing so and come to an agreement with the editor. In some cases, author-editor disagreement arises from a misunderstanding of the paper by the editors or peer reviewers, and this may reflect a poorly written or unclear manuscript. In some cases, editors will ask for further data collection or re-analysis, which may or may not be feasible depending on the accessibility of data. Complete the requested changes as rapidly as possible (prompt responses are viewed as evidence of a conscientious author) and forward the revised manuscript to the decision editor with a brief explanation of what changes were (or were not) made. Frequently, authors will be asked to do a second or third revision before acceptance. If the manuscript concerns can be addressed to the satisfaction of the decision editor or editorial committee, you will ultimately receive a letter of acceptance and the manuscript will move into the publication pipeline. Depending on the timeliness of the subject, the article's priority rating, and the number of articles already in the pipeline, it may still be an additional 2 to 12 months before your article is published.

After acceptance, the senior or decision editor will work with a copy editor to revise the accepted article for clarity, brevity and journal style. Depending on the quality of the initial submission, this sometimes means significant changes to the manuscript and substantial reductions in word count. Authors have the opportunity to review and approve all revisions before publication, but the journal editor holds all the cards. Prior to publication, authors are required to sign transfer-of-copyright forms. Published manuscripts become the property of the journal's copyright holder (likely either the publisher or the sponsoring society), and may not be published or distributed elsewhere, even by the author, without permission. The exception to this is open access publication, in which the author retains copyright and readers are free to reprint, distribute or adapt the work, with proper attribution, in accordance with the particular Creative Commons licence that the journal applies.[f]

Ethical considerations

Various ethical consideration that must be taken into account in the conduct of health research are discussed in Chapter 18 of this guide. The following sections relate to issues of particular relevance to the publishing process.

Criteria for authorship

To qualify for **authorship** credit, a member of the research team should satisfy each of three criteria: contributions to performing the research (i.e., study design, data acquisition or data analysis); drafting or revising the article; and approving the final version for publication.[1] All listed authors should qualify for authorship, and all people who qualify should be listed. Each listed author should feel comfortable taking responsibility for the study content. Other individuals who contributed in some way but do not meet the criteria for authorship should be listed in an Acknowledgments section.

Conflict of interest or competing interests

Authors and their institutions, as well as editors and reviewers, have financial relationships, personal associations and other interests that might influence their actions. Financial interests such as employment income, honoraria, consulting fees and stock ownership present the most obvious conflicts, but personal relationships, academic competition and strongly held beliefs can also compromise scientific and academic objectivity. Authors must declare all potential conflicts of interest at the time of article submission. A standard conflict of interest form is available from the International Committee of Medical Journal Editors;[g] journals frequently have their own forms as part of their online submission process. Editors will publish this information if they feel that it is likely to influence readers' interpretation of the work.

Data access and publication

During the conduct of industry-funded studies, investigators should obtain assurances, in writing, that they will have full access to the study database, will be able to analyze the data independently, and will be able to use their own discretion, free of interference, in preparing and publishing articles derived from the data. Authors should declare the role of the study sponsor in study development, data collection and analysis, and in writing the article—including the absence of any such role. Editors may choose not to publish an article where there is any question about the investigators' access to study data, or evidence suggesting inappropriate involvement of a potentially biased sponsor in the design, analysis or study write-up (see also ch. 18).

Reporting

---

f   See http://creativecommons.ca/index.php?p=explained

g   See www.icmje.org/sample_disclosure.pdf

Confidentiality

The **confidentiality** of people who participate in research must be scrupulously respected. No identifiers, including names, initials or recognizable photographs, should be published without the individual's written informed consent. Non-essential identifying details should be omitted. Informed consent, including a participant's review of the unpublished manuscript, is also warranted if a case description is highly recognizable. When informed consent has been obtained, this should be stated in the submitted manuscript (see also ch. 18).

Authors also have confidentiality rights. Reviewers, editors and other journal staff members must not publicly discuss, present or disseminate study data before publication, except by agreement with the authors. Also, journals editors should not disclose to anyone beyond their staff that they have received a given author's submission; aside from being a breach of the author's privacy, doing so can make them open to undue influence. Reviewers should destroy copies of manuscripts after reviewing them. Reviewer anonymity is variable: some journals offer reviewers the option of being anonymous, and if this is the reviewer's expressed preference at the time of review, journal editors cannot reveal his or her identity to anyone without permission.

Editorial freedom

Journal editors should responsibly exercise full control over the selection of journal content, the review process, the selection and editing of manuscripts, and the timing of publication. Journal owners, whose focus may be commercial success rather than scientific integrity, should neither interfere in the editorial process nor create an environment that unduly influences editorial decision-making. Editors should be free to express opinions or publish materials that conflict with the owner's business goals.

Ethical approval

Authors should include with their submissions a declaration that their work has received all necessary approvals from a Research Ethics Board and/or animal care and use committee.

Trial registration

Investigators should register clinical trials with an appropriate clinical trials registry such as ClinicalTrials.gov as soon as ethics board approval has been obtained. The trial registration number should be included with the manuscript submission.

Conclusion

The natural outcome of research should be the dissemination of new information and the synthesis of evidence-based knowledge. Publishing research articles in peer-reviewed journals remains one of the keystones of knowledge translation in the health sciences, and is supported by extensive databases for indexing and retrieval that enable researchers around the world to benefit from one another's work. However, as natural as the publication of research may seem, it requires a set of skills that are by no means automatic for everyone. This chapter has outlined the key considerations in drafting and submitting manuscripts for publication. Skill in research writing develops with practise, however, and readers are encouraged to seek guidance along the way from the excellent writing guidebooks and workshops that are available, many of which are tailored to the exacting demands of writing up health sciences research. ∎

Reporting

CASE POSTSCRIPT

The emergency physician decides to get a second opinion from a trusted colleague with a modest publication record. Unlike the journal editor, the colleague doesn't have dozens of other manuscripts to read every week, and so takes the time to point out various ways in which both the organization and the writing style make it difficult to follow the methods or gain a clear picture of the findings. Even the research question, she explains, is unclear. After some dicussion, however, she is persuaded that the researcher's method was sound and his results worth reporting. The physician goes back to the drawing board, and after several rounds of rewriting finally produces a manuscript that is clear, logical and concise. He resubmits the paper to the same journal editor, who, this time, agrees that it is worthy of being sent for peer review. A little older and much wiser, he is eagerly awaiting the result.

TEXTBOX 29.2: WRITING TECHNIQUES—SAMPLE SENTENCES FOR REPAIR

Prefer the active voice
In previous studies looking at the management of inflammatory processes such as asthma, community-acquired pneumonia and meningitis, important outcomes such as morbidity, mortality and lengths of hospital stay have been shown to be affected positively by the implementation of early interventions

Better: Previous studies show that early interventions improve outcomes with respect to morbidity, mortality and hospital lengths of stay for inflammatory processes such as asthma, community-acquired pneumonia and meningitis.

Keep structures parallel
Study subjects at the two sites had similar age and gender distributions; however, the inner-city sample included larger proportions of African-Americans and Hispanics, while whites were the predominant ethnic group at the community site.

Better: Age and gender distributions were similar at the two sites; however, inner-city patients were mostly African-American and Hispanic, whereas community patients were predominantly white.

Don't waste words
William Osler, one of the most notable medical teachers, taught using an economy of words. Students marvelled at Osler's teaching style, his clarity and the preciseness of his words on hospital rounds.

Better: William Osler was a remarkable teacher known for his clarity, precision and economy of words.

Use logical groupings
Our data show that, despite high levels of reported pain at discharge and high satisfaction with pain management, subjects reported low rates of analgesic administration.

Better: Our data show that, despite low rates of analgesic administration and high levels of pain at discharge, subjects reported high satisfaction with pain management.

TEXTBOX 29.3: COMMON REASONS FOR REJECTION

- The Title is vague, misleading or uninteresting.
- The Abstract is too long, overly inclusive or disorganized. Results and conclusions reported in the Abstract differ from those in the body of the manuscript. These critical errors often occur because researchers forget to revise the Abstract along with the evolving manuscript.
- The Introduction is boring and does not "hook" the reader. The study does not seem important, novel or intriguing. The authors include too much information that should be incorporated in the Discussion. The research question, hypothesis and study objectives are not specified or are not clear.
- The Methods do not follow the journal's required format or are not clear enough to be reproduced; details are missing or omitted. There are major methodological flaws; the dates of the study are not specified; ethics approval was not obtained. No sample-size calculation is described. The study is underpowered.
- The Results fail to display a patient flowchart, to compare baseline characteristics, or to address potential confounders. Data or patients are missing from the analysis.
- Outcomes are reported only as *P* values or odds ratios, denying readers the opportunity to look at patient counts, rates or proportions. The authors failed to adjust for multiple comparisons or to analyze outcomes by treatment received rather than intention to treat. For subjective observations, no reliability assessment is provided.
- Numbers in tables don't add up. Text and tables are redundant. Authors calculate too many *P* values or fail to recognize the limits and meaning of *P* values. Authors report statistical significance but fail to comment on clinical importance.
- The Discussion is unfocused, expansive or tangential. The key results are not adequately discussed or explained. Study implications and importance are overstated or biased. Important findings are omitted; speculation is not identified as such; and limitations are not described.
- References are outdated, or key papers are not referenced.
- The Conclusion does not answer the study question, does not set limits for generalization, simply restates the results, or merely calls for more study.

Reporting

REFERENCES

1. International Committee of Medical Journal Editors. Updated April 2010. *Uniform requirements for manuscripts submitted to biomedical journals.* Available from: www.icmje.org.

2. Foote M. Some concrete ideas about manuscript abstracts. *Chest.* 2006;129(5);1375–7.

3. Hopewell S, Clarke M, Moher D, Wager E, Middleton P, Altman DG, et al. CONSORT for reporting randomised trials in journal and conference abstracts. *Lancet.* 2008; 371(9609):281–3.

4. Schulz KF, Altman DG, Moher D; CONSORT Group. CONSORT 2010 Statement: updated guidelines for reporting parallel group randomised trials. *Ann Int Med.* 2010;152(11):726–32.

5. Worster A, Rowe BH. Measures of association: an overview with examples from Canadian emergency medicine research. *Can J Emerg Med.* 2001;3(3):219–23.

6. Gilbert EH, Lowenstein SR, Koziol-McLain J, Barta DC, Steiner J. Chart reviews in emergency medicine research: Where are the methods? *Ann Emerg Med.* 1996;27(3):305–8.

7. Schwartz RJ, Boisoneau D, Jacobs LM. The quantity of cause-of-injury information documented on the medical record: an appeal for injury prevention. *Acad Emerg Med.* 1995;2(2):98–103.

8. Higgins JPT, Green S, editors. *Cochrane handbook for systematic reviews of interventions.* Version 5.0.2 [updated September 2009]. The Cochrane Collaboration, 2009. Available from: www.cochrane-handbook.org.

9. Strunk W, White EB. *The elements of style.* 4th ed. Needham Heights (MA): Allyn & Bacon; 2000.

ADDITIONAL RESOURCES

AMA Manual of Style Committee. *AMA Manual of Style.* 10th ed. New York (NY): American Medical Association; 2007.

Equator Network. Resources for authors. Available from: www.equator-network.org/resource-centre/authors-of-research-reports/authors-of-research-reports/#auwrit

- A bibliography, with links, of resources that provide guidance on writing in the health sciences.

Gopen GD, Swan JA. The science of scientific writing: if the reader is to grasp what the writer means, the writer must understand what the reader needs. *Am Scientist.* 1990 Nov-Dec; 78:550–8.

- A classic article describing how scientific writing can be improved and made more effective.

Iles RL. *Guidebook to better medical writing.* Rev. ed. Olathe (KS): Island Press; 2003.

Lang TA. *How to write, publish, and present in the health sciences: a guide for clinicians and laboratory researchers.* Philadelphia (PA): American College of Physicians; 2009.

- A comprehensive guide on scientific writing by an expert in the fields of scientific writing and editing.

Lang TA, Secic M, editors. *How to report statistics in medicine.* 2nd ed. Philadelphia (PA): American College of Physicians; 2006.

- A comprehensive reference on how statistics should be reported in biomedical publications.

Tarshis B. *How to be your own best editor.* New York (NY): Three Rivers Press and Random House; 1998.

Tufte ER. *The visual display of qualitative information.* 2nd ed. Cheshire (CT): Graphics Press; 2001

- A conceptual exploration of how diagrams of various kinds can be used to convey complex data.

Reporting

WRITING EXERCISES

1. Revise this sentence by eliminating unnecessary words.

   Figure 3 shows that changes in emergency department volume in all of the 3 study areas appear to follow the same seasonal fluctuations, and that the ED volume peaks appear to occur during the summer months of May–August.

2. Eliminate unnecessary words and phrases from these sentences.

   All personal identifiers were kept strictly confidential.

   Thus, on average, the data showed that patients spent the majority of their time while in the emergency department (57%) in moderate to severe pain.

3. Strip this sentence to the essentials and use the active voice.

   Emergency departments across the country have often been acknowledged as suffering from profound levels of patient overcrowding, which is the basis of long waiting times, and this challenging situation is not ameliorated by the concurrent inefficient use of time and resources for any given clinical problem.

4. Edit this sentence using a logical progression.

   Furthermore, the decrees required that manufacturers increase public and user awareness of the dangers of motorcycle use through a media campaign, that warning labels be attached to the vehicles and that a training program be provided for those who purchase a motorcycle.

Possible answers

1. Figure 3 shows that emergency department volumes peaked during summer in the 3 study regions.

2a. All personal identifiers were kept confidential.

2b. Patients spent 57% of their emergency department time in moderate to severe pain.

3. Emergency department overcrowding prolongs waiting times. Inefficient use of time and resources aggravates this situation.

4. The decrees required that manufacturers attach warning labels to vehicles, provide training programs for purchasers, and run media campaigns alerting the public to motorcycling hazards

Reporting

SUMMARY CHECKLIST

☐ Prepare for your next publication by doing some personal development, e.g., a writing course, a discussion with a writing mentor, or reviewing a text on effective writing for publication.

☐ Through their websites, familiarize yourself with your target journals of interest, their requirements, and their most popular articles.

☐ Prepare yourself for the fact that many drafts are often needed before an article is suitable for publication.

☐ Consider your target audience for a particular study.

☐ Craft a clear goal for writing this publication.

☐ Draft as much of your article as you can before completing the research.

☐ Review the requirements for your selected target journal.

☐ Revise your manuscript with all of your data and appropriate references.

☐ Revise your manuscript again with a view to enhancing clarity, brevity and impact.

☐ Share your drafts with peers, colleagues, members of your research team, your mentor, and an editor if you can. Revise on the basis of their feedback.

☐ Prepare your submission package.

☐ Submit your manuscript.

☐ Revise and respond to the peer reviews of your draft. Resubmit.

Reporting

30
Knowledge translation

Monika Kastner, PhD

Sharon Straus, MD, MSc, FRCPC

Ian D. Graham, PhD

Jacqueline Tetroe, MA

ILLUSTRATIVE CASE

A Geriatric Medicine resident is struck by the fact that, despite ample evidence demonstrating that routine influenza vaccination is beneficial and safe, many staff working in nursing homes do not receive an annual flu shot. She would like to explore strategies to improve vaccination rates in this group of care providers. She wonders what factors she should take into account in designing and conducting her study to increase its impact. When she mentions this to her project supervisors, they suggest that she first acquaint herself with the principles of "knowledge translation" and think about how they might be applied to her research study.

■ **Knowledge translation (KT) has** been defined by the Canadian Institutes of Health Research as "a dynamic and iterative process that includes synthesis, dissemination, exchange and ethically-sound application of knowledge to improve the health of Canadians, provide more effective health services and products and strengthen the health care system."[1] In basic terms, KT is the process of moving knowledge into action or clinical practice. The concept of KT arose from the realization that it is no longer enough to create, distill or simply disseminate knowledge through traditional strategies such as publishing in peer-reviewed publications and presenting at conferences. Rather, KT aims to foster the application of high-quality knowledge in informed **clinical decision-making**.

An abundance of terms are currently being used to describe the process of KT. These include *implementation science* and *research utilization* (United Kingdom and Europe); *dissemination, diffusion, research use, knowledge transfer* and *uptake* (United States); and *knowledge transfer, knowledge exchange* and *knowledge translation* (Canada).[2] In the course of their work to develop a search strategy for

KT,[3] McKibbon and colleagues identified more than 90 terms that refer to the use of research findings. This plethora of terms is a source of confusion and poses a challenge for those trying to identify relevant literature in the field of KT.

Another source of confusion concerns the domains encompassed by KT. For example, some organizations use *knowledge translation* synonymously with *commercialization*

CHAPTER OBJECTIVES

After reading this chapter, you should be able to:
- define and discuss "knowledge translation";
- discuss "integrated knowledge translation" and how it might provide guidance regarding the membership of a research team;
- discuss the "knowledge-to-action cycle" and its relevance to the design, conduct and reporting of a research study; and
- recognize that research studies can be designed to assess the effectiveness of various knowledge translation strategies.

Reporting

KEY TERMS

Clinical decision making	Knowledge inquiry	Knowledge-to-action cycle
Integrated knowledge translation	Knowledge synthesis	Policy-making
Knowledge creation	Knowledge tools/products	Stakeholders

or *technology transfer.* Although these processes have many similarities, the first two do not usually address the application of knowledge to decision-making. Similarly, the term *continuing medical education* (CME) is sometimes mistakenly used interchangeably with *knowledge translation.* Although CME or continuing professional development interventions (e.g., audit and feedback, journal clubs) can be considered strategies for knowledge implementation, their target audience—health care professionals—is much smaller than that for KT. In contrast, KT strategies vary according to the targeted users (e.g., researchers, clinicians, policy-makers, public, industry) and the type of knowledge being translated (e.g., clinical, biomedical, health services or policy related).[4]

Why is knowledge translation important?

In health care, a failure to use research evidence to inform clinical practice is evident across all settings and decision-making groups: health care providers, patients, informal caregivers, managers and policy-makers. Practice audits performed in a variety of settings have shown that high-quality evidence is not used consistently in practice.[5] For example, despite high-quality evidence that statins are effective in reducing the risk of mortality and morbidity in patients with a history of stroke, these drugs are markedly underprescribed.[6,7] Conversely, antibiotics are, against the evidence on benefits and harms, overprescribed in children with upper respiratory tract symptoms.[8] The importance of KT is also evident in patient participation in decision-making. A synthesis of 14 studies showed that many patients (26%–95%) were dissatisfied with the information they received from their physicians, and that they want to be more involved in treatment decisions.[9]

A failure to use evidence to inform decision-making is also evident in **policy-making** at higher levels. Lavis and colleagues[10] studied 8 provincial health policy-making processes and found that only 4 of these had been informed by citable health science research. Similarly, it has been found that World Health Organization policy-makers infrequently use evidence from systematic reviews.[11] Dobbins and colleagues[12] found that, although public health guidelines in Ontario were developed using systematic reviews, the recommendations were not adopted at the policy level. Increasing recognition of these deficits in translating knowledge into action has led to efforts to change behaviour, practices and policy.

In our illustrative case, the resident will need to ensure that any intervention she develops in her study is guided by appropriate, rigorous and relevant research evidence. She will also need to consider how the research team should be configured, the most appropriate study design to use, and what contextual factors need to be taken into account. For example, she might begin by recruiting research team members who can help identify the barriers to influenza vaccination (e.g., decision-makers concerned with influenza control, vaccine administration, and vaccine uptake). This step may involve conducting informal or formal qualitative interviews or focus groups with physicians and long-term care staff to identify specific barriers to vaccination uptake. She could then conduct a workflow analysis and discussion with staff at the long-term care facility to determine which **stakeholders** should be involved in the development of her study, and which study design might be most suitable. The selection of study design will also depend on available resources and on whether a proposed intervention is ready for a pilot evaluation, such as using an interrupted time-series design (a method more appropriate for interventions that need further refinement and when resources are limited), a randomized controlled trial (RCT) involving staff within one long-term care facility (if the intervention is ready for a more formal evaluation but smaller in scope), or a cluster RCT in which the unit of analysis is at the level of applicable long-term care facilities (if more resources and a larger scope of evaluation are feasible and appropriate).

This example also represents the concept of **integrated knowledge translation** (IKT), which involves active collaboration and exchange among researchers and knowledge end-users throughout the research process—that is, from identifying the research question to collecting and interpreting the data, to disseminating and applying the results.[13,14] IKT is supported by evidence about the collaborative research process, from which it is possible to infer several key factors for success that can be applied to research that addresses a health or health system issue.[15] These factors are as follows:

- a process to develop a shared perspective, common language and common understanding about the problem or issue that the team will address;
- a plan for collaboration that explicitly describes roles and responsibilities and a commitment to regularly assess effectiveness;

Reporting

- a plan for the inclusion of team members who are collaborative; and
- a strategy for ensuring that trusting relationships among team members are maintained and that conflicts are resolved appropriately when they arise.

What are the determinants of knowledge use?

Multiple factors influence the way research findings are applied by decision-makers.[16–20] Indeed, Cabana and colleagues have identified more than 250 barriers to physician adherence to clinical practice guidelines.[16] The challenges faced by clinical decision-makers include the overwhelming amount of research evidence currently produced, barriers to accessing that evidence, a lack of time to read, and the need for specific skills in appraising, understanding and applying research evidence. Twenty years ago, a general internist, for example, would have needed to read 17 articles a day to keep abreast of the primary clinical literature relevant to the field.[21] Today, the challenge of staying current is even more daunting, given that more than 1000 articles are indexed daily in MEDLINE. Lack of skill in the appraisal of published literature has been a challenge for all stakeholder groups: until recently, most educational curricula did not include this competency as a formal component.[19,22] It has also been found that the content of evidence resources does not adequately meet the needs of end users. For example, although there are criteria to enhance the reporting of systematic reviews,[23] these focus mostly on the *validity* of evidence rather than its *applicability*. Glasziou and colleagues[24] found that only 3 out of 25 systematic reviews published during a 1-year period in *Evidence-Based Medicine* contained a description of the intervention that was adequate to enable clinicians to apply the information to clinical decision-making and practice; this was true even of "simple" interventions such as medications.

Although improving the management of knowledge is necessary, this is not enough to ensure that knowledge will be effectively translated. Challenges exist at different levels of the health care system, and it is important to understand the context in which knowledge is being targeted. This includes consideration of determinants of knowledge uptake and behavioural change at the level of the health care system (e.g., financial disincentives), the health care organization (e.g., lack of equipment), health care teams (e.g., misalignment of local standards of care with recommended practice), individual health care professionals (e.g., variations in knowledge, attitudes and skills in critically appraising and using evidence from clinical literature) and patients (e.g. low adherence to recommendations)—as well as of how these determinants influence and interact with one another. Thus, KT strategies that work in one setting may not be immediately transferable to another, especially without adaptation to local factors. For example, findings from the geriatric resident's study may show that delivering an educational intervention aimed at increasing flu awareness is effective in improving vaccination rates when it is delivered using an interactive video presentation in the lunchroom of her local long-term care (LTC) facility. However, the same intervention might not be effective in LTC facilities where the workflow, environment (e.g., space, equipment), or staff attitudes and beliefs are different. These potential barriers to adaptation need to be taken into account in the design of interventions intended for diverse contexts.

The knowledge-to-action framework

The many theories and frameworks for KT that abound can be confusing.[25–29] Graham and colleagues have developed a conceptual framework, termed the **knowledge-to-action (KTA) cycle**,[2] that builds on commonalities identified in a review of more than 30 planned-action theories. The KTA cycle is meant to be iterative and dynamic to reflect the complexities of the KT process, and identifies *knowledge creation* and *the action cycle* (knowledge application) as the two main components of moving knowledge into practice. Although the model is drawn as a cycle (see Fig. 30.1),[30] the phases can be used in any sequence according to the stage of a project that is the most relevant for moving knowledge forward. Integral to the model is the involvement of knowledge end-users (e.g., clinicians, patients, policy-makers) in the process so that the knowledge and its subsequent implementation are relevant to their needs and is more likely to be applied by them.

Knowledge creation. In the centre of the cycle is **knowledge creation**, which can involve three stages of refinement. The first stage is **knowledge inquiry**, which represents the accumulated body of first-generation knowledge and consists largely of a broad base of primary studies and information. When designing and conducting primary studies, researchers should ensure that they select the most

Reporting

appropriate study design to answer their research questions and consider the most appropriate knowledge end-users in the process. The second stage, **knowledge synthesis**, involves identifying, appraising and synthesizing information pertinent to the research question. It attempts to identify patterns within the existing body of research findings on a topic (e.g., through systematic reviews and meta-analyses). Knowledge syntheses are often the base unit of KT activities: the totality of the evidence is considered, rather than the results of individual studies. It is also important to consider the quality of the evidence. For example, if we are considering a disease management issue, ideally we need evidence from a systematic review of good-quality randomized trials. However, information on adverse events may not be fully captured in these studies, in which case findings from observational studies might also need to be considered. The third stage in the cycle involves further synthesizing and refining the best available knowledge into **knowledge tools/products** for decision-making, such as clinical practice guidelines, decision aids or rules (for both clinicians and patients), algorithms, synopses such as those published by the *ACP Journal Club*, and the "Practice Tools" series published by *Canadian Family Physician*. Each stage can be tailored according to the needs of users, identified research questions, and dissemination strategies, which can then facilitate knowledge uptake. As knowledge is refined through each stage in the knowledge creation process, it becomes more clear, the evidence stronger, and the resulting knowledge potentially more useful to end users.

The action cycle. The action cycle is focused on applying the knowledge that has been identified and refined during the knowledge creation stage. The components of this cycle are derived from theories of planned action that focus on deliberately causing change within health care systems and groups.[25,26] Specifically, they involve mapping out a research plan for disseminating knowledge through the following steps:

1. Identifying the problem.
2. Identifying, reviewing and selecting the knowledge to implement (or identifying, reviewing and selecting the knowledge to implement and then identifying whether a problem exists).
3. Adapting or customizing the knowledge to the local context.

4. Assessing barriers to using the knowledge.
5. Tailoring, implementing and monitoring interventions related to KT and resulting knowledge use.
6. Evaluating outcomes or effects of using the knowledge.
7. Determining strategies for ensuring sustained use of the knowledge.

These steps can occur sequentially or simultaneously, and the knowledge creation stages can influence the action steps at any point in the cycle. Integral to the framework is the need to consider the various stakeholders (e.g., patients, clinicians, managers and policy-makers) who are the end users of the knowledge being implemented. Knowledge creation and its action steps can be seen as two separate components undertaken by different stakeholders, or as a unified process involving the same set of participants.

How can the knowledge-to-action cycle be applied?

To illustrate each phase of the knowledge-to-action cycle, we will show how a local group (including researchers, physicians and patient advocates) might address the application of knowledge concerning falls prevention and osteoporosis assessment and follow-up.

Identify, review, select knowledge. A group of clinicians and researchers is aware that systematic reviews have shown that osteoporosis medications such as bisphosphonates can reduce the risk of fractures.[31] Although evidence on the prevention of falls is more controversial,[32] the group is interested in investigating falls prevention and osteoporosis management.

Identify the problem. The group conducts a local audit and finds that less than 40% of patients aged 65 years and older who were admitted to hospital after a fall or with a fracture were subsequently assessed for osteoporosis or risk for falls.[33] They feel that something should be done about this gap between knowledge and practice.

Adapt knowledge to the local context. The group recognizes that, to be applied effectively, evidence in any form—e.g., knowledge syntheses, patient decision aids, and clinical practice guidelines—needs to be adapted to

Reporting

the local context. For example, the ADAPTE tool[a] offers a three-phase process whereby clinical, health service and administrative decision-makers can adapt clinical practices guidelines for local use.[34] The goal of this tool is to engage local stakeholders and preserve the integrity of the evidence that forms the basis for recommendations. Methods such as ADAPTE help users identify potential local barriers, avoid deviations from the evidence base, and align evidence to local contexts.

A useful resource in the context of oncology is the Cancer Guideline Adaptation and Implementation Project (CAN-IMPLEMENT) tool, which consists of a guide, a library science supplement, and a toolkit.[35] This tool was developed as a practical guide to adapting existing guideline recommendations to local contexts, thus facilitating their implementation.

In view of their own local context, where many patients do not have a primary care physician or might not tend to discuss falls and fracture risk with their doctor, the group decides to create tools to help patients implement recommendations for weight-bearing exercise and intake of calcium and vitamin D.

Figure 30.1

The knowledge-to-action cycle.[2,30]

Reproduced by kind permission of The Journal of Continuing Education in the Health Professions

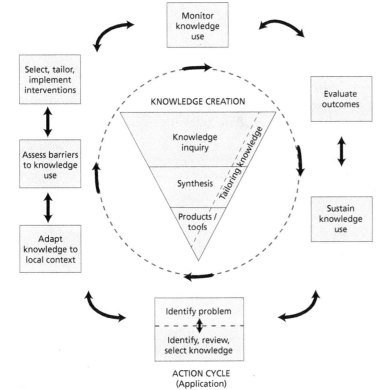

ACTION CYCLE
(Application)

Assess barriers and facilitators to using the knowledge. The group also understands the importance of assessing potential barriers to, and facilitators of, the implementation of their adapted tools. The Clinical Practice Guidelines Framework for Improvement, a conceptual model for investigating barriers to knowledge use in health care, initially identified 293 potential barriers to physician guideline adherence;[16] these were then extended to include facilitators of knowledge use in clinical practice (i.e., factors that promote shared decision-making in clinical practice).[17]

Among the barriers identified by the group are (1) the fragmentation of health records that could be used to identify patients at risk, and (2) the distribution of the target population over a large region. Other barriers are identified at the level of the patient (e.g., lack of understanding that osteoporosis and fractures are linked and that osteoporosis can be prevented) and the provider (e.g., lack of time, and lack of access to bone mineral density testing and interpretation).

Select, tailor and implement interventions. Once factors that can impede or facilitate knowledge use have been identified, KT interventions need to be selected, tailored to specific barriers for change and implemented. The selection of interventions is complex, since current evidence alone cannot be used to guide implementers on the best choice of intervention. Research to date has focused mainly on educational programs, feedback and reminders, and has shown no more than a 10% absolute improvement in selected outcomes (although this change can be clinically or economically relevant). Active educational interventions (e.g., quality circles for professionals), active self-study materials or websites (e.g., for distance learning) are more likely to induce change than passive educational interventions; patient-directed interventions (e.g., decision aids) can support quality improvement in some cases; and interventions that bring evidence to the point of care (e.g., reminders and decision support) are likely to be effective in the areas of prevention and test ordering.[36,37]

In our example, the group developed a multi-component, nurse-led strategy that incorporated patient education, self-management, review of medications, and assessment of homes for fall-related risks.

Reporting

a See www.g-i-n.net/activities/adaptation

Monitor knowledge use. After a KT intervention has been implemented, knowledge use should be monitored to determine how and to what extent it has been disseminated. This will give an indication of whether adjustments to the KT plan are needed. How knowledge uptake is measured depends on the user's perspective, and on how the knowledge is defined and applied. There are two main types of knowledge use, namely instrumental (the concrete application of knowledge and changes in behaviour or practice) and conceptual (changes in understanding or attitude that may inform decision-making but do not change practice). In our example, the use of osteoporosis medications would be an example of instrumental or concrete knowledge use.

Evaluate outcomes or impact. The next step is to determine whether the knowledge use affects patient, provider and system outcomes. This is a point in the cycle when studies can be designed and conducted to evaluate the results of knowledge translation. For example, Tu and colleagues conducted an evaluation that clearly documented the effect of the HOPE study on ramipril prescribing.[38] The group conducts a randomized trial to determine whether their KT strategy is effective. The indicators of knowledge use include appropriate osteoporosis management according to guidelines (e.g., use of medications).[33] The trial also considers quality of life, patient satisfaction and fractures. Another outcome is the strength of the collaboration developed by the group, which grew to include representatives from the provincial government, pharmaceutical companies and insurance companies.

Sustain knowledge use. An important but often overlooked phase of the KTA cycle is sustainability of the knowledge use—that is, the degree to which an innovation continues to be used after initial efforts to secure its adoption have succeeded.[39,40] Scant attention has been given to sustainability, perhaps because many clinical researchers consider system-level change processes to be outside their realm of research. Another barrier is presented by the short-term nature of funding opportunities: follow-up measurements are typically feasible for only 1 or 2 years, allowing only shorter-term change processes to be addressed. Although sustainability is typically not considered until implementation is under way, we recommend that plans to ensure sustainability be made as early as possible in the KTA cycle, when the interventions for knowledge use are being selected and tailored.

Conclusion

Knowledge translation strategies and interventions can close gaps between evidence and practice in many settings and disciplines. Resources must be focused on the use of effective KT strategies, as well as on studying the effectiveness of untested KT interventions. KT interventions must address all aspects of care, including access to and use of valid evidence, patient safety strategies, and organizational and systems issues. However, we must also be cautious of the assumption that all knowledge should be translated, for this depends on whether a mature and valid base of evidence for the knowledge in question exists. Moreover, health care systems have limitations and cannot accomplish every goal, no matter how desirable: researchers must work with stakeholders, including patients, the public, clinicians and policy-makers, to establish an explicit process for prioritizing activities related to knowledge translation. ∎

Reporting

CASE POSTSCRIPT

To enhance all aspects of her proposed study, especially its potential impact on the influenza vaccination rates of staff in long-term care, the geriatrics resident first conducts a systematic review to identify which strategies have the potential to improve vaccination rates. This represents the "knowledge creation" component of the KTA framework. She then uses an IKT (integrated knowledge translation) approach by working with her supervisor to recruit relevant knowledge end-users to become part of the research team, and to determine how the findings of the systematic review could inform the development of an intervention applicable in the context of LTC facilities. The inclusion of a long-term care nurse, a nursing home manager and the local medical officer of health on the research team improved the study's question, design and conduct, greatly enhances the practical applicability and relevance of its results in her local context, and the potential of her intervention to be adapted to other settings.

REFERENCES

1. Canadian Institutes of Health Research (CIHR) definition of KT. Available from: www.cihr-irsc.gc.ca/e/29418.html

2. Graham ID, Logan J, Harrison MB, Straus SE, Tetroe J, Caswell W, et al. Lost in knowledge translation: time for a map? *J Contin Educ Health Prof.* 2006;26(1):13–24.

3. McKibbon KA, Lokker C, Wilczynski NL, Ciliska D, Dobbins M, Davis DA, et al. A cross-sectional study of the number and frequency of terms used to refer to knowledge translation in a body of health literature in 2006: a Tower of Babel? *Implementation Science.* 2010;5:16.

4. Davis D, Evans M, Jadada A, et al. The case for knowledge translation: shortening the journey from evidence to effect. *BMJ.* 2003;327:33–5.

5. McGlynn EA, Asch SM, Adams J, Keesey J, Hicks J, DeCristofaro A, et al. The quality of health care delivered to adults in the United States. *N Engl J Med.* 2003;348(2):2635–45.

6. Majumdar SR, McAlister FA, Furberg CD. From knowledge to practice in chronic cardiovascular disease: a long and winding road. *J Am Coll Cardiol.* 2004;43(10):1738–42.

7. LaRosa JC, He J, Vupputuri S. Effect of statins on risk of coronary disease: a meta-analysis of randomized controlled trials. *JAMA.* 1999;282(24):2340–6.

8. Arnold SR, Straus SE. Interventions to improve antibiotic prescribing practices in ambulatory care. *Cochrane Database Syst Rev.* 2005 Oct 19;(4):CD003539.

9. Kiesler DJ, Auerbach SM. Optimal matches of patient preferences for information, decision-making and interpersonal behavior: evidence, models and interventions. *Patient Educ Couns.* 2006;61(3):319–41.

10. Lavis JN, Ross SE, Hurley JE, Hohenadel JM, Stoddart GL, Woodward CA, et al. Examining the role of health services research in public policymaking. *Milbank Q.* 2002;80(1):125–54.

11. Oxman AD, Lavis JN, Fretheim A. Use of evidence in WHO recommendations. *Lancet.* 2007;369(9576):1883–9.

12. Dobbins M, Thomas H, O'Brien MA, Duggan M. Use of systematic reviews in the development of new provincial public health policies in Ontario. *Int J Technol Assess Health Care.* 2004;20(4):399–404.

13. Graham ID, Tetroe J. How to translate health research knowledge into effective healthcare action. *Healthc Q.* 2007;10(3):20–2.

14. Denis JL, Lomas J. Convergent evolution: the academic and policy roots of collaborative research. *J Health Serv Res Policy.* 2003;8 Suppl 2:1–6.

15. Straus S, Tetroe J, Graham ID, editors. *Knowledge translation in health care: moving from evidence to practice.* Oxford: Blackwell Publishing; 2009. Chapter 5.1. Sustaining knowledge use. p. 240.

16. Cabana MD, Rand CS, Powe NR, Wu AW, Wilson MH, Abboud PA, et al. Why don't physicians follow clinical practice guidelines? A framework for improvement. *JAMA.* 1999;282(15):1458–65.

17. Gravel K, Légaré F, Graham ID. Barriers and facilitators to implementing shared decision-making in clinical practice: a systematic review of health professionals' perceptions. *Implement Sci.* 2006;1:16.

18. Légaré F, O'Connor AM, Graham ID, Saucier D, Côté L, Blais J, et al. Primary health care professionals' views on barriers and facilitators to the implementation of the Ottawa Decision Support Framework in practice. *Patient Educ Couns.* 2006;63(3):380–90.

19. Milner M, Estabrooks CA, Myrick F. Research utilisation and clinical nurse educators: a systematic review. *J Eval Clin Pract.* 2006;12(6):639–55.

20. Grimshaw JM, Eccles MP, Walker AE, Thomas RE. Changing physicians' behaviour: what works and thoughts on getting more things to work. *J Contin Educ Health Prof.* 2002;22(4):237–43.

21. Haynes RB. Where's the meat in clinical journals? [editorial]. *ACP J Club.* 1993;119:A22–3.

22. Lavis JN. Research, public policymaking, and knowledge-translation processes: Canadian efforts to build bridges. *J Contin Educ Health Prof.* 2006;26(1):37–45.

23. Moher D, Liberati A, Tetzlaff J, Altman DG. Preferred reporting items for systematic reviews and meta-analyses: the PRISMA statement. *BMJ.* 2009;339:b2535.

24. Glasziou P, Meats E, Heneghan C, Shepperd S. What is missing from descriptions of treatment in trials and reviews? *BMJ.* 2008;336(7659):1472–4.

Reporting

25. Graham ID, Harrison MB, Logan J and the KT Theories Research Group. A review of planned change (knowledge translation) models, frameworks and theories. Presented at the Joanna Briggs Institute International Convention, Adelaide, Australia, Nov. 28–30, 2005.

26. Graham ID, Tetroe J; KT Theories Research Group. Some theoretical underpinnings of knowledge translation. *Acad Emerg Med.* 2007;14(11):936–41.

27. Estabrooks CA, Thompson DS, Lovely JJ, Hofmeyer A. A guide to knowledge translation theory. *J Contin Educ Health Prof.* 2006;26(1):25–36.

28. McDonald KM, Graham ID, Grimshaw J. Toward a theoretic basis for quality improvement interventions. In: Shojania KG, McDonald KM, Wachter RM, Owens DK, editors. *Closing the quality gap: a critical analysis of quality improvement strategies.* Vol. 1: Series overview and methodology. Technical Review 9.1; 2004 AHRQ Report No. 04-0051-1. Rockville (MD): Agency for Healthcare Research and Quality; 2004. Available from: www.ncbi.nlm.nih.gov/bookshelf/br.fcgi?book=hstechrev&part=A26505

29. Wensing M, Bosch M, Foy R, van der Weijden, Eccles M, Grol R. *Factors in theories on behaviour change to guide implementation and quality improvement in healthcare.* Nijmegen: Centre for Quality of Care Research; 2005.

30. Straus SE, Tetroe J, Graham I. Defining knowledge translation. *CMAJ.* 2009;181(3–4):165–8.

31. Wells GA, Cranney A, Peterson J, Boucher M, Shea B, Robinson V, et al. Alendronate for the primary and secondary prevention of osteoporotic fractures in postmenopausal women. *Cochrane Database Syst Rev.* 2008;(1):CD001155.

32. Gates S, Fisher JD, Cooke MW, Carter YH, Lamb SE. Multifactorial assessment and targeted intervention for preventing falls and injuries among older people in community and emergency settings: systematic review and meta-analysis. *BMJ.* 2008;336(7636):130–3.

33. Ciaschini PM, Straus SE, Dolovich LR, Goeree RA, Leung KM, Woods CR, et al. Community-based randomised controlled trial evaluating falls and osteoporosis risk management strategies. *Trials.* 2008;9:62.

34. Fervers B, Burgers JS, Haugh MC, Latreille J, Mlika-Cabanne N, Paquet L, et al. Adaptation of clinical guidelines: literature review and proposition for a framework and procedure. *Int J Qual Health Care.* 2006;18(3):167–76.

35. Harrison MB, van den Hoek J; Canadian Guideline Adaptation Study Group. *CAN-IMPLEMENT: guideline adaptation and implementation planning resource.* Available from: www.cancerview.ca/idc/groups/public/documents/webcontent/canimp_toolkit.pdf

36. Grimshaw JM, Thomas RE, MacLennan G, Fraser C, Ramsay CR, Vale L, et al. Effectiveness and efficiency of guideline dissemination and implementation strategies. *Health Technol Assess.* 2004;8(6):iii–iv, 1–72.

37. Straus SE, Tetroe, J, Graham ID, editors. *Knowledge translation in health care: moving from evidence to practice.* Oxford: Blackwell Publishing; 2009. Chapter 3.5. Selecting KT interventions. p. 94–150.

38. Tu K, Mamdani MM, Jacka RM, Forde NJ, Rothwell DM, Tu JV. The striking effect of the Heart Outcomes Prevention Evaluation (HOPE) on ramipril prescribing in Ontario. *CMAJ.* 2003;168(5):553–7.

39. Rogers EM. *Diffusion of innovations.* 5th ed. New York: Free Press; 2005. p. 429.

40. Straus Se, Tetroe J, Graham ID, editors. *Knowledge translation in health care: moving from evidence to practice.* Oxford: Blackwell Publishing; 2009. Chapter 3.7. Sustaining knowledge use. p. 165–73.

Reporting

SUMMARY CHECKLIST

- ❑ In the context of your study, describe why knowledge translation is relevant and important.
- ❑ List the stakeholders of your study.
- ❑ Using the knowledge-to-action cycle, develop a plan to enhance the adoption of any results of your work.

31
Responsibility and integrity: Disseminating research findings to the public

Robert L. Reid, MD, FRCSC

ILLUSTRATIVE CASE

A final-year resident in Internal Medicine has collaborated on a research project in which umbilical cord stem cells have been induced to differentiate into what appear to be primitive renal glomeruli. To generate enthusiasm for his research presentation at a national meeting, he titles it "Kidneys from a dish: advances in stem cell research." After the presentation he is approached for a story by a local science reporter. He is surprised and embarrassed the next day when his supervisor calls him to ask what he was thinking when he spoke to the reporter. His presentation and interview resulted in headlines across the country, and he was quoted as saying, "This breakthrough has opened the door for us to grow artificial kidneys from stem cells." Apparently the phone at the hospital has been ringing constantly with calls from anxious parents of children on dialysis wanting to know when their child can get a kidney. What went wrong?

■ **Knowledge translation has been** defined by the Canadian Institutes of Health Research as "a dynamic and iterative process that includes synthesis, dissemination, exchange and ethically-sound application of knowledge to improve the health of Canadians, provide more effective health services and products and strengthen the health care system."[1]

Successful clinician-researchers are very busy people, many of whom feel that their duty to disseminate research findings ends with publishing their studies in peer-reviewed health science journals. Some tend to avoid the lay media entirely. There can be many reasons to be media-shy (Textbox 31.1), not the least of which is the difficulty of explaining complex scientific principles or new findings to a reporter with little scientific training. And then there are the horror stories of articles or broadcasts in which the researcher's comments are misquoted or taken out of context, or his or her work is ridiculed by an outspoken antagonist in the name of "balance" or "debate."[2–4]

For their part, journalists frequently express concerns about health researchers and how they respond to legitimate enquires about health and scientific matters (Textbox 31.2). Given these perceptions and misgivings on both sides, it is not surprising that a mutual mistrust has developed between these two professional cultures.

CHAPTER OBJECTIVES

After reading this chapter, you should be able to:
- describe the role of the media in the dissemination of research
- describe sources of misunderstanding between researchers and the media
- list occasions when it is appropriate for researchers to interact with the media
- cite common errors that have an adverse impact on researchers' interactions with the media
- describe key strategies to deliver an effective health science message

Reporting

KEY TERMS		
Absolute and relative risks	Convenience sample	Media interview
Bias	Fraud	Peer review
Competing interests	Knowledge translation	Pitfalls of reporting
Context	Lay media	Redundant publication

TEXTBOX 31.1 HEALTH RESEARCHERS' NEGATIVE PERCEPTIONS OF JOURNALISTS AND THE MEDIA

Journalists

- Often lack health and scientific knowledge
- Are ill informed about critical appraisal and the principles of evidence-based medicine
- Prefer to report relative versus absolute risks and benefits
- Often fail to distinguish between association and causation
- May fail to put risks into context
- Report "latest news" from scientific meetings without appreciating that these data have had only preliminary analysis and peer review

The media

- Are profit-driven and highly competitive
- Prefer sensational articles to true ones ("If it bleeds it leads.")
- Concentrate on bad news and weird events
- Have a bias toward controversy and conflict
- Believe "balance" is achieved when two opposing views are presented without consideration of the validity of those views
- Have a short time frame for comment
- Distill complex issues into simple "Yes" or "No" answers for the public
- Allow unadjudicated "Letters to the editor" by lay public that frequently castigate health professionals and misinform the public

TEXTBOX 31.2 JOURNALISTS' NEGATIVE PERCEPTIONS OF HEALTH RESEARCHERS

Health researchers

- Work in a highly competitive "publish or perish" culture; some go so far as to fake their data
- Sometimes try to use the media for self-promotion
- Are often elitist and unapproachable (won't return calls)
- Are poorly trained to be knowledge translators (don't speak in plain language)
- Give complex answers to simple questions
- Cannot agree: different experts often give conflicting answers and explanations
- May have financial conflicts of interest (e.g., pharmaceutical sponsorship or industry ties)
- Lack understanding of the constraints of journalism (e.g., timelines and space limitations)

As health researchers, we need to improve the way we translate knowledge arising from our research findings. Doing so involves developing skills in working effectively with the media. The sooner we recognize that the media represent a critical bridge to the public, and to the policy-makers who support our research, the better off we will be. Although it is important to be aware of the potential pitfalls of communicating research findings through the **lay media**, it is also important to appreciate the potential benefits (Textbox 31.3).

Common errors in reporting scientific findings

This section will examine common errors that can lead to misleading conclusions or interpretations being reported to the public. These errors can arise from the original research report, its translation to the media through news releases, an inaccurate representation of the work by the researcher in interviews, or a lack of understanding on the part of the journalist of research practices and their limitations or the meaning of statistical analyses. In their communications with the media, researchers and their communications staff can be alert to these **pitfalls of reporting** and present findings in a clear way that will help to avert misunderstanding.

TEXTBOX 31.3 REASONS FOR HEALTH EXPERTS AND RESEARCHERS TO WORK WITH THE MEDIA

- To address important public health issues or respond to public concerns about health issues
- To respond to inaccurate or incomplete media coverage of important issues
- To provide information during a health crisis (medication shortage, SARS, H1N1, etc.)
- To discuss new research findings after there has been an opportunity for peer review through formal presentation and publication

Reporting

- To draw the attention of funding agencies and policy-makers to a promising line of research in order to facilitate grant support
- To raise public awareness about a research centre and its programs, attracting potential research participants and those wishing to make donations to support the centre's research
- To respond to a request for expert opinion about a new research finding

Extrapolating results from convenience samples to the general population

Researchers often choose a readily accessible research target population without considering, or making it clear, that this **convenience sample** does not necessarily represent the true population at large and that the results might not, therefore, be widely applicable.

Example: A health researcher decides to study the rates of *Chlamydia* infection in the community by examining the available test results of an infertility clinic. Of 100 swabs, 8 are positive for *Chlamydia*. The researcher reports that *Chlamydia* is on the rise in the local community because a public health survey five years earlier found only a 2% positive rate in women attending for annual Pap smears. Clearly, the convenience of using results that were readily available needed to be balanced with caution about extrapolation to a different population: no conclusions about a rise or fall in the prevalence of *Chlamydia* would be warranted. This error is repeated in media reports on the research.

Reporting risks and benefits reported as relative risk rather than as absolute or attributable risks

A common marketing tool is to report a benefit as a percentage (or relative) change because this often magnifies the apparent effect. Journal articles often report **absolute and relative risks**, and authors and editors need to take care that these two categories are distinct and clear. Similarly, media reports frequently fail to make this distinction, reporting relative risks and benefits as if they were absolute or attributable, thus presenting an exaggerated and even misleading picture of the research results.

Example: A newspaper reported that a medication reduces the risk of heart attack by 50%. Your patient, a 40-year-old man with a family history of heart disease, asks to be started on the medication. You read the research paper on which the news item was based and discover that, given his age and his few personal risk factors for heart disease, your patient would need to take the medicine for 10 years to achieve a reduction in myocardial infarction risk from 1/1000 to 0.5/1000. (You advise instead that he increase his physical activity!)

Example: The Results section of the first report from the Women's Health Initiative announced that women who used combined estrogen/progestin hormone therapy had a 26% increase in the risk for breast cancer.[5] Not surprisingly, many media outlets used this worrisome statistic in subsequent reports. In fact, the published data actually showed that no increase in breast cancer risk had been observed in the 75% of women who had never used hormone therapy before study entry, and that among those women who had received hormone therapy in the past, breast cancer was detected in 30/10 000 of those who received placebo versus 38/10 000 who received hormone therapy. The "absolute" increase was thus 8/10 000 users per year, giving an attributable risk of 0.08%—a level classified as "rare" by the World Health Organization.[6]

Failing to put risks and benefits in context.

"By underestimating common risks while exaggerating exotic ones we end up protecting ourselves against the unlikely perils while failing to take precautions against those most likely to do us in."

—Larry Laudan, *The Book of Risks*[7]

A number of factors determine how the general public perceives and assesses risk. The perception of risk varies according to whether the risk is natural or artificial (exposure to sun is perceived as less worrisome than exposure to asbestos), voluntary or involuntary (smoking is seen as less worrisome than exposure to pesticides or nuclear power plants), offers significant benefits (heart surgery has risks, but the potential benefit is thought to outweigh the risk for most patients), or has affected a personal acquaintance (having a relative with osteoporosis or Alzheimer's disease engenders increased worry about these conditions). Finally, and probably most importantly, risk is perceived relative to other risks of daily living—that is, in **context**.[8–11]

Reporting

Example: The risk of breast cancer in postmenopausal women using combined hormone therapy for 5 years is comparable to the risk resulting from early menarche, delayed menopause, postmenopausal obesity, failure to exercise, and daily ingestion of alcohol.[12] It is less than the risk that results from delayed first pregnancy and failure to breastfeed. When the risks are considered in this context, many women are less fearful than they might otherwise be of using short-term hormone therapy for the relief of distressing vasomotor symptoms.

Failing to properly examine correlations to determine whether a finding represents association, or causation.

This is perhaps one of the most common mistakes in media reporting. In evaluating causation, the Bradford-Hill criteria[13] should be used. These stipulate that the case for a causal association is strengthened by a demonstration of consistency, the strength of the association, specificity, a temporal relationship, biological plausibility, coherence, a dose–response relationship, and experimentation.

Example: The rising incidence of autism has occurred over the same time frame as the increasing use of vaccines containing the preservative thimerosal. The resulting speculation that the two might be causally linked has led to fear and the under-utilization of vaccines, resulting in recent outbreaks of measles and mumps.

Reporting (non peer-reviewed) preliminary findings without subsequent confirmation

Journalists, eager to give their readership the latest scientific news, describe new breakthroughs described in the program of a health science meeting. Unfortunately, these findings have not undergone the scrutiny of **peer review** and publication in a scientific journal, the methods may not be mature and reproducible, and the suggested results may never pan out. Unfortunately, this misleads the general public, raising false hope about new tests and treatments.

Example: In September 2009, in the midst of the H1N1 influenza pandemic, the media reported on preliminary research suggesting that the seasonal flu shot may put people at greater risk for getting pandemic flu.[14] Although they had not been validated at the time, these reports resulted in increased uncertainty and anxiety about

whether Canadians should receive the seasonal influenza vaccine. The results of the implicated studies were ultimately published in April 2010,[15] after the H1N1 pandemic had subsided.

Advocating the use of certain medications, procedures or products without acknowledging vested interests

The issue of vested interests arises in various contexts of knowledge translation. Medical journals require that financial and other **competing interests** be declared, and contemporary guidelines for continuing medical education require presenters to disclose their industry ties. It is hardly surprising, however, that medical experts are called on to act as advisors or consultants for pharmaceutical or device manufacturing companies. Indeed, such collaborations are needed. In Canada, a lack of collaboration between academic researchers and industry, particularly in phase 1 trials, has led to the loss of opportunities for researchers and their institutions.[16] The acknowledgement of a competing interest should not be seen as an indication that **bias** or undue influence necessarily exists; however, to alert the media audience to the *potential* for bias, competing interests—both for the researchers whose findings are reported, and for any experts asked to comment on that research—should be stated transparently. Further, the potential effects of industry conflict of interest have been documented in at least two studies, one finding that 98% of papers based on industry-sponsored studies reflected favourably on the industry's products[17] and another concluding that industry-funded studies were 8 times less likely to reach conclusions unfavourable to their drugs than were independently funded studies.[18] This issue was highlighted recently by the controversy caused by revelations that the increased cardiovascular risks caused by the use of selective cyclo-oxygenase-2 (COX-2) inhibitors were deliberately concealed by the manufacturer.[19]

Portraying a visionary interpretation of preliminary findings a state-of-the-art

The health sciences need visionaries: individuals who are forward-looking and can picture exciting new applications for emerging technologies. This is the basis for research and clinical experimentation. However, when such individuals talk to reporters they must clearly identify when their ideas are conjectural and when they are backed by sound scientific evidence.

Reporting

Example: See the illustrative case at the beginning of this chapter!

Publishing duplicate or fraudulant data

There are numerous examples of situations in which a scientist has published a case series involving a new treatment and has had a second publication at a later date in which the original cases were reported again. Unless this is explicitly stated in the methods, it gives the impression that the method is more mature and valid than is justified by the clinical experience. There are also a surprising number of cases of research reports wherein data were fabricated or falsified. Media accounts of the original reports garnered worldwide attention because of the striking claims made by the investigators. Although subsequent revelations that the reports were fraudulent have set the record straight, such cases undermine the credibility of scientists in general and heighten public skepticism about the role and value of research.

In 1997 an organization called COPE (Committee on Publication Ethics) was founded by medical editors in the United Kingdom in response to growing anxiety about the integrity of research submissions. The members—including those of the *British Medical Journal, Gut* and The *Lancet*—advise on cases of suspected **redundant publication** or **fraud** brought to them by other editors. Of 212 issues discussed by COPE between 1997 and 2004, 58 involved undeclared duplicate or redundant publication, 26 involved authorship issues, 25 involved a lack of ethics approval, 22 involved the absence or inadequacy of informed consent, and 19 involved fabrication or falsification.[20,21]

The implications of research fraud are enormous.[22,23] Its victims include other researchers, who may base current or future research on findings that are impossible to replicate, funding agencies that invest valuable resources on fraudulent research, pharmaceutical companies that may invest millions into developing a promising medication when adverse side effects are hidden, and, most importantly, the public who may receive interventions with little or no benefit and undisclosed risks.

Examples: See Textbox 31.4.

TEXTBOX 31.4   EXAMPLES OF FALSIFICATION OF RESEARCH FINDINGS

1. Jon Sudbø and 13 coauthors from Denmark reported in *The Lancet* that nonsteroidal anti-inflammatory drugs reduced the risk of oral cancers. This "finding" was based entirely on fabricated data on the lives and lifestyles of 900 people.[24] A retraction was published by the journal's editor in 2006 when the data were discovered to be false.

   Penalty: Sudbø's authorization as physician and dentist was revoked by the Norwegian Board of Health, his PhD was revoked by the University of Oslo, and his papers were retracted from journals, including *The Lancet*.

2. Malcolm Pearce (then associate editor of the *British Journal of Obstetrics and Gynaecology* [*BJOG*]) authored two papers in one issue of the *BJOG*.[25,26] In one article the claim was made that an ectopic pregnancy was moved from the fallopian tube into the uterus, resulting in survival of the offspring. The other was a randomized clinical trial involving a new treatment to prevent recurrent miscarriage in women with polycystic ovary syndrome. Both reports were later proven to have been falsified.

   Penalty: Pearce was found guilty of serious professional misconduct and struck from the medical register. Geoffrey Chamberlain (then editor of the *BJOG* and President of the Royal College of Obstetrics and Gynaecology in the United Kingdom, and whose name appeared on one of the papers (a "gift" authorship), resigned as editor of *BJOG* and president of the College. The medical school identified other publications by Pearce to be dubious, and a total of six publications were retracted, including two in *BMJ*.

3. Woo-Suk Hwang was acclaimed as a national hero in his native South Korea after he published a report in the journal *Science* describing the first cloning of human embryonic stem cells.[27] Other researchers could not replicate his work, and the findings were subsequently shown to have been falsified.

   Penalty: Hwang was dismissed by Seoul National University and expelled from the Korean Society for Molecular and Cellular Biology; his licence on embryonic stem cell research was revoked by the South Korean government, he was convicted of fraud and embezzlement, and his papers were retracted from *Science*.

Reporting

Giving an effective media interview

If your professional role exposes you to the media, the most important preparation you can make is to take a media training course. A one-day training program for Canadian residents in Obstetrics and Gynecology was shown to significantly improve residents' ability to deliver medical messages effectively.[28]

When asked for a **media interview**, remember to respect the reporter's timelines. You do have the opportunity to control the interview, but only if you come prepared. To do this you should understand the reporter's angle on the story and determine who else will be interviewed, to see what opposing or contradictory viewpoints may be aired. Your audience is the general public—not the reporter—and so you should speak in short, manageable "sound bites" that will be clear to non-scientists. Be sure to express your views in a way that is sympathetic to the concerns of the general public. For example, don't say: "The cutbacks in operating room time are upsetting the cardiac surgeons." This sounds as if the main problem with cutbacks is lost income for doctors—a view that will gain little sympathy from the public. A more appropriate concern to express would be: "Cutbacks in operating room time are raising fears of longer waiting lists and the possibility of needless deaths while people wait for life-saving cardiac surgery."

The telephone interview

If you have a receptionist, it may be advisable for him or her to field calls from the media so that, rather than agreeing to speak to a reporter immediately, you will have a little time to prepare. Train your receptionist to ask for the reason for the interview, the "angle" for the story, who else will be interviewed, and the deadline. If the reporter is seeking comments about a newly published article , have him or her fax a copy to your office. This will give you a chance to read the article and seek advice from other experts so that your critique is well-informed and thorough. Prepare a "bottom-line message" in advance of the interview and seek opportunities to bridge your answer to that point. If you are asked whether you have anything else to add at the end of the interview, return to your key point. Media people also know that a catchy phrase or quotation that supports their viewpoint will often feature prominently in the next day's paper.

Example: Imagine you are the head of Geriatrics at a regional hospital and you have been lobbying the administration to expand facilities to allow better local care for elderly people in your community. At last night's hospital board meeting a community member put forward a motion to spend the money on a much-needed facelift for the hospital, which would delay the expansion of the geriatrics department for three years. A reporter calls to get your viewpoint.

You prepare your bottom-line message before calling the reporter: "While there is no doubt that a cosmetic facelift of the whole facility is needed, our resources are limited and every year that we delay the upgrade to our geriatric facilities more families with ageing parents in this community will have to travel great distances to get the care that should be available locally."

During the interview the reporter asks, "Aren't you just opposing the overall hospital facelift because you are a geriatrician who wants nicer facilities to work in? Shouldn't all hospital staff benefit from renovation dollars?"

At this point you need to take the heat off yourself, focus on the perspective of the general public, and "bridge" to your bottom line. You reply: "The debate is not about who is going to enjoy the renovations more. Rather, the real issue is that if we do not upgrade our geriatric facilities, many families will experience significant disruption to their lives when referrals to other centres are needed to get basic care for their ageing parents—care that should be available right here in our community!"

You then add a catchy sound-bite: "As geriatricians our goal is not just to add years to life; we realize the importance of adding life to years!"

The television interview

A live television interview is generally a "safer" bet than a prerecorded interview, from which selected comments can be edited to suit a reporter's agenda. In a live interview it is critical to prepare as you would for a telephone interview: know the agenda and have a prepared, bottom-line message. Practice bridging to your message from a variety of angles. Remember to dress neatly and professionally, look at the camera, don't fidget, and do not respond with hostility, as this can make you look nervous or "guilty as charged."

You should avoid saying "No comment" when asked about something of a sensitive nature: this may give the appearance of a cover-up. For example, a newborn baby disappears during your shift on call at the hospital. The reporter asks: "Is it true that the hospital doesn't know where baby X was taken last night?" Rather than say "No

Reporting

comment," you could state: "While I am not at liberty to comment on a specific situation, I can assure you that if a baby has gone missing at our hospital there will be a thorough investigation and appropriate action taken."

It is entirely appropriate to decline to answer "what if" questions (e.g., "If your hospital burned down, what would happen to cardiac surgery?") by stating that you are not prepared to address hypothetical issues: "Let's stick to the real problem today [bridge], which is …. [bottom line message]." It is also appropriate to decline to answer questions of a personal nature (e.g., "Would you allow your daughter to have an abortion?") by responding, "What I would or wouldn't do is not the issue. What needs to be remembered [bridge] is the fact that … [bottom-line message]."

In a recorded interview, it is appropriate to "stop and reload" if you stumble on an answer: "Let me rephrase that …". The editor will usually only use a very short sound bite after what may seem like an hour of actual taping.

Don't ramble on in an interview. Await a specific question and stop after giving a succinct answer. Some reporters will look at you and nod or say "Uh-huh" as a way to get you to keep talking, but don't be lured into saying more than you intended.

Follow-up

If you see an article with faulty health information in your local newspaper, you may wish to write to the editor of the paper with a correction. You need to sound professional in both the tone and the content of your letter.

Example: "In the interest of clarity and accuracy I wanted to set the record straight about the number of knee replacements that we do and our complication rate …"

Unfortunately, letters of this nature often incite disgruntled patients to write with their horror stories of bungled knee operations, and so forth, and so it's wise to reserve your letters to the editor for extremely important points. Alternatively, you can send a letter or email directly to the reporter to help him or her get the facts straight. This is par-

ticularly important when an article lacks balance or perspective. Provide references so that your position is well substantiated. Rarely will this cause the reporter to write a retraction or correction. However, he or she may appreciate your expertise in the subject area and call you in advance of a future report on a similar topic.

If you read or see an excellent report on a health topic, this might be an excellent opportunity to build rapport with the reporter by sending a short congratulatory email on the quality or balance of the story. Positive feedback can be a factor in how journalists interact with you and the medical profession in the future.

Conclusion

As health care researchers, we need to appreciate our vital responsibility to share our discoveries with colleagues in the health sciences, with the public, and with policy-makers, who may use these findings to improve health care. Health care researchers are held in high regard: this respect carries with it a responsibility to ensure that the messages we deliver are well reasoned and balanced. Although presentations at scientific meetings and publications in peer-reviewed journals provide a microscope under which the quality of research is examined, history has shown that these filters alone are not foolproof. We must be vigilant in our scrutiny of others' research claims and have the integrity to acknowledge the potential and real shortcomings in our own research. The media play a powerful role in public education. As an example, it was an article in Reader's Digest[29] that did more to promote internal mammary artery ligation for coronary artery disease in the 1950s than the technical publication that first described the proposed surgical technique.[30,31] Health practitioners and researchers need to understand how media work and how to deliver a health science message effectively. This chapter has highlighted the opportunities and perils inherent in health researchers' interactions with the media and should be seen as a stepping-stone toward becoming a more capable and confident communicator. ■

Reporting

REFERENCES

1. Canadian Institutes of Health Research (CIHR) definition of KT. Available from: www.cihr-irsc.gc.ca/e/29418.html

2. Pribble JM, Goldstein KM, Fowler EF, Greenberg MJ, Noel SK, Howell JD. Medical news for the public to use? What's on local TV news. *Am J Manag Care.* 2006;12(3):170–6.

3. Motl SE, Timpe EM, Eichner SF. Evaluation of accuracy of health studies reported in mass media. *J Am Pharm Assoc.* 2003;45(6):720–5.

4. Zuckerman D. Hype in health reporting: "checkbook science" buys distortion of medical news. *Int J Health Serv.* 2003;33(2):383–9.

5. Rossouw JE, Anderson GL, Prentice RL, LaCroix AZ, Kooperberg C, Stefanick ML, et al. Risks and benefits of estrogen plus progestin in healthy postmenopausal women: principal results from the Women's Health Initiative randomized controlled trial. *JAMA.* 2002;288(3):321–33.

6. Council of International Organizations of Medical Sciences. *Guidelines for preparing core clinical-safety data on drugs.* 2nd ed. Geneva: CIOMS; 1998.

7. Laudan L. *The book of risks: fascinating facts about the chances we take everyday.* New York: John Wiley; 1995.

8. Moore RA, Derry S, McQuay HJ, Paling J. What do we know about communicating risk? A brief review and suggestion for contextualising serious, but rare, risk and the example of cox-2 selective and non-selective NSAIDs. *Arthritis Res Ther.* 2008;10(1):R20.

9. Gigerenzer G, Gaissmaier W, Kurz-Milcke E, Schwartz LM, Woloshin S. Knowing your chances: what health stats really mean. *Sci Am Mind.* 2009;1 April: 44–51.

10. Sandman PM. The Peter Sandman risk communication website. Available at: www.psandman.com.

11. Weinstein ND, Sandman PM, Hallman WK. Testing a visual display to explain small probabilities. *Risk Anal.* 1994;14(6):895–7.

12. Singletary SE. Rating the risk factors for breast cancer. *Ann Surg.* 2003;237(4):474–82.

13. Hill AB. The environment and disease: Association or causation. *Proc R Soc Med.* 1965;58:295–300.

14. CBC news. Seasonal flu shot may increase H1N1 risk. 2009; Sept 23. Available from: www.cbc.ca/news/health/story/2009/09/23/flu-shots-h1n1-seasonal.html

15. Skowronski DM, De Serres G, Crowcroft NS, Janjua NZ, Boulianne N, Hottes TS, et al. Association between the 2008-09 seasonal influenza vaccine and pandemic H1N1 illness during Spring-Summer 2009: four observational studies from Canada. *PLoS Med.* 2010;7(4):e1000258.

16. Silversides A. Clinical trials: the muddled Canadian landscape. *CMAJ.* 2009;180(1):20–2.

17. Rochon PA, Gurwitz JH, Simms RW, Fortin PR, Felson DT, Minaker KL, et al. A study of manufacturer-supported trials of nonsteroidal anti-inflammatory drugs in the treatment of arthritis. *Arch Intern Med.* 1994;154(2):157–63.

18. Campbell EG, Louis KS, Blumenthal MD. Looking a gift horse in the mouth. *JAMA.* 1998;279(13):995–9.

19. Faunce T, Townsend R, McEwan A. The Vioxx pharmaceutical scandal: Peterson v Merke Sharpe & Dohme. *J Law Med.* 2010;18(1):38–49.

20. Mary C. Tackling fraud in medical research and scientific communication: A report of the lecture by Dr Frank Wells at the 28th EMWA Conference. *The Write Stuff* [Journal of the European Medical Writers Association] 2009;18:28–9. Available from: www.avicenne-sciences.com/IMG/pdf/Fraud.pdf

21. Fraud Advisory Panel. Fraud in Research: Is it new or just not true? Occasional Paper 01/07. Available from: www.fraudadvisorypanel.org/newsite/pdf_show.php?id=71

22. Smith R. Research misconduct: the poisoning of the well. *J R Soc Med.* 2006;99(5):232–7.

23. Jaffer U, Cameron A. Deceit and fraud in medical research. *Int J Surg.* 2006;4(2):122–6.

24. Sudbø J, Lee JJ, Lippman SM, Mork J, Sagen S, Flatner N, et al. Non-steroidal anti-inflammatory drugs and the risk of oral cancer: a nested case-control study. *Lancet.* 2005;366(9494):1359–66. Retraction in: Horton R. *Lancet.* 2006;367(9508):382.

25. Pearce JM, Manyonda IT, Chamberlain GVP. Term delivery after intrauterine relocation of an ectopic pregnancy. Br J Obstet Gynaecol. 1994;101(8):716–7. Retraction in: *Br J Obstet Gynaecol.* 1995;102(11):853.

Reporting

26. Pearce JM, Hamid RI. Randomised controlled trial of the use of human chorionic gonadotrophin in recurrent miscarriage associated with polycystic ovaries. *Br J Obstet Gynaecol*. 1994;101(1):685–8. Retraction in: *Br J Obstet Gynaecol*. 1995;102(11):853.

27. Hwang WS, Ryu YJ, Park JH, Park ES, Lee EG, Koo JM, et al. Evidence of a pluripotent human embryonic stem cell line derived from a cloned blastocyst. *Science*. 2004;303(5664):1669–74. Retraction in: Kennedy D. *Science*. 2006;311(5759):335.

28. Tessier J, Hahn P, Reid RL. Media training for residents in Obstetrics and Gynecology: Improving communication skills and advocacy for women's health. *J Soc Ob Gyn Can*. 2001;23(6):495–500.

29. Ratcliff J. New surgery for ailing hearts. *Reader's Digest*. 1957;71:70–3.

30. Kitchell JR, Glover RP, Kyle R. Bilateral internal mammary artery ligation for angina pectoris: preliminary clinical considerations. *Am J Cardiol*. 1958;1(1):46–50.

31. Glantz SA. *Primer of biostatistics*. 6th ed. New York: McGraw-Hill Medical Publication Division; 2005:448.

SUMMARY CHECKLIST

- ❏ Thinking about your study, list the potential benefits of sharing the findings in the lay media. List any pitfalls.
- ❏ Prepare a list of key messages arising from your study that you would like to disseminate.
- ❏ List the forms of media that you would like to use (e.g., web page, blog, Twitter, radio, TV, newspapers).
- ❏ If you have arranged a media interview, prepare and practise the delivery of your key messages.
- ❏ List key findings from your study that could be misunderstood if taken out of context. Prepare explanations that convey these findings simply and clearly.

Reporting

32

So, you've finished your first research project ... now what?

Ross Upshur, MD, MA, MSc, CCFP, FRCPC

ILLUSTRATIVE CASE

After completing a research project exploring whether the introduction of a computer-based reminder system actually increased the provision of selected preventive services in a General Internal Medicine ambulatory clinic, a third-year Internal Medicine resident considers what, if any, further research experiences she should pursue during the remainder of her residency training. She also wonders whether it would be possible to pursue clinical research as a component of her career after the completion of specialty training and, if so, what additional research training she might require.

■ **So, you've just completed your first** health sciences research project. Now what? Including research activities as one component of your career as a health professional is an excellent way to keep your interests diversified, to contribute to knowledge generation in your field and, perhaps most importantly, to engage in a wide range of collaborations on interesting issues relevant to your practice. Many health professionals finish their training with a desire to acquire clinical mastery and to be a researcher, but feel that it is impossible to combine these two paths, especially in view of the time involved not only in conducting research but also in acquiring the methodological expertise necessary to do so. Balancing multiple competing obligations is a recognized difficulty in the transition from supervised to independent practice. This chapter makes the case that all health professionals should play some role in research in their field, and that it is possible to participate in research at different levels, and at any point in one's career.

Few descriptions of **medical research careers** account for the wide range of projects that a health professional can become involved with, or the various degrees of involvement that are possible. Each type of engagement entails a different level of skill development (which can include study design, statistics, research ethics, database construction and management, and manuscript and grant writing), time commitment, responsibilities and rewards. The following sections describe six variants of research involvement.

CHAPTER OBJECTIVES

After reading this chapter, you should be able to:

- discuss various paths to further involvement in research after the completion of your first research project
- describe the merits of including research activities as a component of your professional career

---

KEY TERMS

Co-investigator

Collaborator

Critical appraisal skills

Medical research careers

Mentor

Principal investigator

Recruiter

Reflecting

The critical consumer

Although you might not wish to be an actively participating researcher, all health professionals should, at a minimum, become and remain critical consumers of the published literature relevant to their practice. Completing a research project gives you an appreciation of the challenges inherent in bringing a health research project through all of its stages: from the initial idea to the formulation of a clear research question, to the marshalling of a research team, the creation of data collection instruments, the collection, analysis and interpretation of data, and their synthesis into a completed project report, presentation and perhaps a peer-reviewed publication. Having first-hand experience of these steps and of the ways in which a project can run into difficulties gives you a practical understanding of the research process that can help you to read between the lines of published studies. This insight will undoubtedly complement the **critical appraisal skills** you will need to be a capable, critical consumer of the health care literature, and will enhance your appreciation of unbiased and rigorous research results. This level of engagement involves keeping up with the literature and maintaining critical appraisal skills. Participating in a journal club that rewards participation with continuing professional development credits is an excellent way to facilitate this. If such a club does not exist where you practise, create one!

The recruiter

A second way in which you can become involved in research is as a **recruiter**. In this role you are plugged into clinical trials networks or other structures for ongoing health research to see whether patients in your practice would be eligible for enrolment in an appropriate study. Although recruiters are not major players on the research team, it is clear that, without the broad-based support of these front-line practitioners, clinical trials would never attain the sample sizes they need to obtain meaningful results. Identifying and referring potential participants to applicable clinical trials and other health research studies can be rewarding: it links you to research projects through frequent communications from the principal investigator and the study team and through access to preliminary research results. This level of involvement also provides insight into the research process, including any challenges leading up to the synthesis of the research results; can help you to forge links with active researchers; and, can alert

you to advances in the field before they are more broadly known. No further research training is required for this type of involvement, and study co-ordinators and hired research assistants tend to provide support for recruiters with regard to study procedures.

The occasional collaborator

The third way to be engaged in health research is as an occasional **collaborator**. This would mean that you are not actively involved with health research projects at all times, but occasionally collaborate actively in projects that come to your attention and are related to your area of practice. Being an occasional collaborator can include the opportunity to be a coauthor of published results. The best place to formulate important new questions is in the front lines of health care: questions arise every day in clinical practice that might be answered by a structured research project. Being an occasional collaborator might lead you to the next level of research engagement, which is that of a research collaborator with a mentor.

The research collaborator with a mentor

Chapter 5 of this guide stresses the importance of finding a research **mentor**. If you want to become more engaged in research, you will need—at least in the early part of your research career, whether in the community or in close association with an academic health sciences centre—a mentor to foster the growth of your methodological skills and to open up opportunities for you to gain research experience. It often helps to start as a collaborator on a project under the supervision and guidance of a more experienced researcher. This way, you can learn where your methodological strengths and weaknesses lie and figure out how best to tailor your interests to the range of possible studies and principal investigators available. Although it is to your advantage to find a mentor who is an experienced and accomplished investigator, it is equally important for this person to have a genuine interest in helping you—and the time to do so. At this stage of engagement you might wish to acquire more advanced research skills. Part- or even full-time study in a graduate program, or in short courses, weekend or summer courses, or online courses can enhance your methodological and analytical skills. In addition, specialized health research training programs are available

Reflecting

through the Royal College of Physicians and Surgeon of Canada's Clinical Investigator Program[1] and the College of Family Physicians of Canada's Clinical Scholars Program.[2] As a collaborator, you should also become engaged in the process of writing and submitting manuscripts for publication in peer-reviewed journals.

The co-investigator

The next level of research engagement is that of **co-investigator**. Co-investigators are an important component of a multiprofessional or interdisciplinary research team and assume substantial responsibility for the execution and oversight of the project. They help with formulating the research question, writing the protocol, and building, structuring and supervising the research team, and typically bring a fairly high level of expertise to the project. Additionally, co-investigators should play a role in the dissemination of results, including by co-authoring manuscripts, preparing abstracts and posters, and presenting results at conferences. Most researchers make the step to co-investigator after having been a mentored collaborator for some time, and typically first serve as a co-investigator with their research mentor. Attaining this level of engagement usually involves formal graduate training in research methodology.

The principal investigator

Finally, in the role of **principal investigator**, you are in charge of the whole show. You take the lead in formulating the research question, recruiting the research team, and writing the protocol and grant application. You shepherd the project through the ethics review process, take charge of the recruitment and supervision of the support staff, and mentor and lead the research team. I have found being a principal investigator to be among the most rewarding roles of my professional life. The opportunity to work with collaborators and co-investigators from a wide range of professions and disciplines on health-related questions is continually refreshing and challenging. One learns not only new methods but is in contact with talented graduate students who push one's understanding and knowledge and ask questions that frequently expose flaws in one's own reasoning or room for development in one's own skills.

The rewards of a research career

Why do research? What does it bring to a health professional's career? The rewards are numerous, as the following reflections show.

- The knowledge that informs health practice is best created when practising health professionals have the opportunity to ask questions and look for solutions that aim to provide better health care for future generations of patients and populations, or to develop diagnostic and prognostic tools that help us to better inform our patients about their situation.

- Research is endlessly challenging. One must frequently overcome obstacles that were not foreseen in the protocol phase. This requires patience and ingenuity. I have often referred to grant writing as a form of creative non-fiction in which one must project one or more years into the future things that one wishes to see happen, even though the world in which one does research is not necessarily aligned with those goals. Indeed, perhaps one of the best reasons to persevere with a research career is to see the multiplicity of ways in which the real world can thwart the most beautifully created protocol. This may be frustrating to some, but with a little humour you can come to appreciate these unexpected turns as one of the more fascinating aspects of research.

- A research career permits you to meet, work with and learn from many interesting, bright and engaging colleagues, including graduate students, research coordinators, research associates, not to mention the patients recruited into your studies. I have learned a great deal from the participants in our studies and recently added patients to our Research Advisory Committee: they bring a perspective that is often overlooked in the planning and conduct of study protocols. In addition, research provides opportunities to meet and interact with other researchers by attending and giving presentations at local, national and international meetings.

- Research also offers some more direct personal rewards. It still gives me great pleasure to see a letter of acceptance from a peer-reviewed journal or a letter of congratulations from a funder. These are by no means taken for granted. People who do not engage in research as part of their professional life do not see the immense amount of work it takes to get from a

Reflecting

grant proposal to a peer-reviewed publication. It truly is an accomplishment worth celebrating. Even if most of the world ignores your paper, family members are bound to be pleased to receive a copy of a paper with your name listed among the authors. And— more seriously—publishing in the peer-reviewed literature establishes your credibility and may lead to invitations as a peer reviewer or to participate on expert advisory boards locally and internationally.

- Last but by no means least, your research may contribute to the development of best practices and the improvement of patient outcomes.

Conclusion

There are many paths to engagement in the research process. Increasingly, the more I do research the more I think it should be integral part to every health professional's activities. In this chapter I have tried to point to some of the ways in which health professionals can integrate research into their day-to-day practice. I hope all readers who are in the midst of or have already completed their health training will find ways to become involved in research in some way in their professional lives. ■

REFERENCES

1. Royal College of Physicians and Surgeons of Canada. *Specific standards of accreditation for clinical investigator programs.* Ottawa: The College; 2009. Available from: http://rcpsc.medical.org/residency/accreditation/ssas/CIP_e.pdf

2. College of Family Physicians of Canada. *Clinical Scholar Program.* Mississauga (ON): The College; 2009. Available from: www.cfpc.ca/local/files/Education/Clinician%20Scholar%20Program%20-%20Final%20January%202009%20(2).pdf

ADDITIONAL RESOURCES

Hayward AR. Making clinical research a robust career path. *Acad Med.* 2009;84(4):409–10.

- This brief editorial describes initiatives to enhance the attractiveness of research to clinicians.

Jarvis P. *The practitioner-researcher: developing theory from practice.* New York (NY): Jossey-Bass Publishers; 1999.

- Although not focused on medical practice, this book contains a comprehensive account of what is required to do research in practice-based locations.

Melnick A. Transitioning from fellowship to a physician-scientist career track. *Hematology Am Soc Hematol Educ Program.* 2008:16–22.

- This paper contains excellent practical advice on getting a research career started in academic settings.

Teo AR. The development of clinical research training: past history and current trends in the United States. *Acad Med.* 2009;84(4):433–8.

- This paper highlights the development of clinical research career paths in the United States and outlines current trends.

Reflecting

SUMMARY CHECKLIST

❑ Thinking about your experiences with research and your career interests, describe the role you would like research to play in your career. Describe how you expect this to change over time.

❑ Develop your strategy for a successful role in research, as outlined above. Be sure to list:
  — experience you wish to have
  — training you wish to obtain
  — mentors you would like to work with
  — levels of involvement in proposed studies

Reflecting

Reviewers

Katherine Boydell, PhD
Department of Psychiatry
University of Toronto
Toronto, Ontario

Antoinette Colacone, BSc, CCRA
Emergency Multidisciplinary Research Unit–FMRU
Sir Mortimer B. Davis-Jewish General Hospital
Montreal, Quebec

Donald Cole, MD, MSc, FRCPC
Department of Public Health Sciences
Dalla Lana School of Public Health
University of Toronto
Toronto, Ontario

Scott Compton, PhD
Dept of Emergency Medicine
New Jersey Medical School–The University Hospital
Newark, New Jersey

David C. Cone, MD
Department of Emergency Medicine
Yale University
New Haven, Connecticut

Neil Drummond, BA, MFPHM (UK), PhD
Department of Family Medicine and Community Health
University of Calgary
Calgary, Alberta

Nancy Feeley, RN, PhD
School of Nursing
McGill University
Montreal, Quebec

Dionne Gesink, PhD
Dalla Lana School of Public Health
University of Toronto
Toronto, Ontario

Corinne Hohl, MD, FRCPC
Department of Emergency Medicine
University of British Columbia
Vancouver, British Columbia

Tanya Horsley, PhD
Centre for Learning in Practice
Royal College of Physicians and Surgeons of Canada
Ottawa, Ontario

Thomas A. Lang, MA
Tom Lang Communications and Training International
Kirkland, Washington

Trevor Langhan, MD, FRCPC
Division of Emergency Medicine
University of Calgary
Calgary, Alberta

A. Curtis Lee, PhD
Education and Evaluation and Analysis Unit
Royal College of Physicians and Surgeons of Canada
Ottawa, Ontario

Jacques S. Lee, MD, MSc, FRCPC
Department of Emergency Medicine and
    Clinical Epidemiology Unit
Sunnybrook Health Sciences Centre
Toronto, Ontario

Marilyn MacDonald, RN, PhD
School of Nursing
Dalhousie University
Halifax, Nova Scotia

Jessie McGowan, BMus, MLIS, PhD
Departments of Medicine and Family Medicine
University of Ottawa
Ottawa, Ontario

Index

Note: (f) after a page reference denotes a figure, (t) a table.

Notes

CPSIA information can be obtained
at www.ICGtesting.com
Printed in the USA
LVHW061617221020
669548LV00009B/845